Acute coronary syndromes

A handbook for clinical practice

THE ESC EDUCATION SERIES

EUROPEAN
SOCIETY OF
CARDIOLOGY®

Acute coronary syndromes

A handbook for clinical practice

A publication based on ESC Guidelines
(www.escardio.org/knowledge/guidelines)

EDITED BY

Michel E. Bertrand
Spencer B. King III

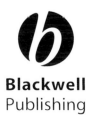

Blackwell
Publishing

©2006 European Society of Cardiology
2035 Route des Colles-Les Templiers, 06903 Sophia-Antipolis, France
For further information on the European Society of Cardiology:
www.escardio.org

Published by Blackwell Futura, an imprint of Blackwell Publishing
Blackwell Publishing, Inc., 350 Main Street, Malden, Massachusetts 02148-5020, USA
Blackwell Publishing Ltd, 9600 Garsington Road, Oxford OX4 2DQ, UK
Blackwell Science Asia Pty Ltd, 550 Swanston Street, Carlton, Victoria 3053, Australia

First published 2006

Library of Congress Cataloging-in-Publication Data

Acute coronary syndromes: a handbook for clinical practice/edited by
   Michel E. Bertrand, Spencer B. King III.
      p. ; cm.
   Includes bibliographical references and index.
   ISBN-13: 978-1-4051-3501-6 (alk. paper)
   ISBN-10: 1-4051-3501-8 (alk. paper)
   1. Coronary heart disease–Handbooks, manuals, etc. I. Bertrand, M. II. King, Spencer B.,
1937–.
   [DNLM: 1. Myocardial Ischemia. 2. Acute Disease. WG 300 A185815 2006]
RC685.C6A2885 2006
616.1'23–dc22

                                                                              2005015933

ISBN-13: 978-1-4051-3501-6
ISBN-10: 1-4051-3501-8

A catalogue record for this title is available from the British Library

Set in 9.5/12 Meridien by Newgen Imaging Systems (P) Ltd, Chennai, India
Printed and bound in Singapore by Fabulous Printers Pte Ltd

Commissioning Editor: Gina Almond
Development Editor: Vicki Donald

For further information on Blackwell Publishing:
www.blackwellcardiology.com

Contents

Section nine: Secondary prevention

List of contributors

Editors

Michel E. Bertrand, MD, Lille Heart Institute, Lille, France
Spencer B. King III, MD, Fuqua Heart Center of Piedmont Hospital, Atlanta, GA, USA

Contributors

A.A. Jennifer Adgey, MD, Royal Victoria Hospital, Belfast, UK
Lina Badimon, MD, PhD, Hospital della Santa Creu i Sant Pau, Barcelona, Spain
Jean-Pierre Bassand, MD, CHU Jean Minjoz, Besançon, France
Alexander Battler, MD, Rabin Medical Center, Petach-Kiva, Israel
Christophe Bauters, MD, PhD, Hopital Cardiologique, Lille, France
Dirk Boese, MD, Universität GHS, Essen, Germany
Piero O. Bonetti, MD, University Hospital, Basel, Switzerland
Raphaelle Dumaine, MD, Pitié Salpétrière University Hospital, Paris, France
Raimund Erbel, MD, Universität GHS, Essen, Germany
Erling Falk, MD, PhD, Skejby University Hospital, Aarhus, Denmark
Pim J. de Feyter, MD, PhD, Thorax Center of the University Hospital Rotterdam, Rotterdam, The Netherlands
Keith A.A. Fox, MD, Edinburgh Royal Infirmary, Edinburgh, UK
Christian W. Hamm, MD, Kerckhoff Clinic, Bad Nauheim, Germany
David Hasdai, MD, Rabin Medical Center, Petach-Kiva, Israel
Christopher Heeschen, MD, Ludwig Maximillian University, Munich, Germany
Christoph Kaiser, MD, University Hospital, Basel, Switzerland
Victor Legrand, MD, CHU Sart Tilman, Liege, Belgium
David McCarty, MB, Royal Victoria Hospital, Belfast, UK
Eugene McFadden, MD, PhD, Cork University Hospital, Cork, Ireland
Bernhard Meier, MD, Swiss Cardiovascular Center, Bern, Switzerland
Nicolas Meneveau, MD, PhD, CHU Jean Minjoz, Besançon, France
Nico R.A. Mollet, MD, Thorax Center of the University Hospital Rotterdam, Rotterdam, The Netherlands
Gilles Montalescot, MD, Pitié Salpétrière University Hospital, Paris, France
Colum G. Owens, MB, Royal Victoria Hospital, Belfast, UK
Matthias E. Pfisterer, MD, University Hospital, Basel, Switzerland
Evelyne Regar, MD, Thorax Center of the University Hospital Rotterdam, Rotterdam, The Netherlands

Jaydeep Sarma, MD, Edinburgh Royal Infirmary, Edinburgh, UK
François Schiele, MD, CHU Jean Minjoz, Besançon, France
Luigi Tavazzi, MD, Policlinico San Matteo IRCCS, Pavia, Italy
Pierre Théroux, MD, Montreal Heart Institute, Montreal, Canada
Mario Togni, MD, Swiss Cardiovascular Center, Bern, Switzerland
Eric Van Belle, MD, PhD, Hopital Cardiologique, Lille, France
Lars Wallentin, MD, Uppsala Cardiothoracic Center, Uppsala, Sweden
Michael J. Zellweger, MD, University Hospital, Basel, Switzerland

Preface

Within the last ten years, acute coronary syndromes have become a major health care problem with millions of patients hospitalized annually around the world.

Acute coronary syndromes, namely unstable angina and evolving myocardial infarction, share a common anatomic substrate. Pathological, angioscopic, and biological observations have demonstrated that unstable angina and myocardial infarction have different clinical presentations that result from a common underlying pathophysiological mechanism, namely atherosclerotic plaque rupture or erosion, with differing degrees of superimposed thrombosis and distal embolization.

Complete thrombotic occlusion is characterized by a typical electrocardiographic profile, defined by ST-segment elevation (STE-ACS). This finding is a true emergency and implies immediate recanalization of the vessel with primary percutaneous coronary intervention or fibrinolytic treatment.

Other patients presenting with acute chest pain may have different electrocardiographic characteristics: ST-segment depression or T-wave inversions. These cases characterize the non-ST-segment elevation acute coronary syndromes (NSTE-ACS) and represent 52–57% of all acute coronary syndromes. More importantly, the prognosis of these patients, in terms of death and myocardial infarction is still poor despite modern therapeutic approaches.

The management of NSTE-ACS has been rapidly evolving over recent years. Since 2000, the European Society of Cardiology, American Heart Association, and American College of Cardiology have provided guidelines concerning the management of NSTE-ACS and these guidelines have already been updated.

Although this topic is well addressed in the major textbooks of cardiology, this is a rapidly changing field and this succinct handbook serves to provide the reader with current information on the therapeutic options and strategies for the management of ACS patients.

This handbook is edited under the aegis of the European Society of Cardiology. The different aspects of NSTE-ACS are addressed by famous European and international experts in the field. We do hope that it will bring interesting information for those who, as clinicians, urgentists, or surgeons are involved in the difficult management of these patients.

Michel E. Bertrand, MD
Spencer B. King III, MD

Section one:
Epidemiology

CHAPTER 1

Epidemiology of non-ST-segment elevation acute coronary syndromes: Euro Heart Survey, GRACE, CRUSADE

David Hasdai and Alexander Battler

The term "acute coronary syndromes" (ACSs) is used to denote episodes of acute myocardial ischemia due to impaired coronary flow. Although there are several ancillary examinations that may influence the clinician contemplating a diagnosis of ACS, the diagnosis of ACS is, above all, based on clinical judgment. Because there is no strict and binding definition of ACS, there may be significant variance in its use, with some using it more loosely and others on a more reserved basis. Therefore, when one examines the epidemiology of ACS, and more so particular types of ACS [1], there are several caveats that must be taken into account.

Non-ST-elevation ACS – electrocardiographic caveats

Clinicians prefer to divide the ACS based on the initial electrocardiographic presentation – ACS with ST segment elevation and ACS without ST-segment elevation. The latter group usually includes patients with normal electrocardiographic patterns, T-wave changes, or ST-segment depression. The distinction based on the presence of ST-segment elevation bears therapeutic ramifications, because ACS with ST-segment elevation usually mandates immediate reperfusion therapy, as opposed to most other types of ACS. However, even this simple distinction may be flawed. The general approach to a patient with ST-elevation ACS applies to a patient with *persistent* ST-segment elevation. It is well known that a substantial minority of ACS patients presenting with ST-segment elevation have a rapid resolution of symptoms and ST-segment elevation either spontaneously or more commonly after simple pharmacological therapy (i.e. aspirin, nitrates). If an ensuing electrocardiogram is not performed, these patients are treated as ST-elevation ACS, and are clinically and epidemiologically considered as having had ST-elevation ACS. However, if the rapid resolution of ST-segment elevation is documented, then the patients are often treated similarly as patients without ST elevation. Indeed, many of the randomized studies examining different pharmacological and mechanical means for the treatment of ACS without ST elevation have included patients with *transient* ST-segment elevation (usually ST-segment elevation lasting less than 20–30 min). Likewise, several of the ongoing registries of patients with non-ST-elevation ACS (NSTE-ACS) have included patients with transient ST-segment elevation ACS [1]. In this case, these patients would be clinically and epidemiologically considered as having had NSTE-ACS. Thus, the incidence of NSTE-ACS depends on the epidemiological definition of ST elevation.

Although it is convenient to divide the ACS population into those with and without ST-segment elevation in their initial electrocardiogram, there is a small proportion of ACS patients who have electrocardiograms that are difficult to interpret, due in part to severe intraventricular conduction defects, paced rhythms or other arrhythmias, and repolarization abnormalities (i.e. left ventricular hypertrophy, digitalis effect, etc.). These patients, who often have high-risk clinical features and an ominous clinical course, are usually classified as having an "undetermined-electrocardiogram" ACS [2]. However, there are some clinicians who lump this small group of patients along with the bigger NSTE-ACS group, thus influencing the evaluation of the incidence of NSTE-ACS and its prognosis.

Definition of ACS

The classic clinical presentation of ACS is the typical retrosternal pain or heaviness radiating to the neck, jaw, or left arm, and often accompanied by other symptoms such as diaphoresis, nausea, and dyspnea. In recent years, it has become apparent that patients, more commonly diabetic or elderly patients, may manifest myocardial ischemia with atypical or very subtle symptoms. The diagnostic and therapeutic challenges arise especially when the electrocardiogram is normal or nearly normal. Such patients may be diagnosed as having NSTE-ACS based on ancillary laboratory tests, such as tests for serum cardiac biomarker levels. However, there are several problems when relying on cardiac biomarkers for the diagnosis of NSTE-ACS. Cardiac biomarkers may rise in situations associated with myocardial injury other than ACS, such as myocarditis, sepsis, trauma, heart failure, etc. Elevated cardiac biomarkers do not necessarily denote ACS, and the reported incidence of NSTE-ACS may depend on the clinician's subjective assessment. Thus, one physician may categorize a patient with known coronary artery disease and left ventricular dysfunction who presents with pulmonary edema, elevated biomarker levels, and nonspecific electrocardiographic changes as having had NSTE-ACS, whereas another would report this scenario as acute heart failure with nonspecific myocardial injury. Moreover, there are several biomarkers in clinical use to detect myocardial injury, with cardiac troponin assays being the most specific and sensitive. However, cardiac troponin assays are not widely available, even in Western societies [3]. Therefore, the reported incidence of NSTE-ACS in different regions may also be affected by the availability of different biomarkers.

On September 4, 2000, the European Society of Cardiology and the American College of Cardiology issued a joint consensus document, redefining acute myocardial infarction (AMI) [4]. The new definition of AMI emphasizes the role of more sensitive and specific serologic biomarkers of myocardial necrosis, in particular the cardiac troponins. Thus, the diagnosis of acute, evolving, or recent AMI, based on the new definition of AMI, primarily relies on the typical rise and fall of biochemical markers of myocardial necrosis. One of the most controversial aspects of this redefinition was the determination that an elevation in cardiac biomarkers after percutaneous coronary interventions is considered an AMI. Given that cardiac biomarker levels – especially of sensitive biomarkers, such as troponin – may rise in up to 50% of patients undergoing percutaneous coronary interventions, and given that the number of percutaneous coronary interventions is steadily increasing, the reported incidence of ACS would be expected to rise dramatically. However, there is great variation in the adherence to the redefinition of AMI, especially with regard to the aspect of postintervention AMI. In addition, cardiac biomarker levels are not routinely measured among asymptomatic postintervention patients in most institutions. Therefore, the reported incidence of postintervention AMI depends on the attitude of the physicians to the redefinition of AMI and the application of an approach of routine cardiac biomarker measurements. Because the vast majority of postintervention AMIs falls under the category of NSTE-ACS, the epidemiology of NSTE-ACS is greatly affected by the implementation of this redefinition.

Initial versus discharge diagnosis

Traditionally, patients discharged after having had an ACS receive a diagnosis of unstable angina or AMI. Moreover, the patients with a diagnosis of AMI are classically divided into those with and without Q waves. This classic distinction arose from the erroneous notion that Q waves represent transmural infarcts. Although the distinction between NSTE-ACS and ST-elevation ACS was once primarily used as an initial diagnosis with therapeutic ramifications, it has become increasingly popular to discharge patients using the definition based on the ST segment. Because the diagnosis of ST-elevation ACS does not necessarily denote Q-wave AMI, especially in the era of early reperfusion, these different diagnoses cannot be used interchangeably. Nevertheless, there is no standard diagnostic code for discharging ACS patients. Thus, the reported incidence of NSTE-ACS may be greatly affected by the diagnostic code used.

Source of data

One of the major factors determining the incidence of ACS, and more so the different types of ACS, is the source of the database. In order to determine the true incidence of a phenomenon in a particular population, one must either sample a subgroup that represents the general population or sample the whole population. Any such evaluation must ensure that all patients are captured in the database and that biases are kept to a minimum. For example, if an ACS survey were performed in a hospital that admits ACS patients to cardiology and general internal medicine wards, it would only be accurate in determining the incidence of ACS if patients in both types of wards are sampled.

Several countries have been successful in establishing periodic surveys or ongoing registries of ACS patients that encompass the greater part of the country. For example, the Swedes have established an ongoing registry of ACS patients admitted to almost all coronary care units in Sweden. Although this would offer a fairly accurate assessment of ACS incidence in Sweden, this assessment is biased by the fact that ACS patients, usually those with NSTE-ACS, may be admitted to wards other than coronary care units.

In February–March, 2000 a unique survey was performed in Israel. The survey encompassed all 26 hospitals in Israel and their cardiology wards (coronary care and step-down units). In addition, 82 of the 99 internal medicine wards in Israel participated in this survey of patients receiving a discharge diagnosis of ACS, either unstable angina or AMI. Thus, the database offers a fairly accurate estimate of the incidence of ACS admissions in a single country. The survey included 3656 patients, of whom only 1508 were admitted to cardiology wards. Of these 3656 patients, 1048 had ST-elevation AMI and the rest had either NSTE-ACS or undetermined electrocardiogram ACS. Thus, approximately 2500 admissions were due to NSTE-ACS over 2 months, suggesting 15 000 admissions over 12 months. Assuming that the population of Israel was approximately 5 million inhabitants in 2000, the estimated per capita annual incidence of NSTE-ACS admissions would be 0.003. In other words, of every 1000 inhabitants in Israel in 2000, about three were admitted due to NSTE-ACS.

In the United States, approximately 8 million people visit the emergency room each year because of chest pain, but only some have ACS. The National Center for Health Statistics reported that in 1996 alone there were 1 433 000 hospitalizations for unstable angina and NSTE myocardial infarction.

International surveys

In recent years, several ACS surveys have been conducted in different regions of the world. The first Euro Heart Survey of ACS, conducted from September 4, 2000 until May 15, 2001, included over 10 000 patients from 25 countries across Europe and the Mediterranean basin with a discharge diagnosis of ACS [5]. The survey was designed to screen consecutive patients with suspected ACS, but only patients with a final diagnosis of ACS were analyzed. There were no rigid criteria for the diagnosis, and in fact all diagnoses were made at the discretion of the attending physician, indicating that this survey encompassed a wide spectrum of ACS patients. About 3800 patients who were admitted due to suspected ACS, the vast majority of whom did not have ST elevation, were subsequently discharged with another diagnosis, emphasizing the difficulty in making the accurate diagnosis of NSTE-ACS and its dynamic nature. Altogether, of the 10 484 patients in the survey, 51.2% were admitted with NSTE-ACS. Although this survey offers unique insight into the proportion of the different types of ACS, their treatment approaches, and their outcomes, it does not specifically address the issue of epidemiology of ACS. This notion is reinforced by the characteristics of the participating 103 medical centers: 65% were academic, 77% had catheterization laboratories, and 57% had cardiac surgery facilities [5]. Clearly, these centers do not represent the average hospital in this part of the world, and hence the patient characteristics may also be biased. Currently, the second Euro Heart Survey of ACS is being conducted in 32 countries throughout this region.

The American counterpart to this survey is the Can Rapid Risk Stratification of Unstable Angina Patients Suppress Adverse Outcomes with Early Implementation of the ACC/AHA Guidelines (CRUSADE) Quality Improvement Initiative [1]. This ongoing survey includes patients with ischemic symptoms at rest and high-risk features including ST-segment depression, transient ST-segment elevation, or positive cardiac markers. By September 30, 2002, 30 295 patients from 248 hospitals in the United States had been enrolled. Once again, this ongoing survey sheds light on the treatment of NSTE-ACS in this important part of the world, and more so on the adherence to published guidelines, but is not suited to address the incidence of NSTE-ACS, because only high-risk NSTE-ACS patients are enrolled and the reported incidence is pertinent to a small number of hospitals across this country.

A more global initiative is the Global Registry of Acute Coronary Events (GRACE) project, an ongoing, multinational, observational study of patients hospitalized with suspected ACS [6]. The original project involved 14 countries across four continents. Data collection began in 1999, with the aim of collecting data from around 10 000 patients per year. Special care was exercised to choose clusters of hospitals with different demographic, clinical, and treatment characteristics. Patients included in the study must have electrocardiographic changes consistent with ACS, elevated cardiac biomarker levels, or documented coronary artery disease, thus narrowing the spectrum of patients by excluding patients with NSTE-ACS who do not have these features. Although this ambitious endeavor provides an abbreviated glimpse of ACS patients throughout vast regions of the world, it is presumptuous to conclude that these patients represent the "global" patient, given the great variability in patient characteristics, treatment, and diagnostic modalities, and comorbidities in different regions of the world. Moreover, although great care was exercised in choosing representative clusters, these centers probably are more academic and well equipped than the average hospital in the specific regions. Lastly, although GRACE provides us with unique knowledge regarding the management and outcomes of ACS patients in these 14 representative countries, it clearly does not offer insight into the epidemiology of ACS in these countries or elsewhere.

Conclusions

The diagnosis of NSTE-ACS is difficult to make, given the relative weight of subjective clinical judgment, the influence of ancillary examinations, the variability in adherence to recommended definitions, and the nonuniform coding of ACS events. Most of the current surveys and registries provide important insight into the treatment and outcomes of selected ACS patients, although these data may be biased by the strict criteria defining NSTE-ACS in some of these surveys/registries, as well as by the profile of the participating medical centers, which may be more academic and invasive than the average hospital in each region. Finally, because these surveys and registries sample only a proportion of ACS patients, it is difficult to determine the true incidence over a period of time of each type of ACS. The Israeli survey of ACS in 2000, being a uniquely comprehensive survey of almost all the relevant wards in Israel attending to ACS patients, suggests that the annual incidence of an admission due to NSTE-ACS is three per thousand inhabitants. These data should serve as a benchmark for the incidence of NSTE-ACS in most Western societies.

References

1. Hoekstra JW, Pollack CV Jr, Roe MT *et al*. Improving the care of patients with non-ST-elevation acute coronary syndromes in the emergency department: the CRUSADE initiative. *Acad Emerg Med* 2002; **9**: 1146–1155.
2. Lev EI, Battler A, Behar S *et al*. Frequency, characteristics and outcome of acute coronary syndrome patients admitted with undetermined ECG. *Am J Cardiol* 2003; **91**: 224–227.
3. Hasdai D, Behar S, Boyko V, Danchin N, Bassand JP, Battler A. Cardiac biomarkers and acute coronary syndromes – the Euro-Heart Survey of Acute Coronary Syndromes experience. *Eur Heart J* 2003; **24**: 1189–1194.
4. Myocardial infarction redefined – a consensus document of the Joint European Society of Cardiology/American College of Cardiology Committee for the redefinition of myocardial infarction. *Eur Heart J* 2000; **21**: 1502–1513.
5. Hasdai D, Behar S, Wallentin L *et al*. A prospective survey of the characteristics, treatments and outcomes of patients with acute coronary syndromes in Europe and the Mediterranean basin: the Euro Heart Survey of Acute Coronary Syndromes (Euro Heart Survey ACS). *Eur Heart J* 2002; **23**: 1190–1201.
6. The GRACE Investigators. Rationale and design of the GRACE (Global Registry of Acute Coronary Events) project: a multinational registry of patients hospitalized with acute coronary syndromes. *Am Heart J* 2001; **141**: 190–199.

Section two: Pathophysiology

CHAPTER 2

Pathologic findings in acute coronary syndromes

Erling Falk

Atherosclerosis is by far the most frequent cause of coronary artery disease, carotid artery disease, and peripheral artery disease. Life-threatening manifestations of atherosclerosis such as the acute coronary syndromes (ACSs) are usually precipitated by acute thrombosis, superimposed on a ruptured or eroded atherosclerotic plaque, with or without concomitant vasoconstriction, causing a sudden and critical reduction in blood flow [1–3]. In rare cases, ACS may have a nonatherosclerotic cause such as arteritis, trauma, dissection, thromboembolism, congenital anomaly, cocaine abuse, and complications of cardiac catheterization.

Atherothrombosis

Atherosclerosis is a chronic and multifocal immunoinflammatory, fibroproliferative disease of medium-sized and large arteries mainly driven by lipid accumulation [4–6]. Atherosclerosis begins to develop early in life and progresses with time, but the speed of progression is unpredictable and varies markedly among different subjects. At every level of risk factor exposure, there is substantial variation in the resulting atherosclerotic plaque burden, probably because the individual susceptibility to atherosclerosis and its risk factors varies greatly. However, even in susceptible individuals, it usually takes several decades to develop obstructive or thrombosis-prone plaques, so there should in principle be ample time to inhibit plaque development and its complications by timely screening and, where necessary, risk-reducing interventions [7,8].

Serial angiographic and pathoanatomical observations indicate that the natural progression of coronary artery disease involves two distinct processes: a fixed and hardly reversible process that causes gradual luminal narrowing slowly over decades (atherosclerosis), and a dynamic and potentially reversible process that punctuates the slow progression in a sudden and unpredictable way, causing rapid coronary occlusion (thrombosis or vasospasm, or both). Thus, symptomatic coronary lesions contain a variable mix of chronic atherosclerosis and acute thrombosis, but because the exact nature of the mix is unknown in the individual patient, the term *atherothrombosis* is frequently used. Generally, atherosclerosis predominates in

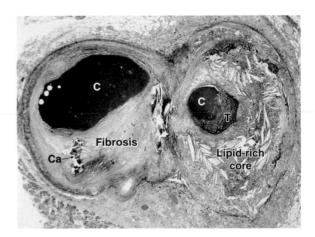

Figure 2.1 Atherothrombotic plaque, consisting of a variable mix of chronic atherosclerosis and acute thrombosis. Cross-section of a coronary artery bifurcation illustrating a collagen-rich plaque in the circumflex branch (left), and a lipid-rich and ruptured plaque with a nonocclusive thrombus superimposed in the obtuse branch (right). Ca = calcification; T = thrombus; C = contrast in the lumen.

lesions responsible for chronic stable angina, whereas thrombosis constitutes the critical component of culprit lesions responsible for the ACS [1–3].

Abnormal coronary vasomotion is common in ACS, but "spasm" is usually confined to the culprit lesion, suggesting that it is caused by locally released vasoactive substances [9]. The plaque, particularly the inflamed and disrupted plaque responsible for an ACS, may contain potent vasoconstrictors such as endothelin-1, and superimposed thrombosis may also contain or generate vasoconstrictors such as thrombin and platelet-derived serotonin and thromboxane A.

Vulnerable plaques

Coronary atherosclerotic plaques are very heterogeneous structurally as well as biologically, and even neighboring plaques in the same artery may differ markedly (Figure 2.1). The vast majority of coronary plaques are and will remain quiescent, at least from a clinical point of view. In fact, during a lifetime, none or only few coronary plaques become complicated by clinically significant thrombosis, and these rare but dangerous thrombosis-prone plaques are called vulnerable. Thus, a vulnerable plaque is a plaque assumed to be at high short-term risk of thrombosis, causing an ACS [10,11]. The challenge is to find the thrombosis-prone plaques, treat them (or rather the patients harboring them), and thus avoid ACS [12].

Approximately 75% of all coronary thrombi responsible for ACS are precipitated by *plaque rupture* [1,2]. In plaque rupture, there is a structural defect – a gap – in the fibrous cap that separates the lipid-rich core of an inflamed

Table 2.1 Features of ruptured plaques[a].

Thrombus
Large lipid-rich core (>30–40% of plaque)
Fibrous cap covering the lipid-rich core
    Thin (thickness <100 μm)
    Many macrophages (inflammation)
    Few smooth muscle cells (apoptosis)
Outward remodeling preserving the lumen
Neovascularization from vasa vasorum
Adventitial/perivascular inflammation

---

[a] By inference, the same features, except thrombus, are assumed to characterize rupture-prone (vulnerable) plaques.

plaque from the lumen of the artery [11]. Based on the morphological appearance of ruptured plaques, it is assumed that a rupture-prone plaque will possess the features outlined in Table 2.1 and illustrated in Figure 2.2. Lipid accumulation [13], thinning of the plaque's fibrous cap with local loss of smooth muscle cells [14] and inflammation with many macrophages and few mast cells and neutrophils [3,15,16], and intraplaque hemorrhage [17] destabilize plaques, making them vulnerable to rupture. In contrast, smooth muscle cell mediated healing and repair processes stabilize plaques, protecting them against rupture [18]. Plaque size or stenosis severity reveals nothing or only little about a plaque's vulnerability [19]. Many rupture-prone plaques are invisible angiographically, due to compensatory vascular remodeling, and they appear to be highly thrombogenic after rupture, probably because of a high content of tissue factor [20].

Clinical observations suggest that culprit lesions responsible for ACS generally are less calcified than plaques responsible for stable angina, indicating that calcium confers stability to plaques rather than the opposite [21]. The total amount of coronary calcification – the coronary calcium score – is a marker of plaque burden (and thus a marker of cardiovascular risk) rather than a marker of risk conferred by the individual calcified plaque [22].

The term *plaque erosion* is generally used for intact plaques with superimposed thrombosis, that is, there is no underlying plaque rupture but the endothelium is missing at the plaque–thrombus interface [23]. These plaques have identified themselves as being relatively thrombogenic, but the precipitating factor or condition may, in fact, be found outside rather than inside the plaque (e.g. a hyperthrombotic tendency or so-called vulnerable blood) [12].

Plaque vulnerability and remodeling

Arterial remodeling is bidirectional. Plaques responsible for ACS are usually relatively large and associated with compensatory enlargement that tends to

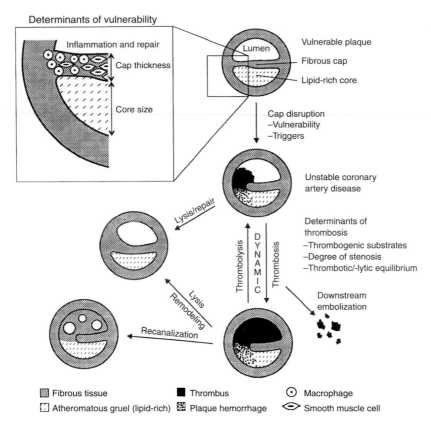

Figure 2.2 Plaque vulnerability, rupture, and thrombosis. Lipid accumulation, cap thinning, macrophage infiltration, and local loss of smooth muscle cells destabilize plaques, making them vulnerable to rupture. It is unknown whether rupture of a vulnerable plaque is a random (spontaneous) or triggered event. The thrombotic response to plaque rupture is dynamic and depends on local (e.g. exposed substrate and shear forces) as well as systemic factors (e.g. platelets, coagulation, and fibrinolysis).

preserve a normal lumen despite the presence of significant, and potentially dangerous, vessel wall disease [19,24]. Such lesions, hidden in the arterial wall, may not be seen by angiography. As many as three-fourths of all infarct-related thrombi appear to evolve over plaques causing only mild-to-moderate stenosis prior to infarction, partly because of their propensity for outward remodeling and their much greater prevalence compared with stenotic plaques [1]. Thus, the great majority of myocardial infarctions originate from atherosclerotic lesions that, prior to the acute events, were hemodynamically insignificant and probably asymptomatic. In contrast, plaques responsible for stable angina are usually smaller but, nevertheless, may cause more severe luminal narrowing because of concomitant local shrinkage of the artery (inward remodeling).

Onset of ACS: vulnerability versus triggers

Sudden rupture of a thin and inflamed fibrous cap may occur spontaneously but triggering could also play a role and thus help explain the nonrandom onset of ACS [25]. Potential triggers may include extreme physical activity – especially in someone unaccustomed to regular physical activity, severe emotional trauma, sexual activity, exposure to illicit drugs such as cocaine or amphetamines, cold exposure, and acute infections – or simply normal daily activities [25]. The fact that exercise stress testing in individuals with advanced coronary atherosclerosis rarely triggers an ACS suggests that plaque vulnerability ultimately plays a more important role in plaque rupture than physiologic stresses or other potential triggers.

After an ACS, the risk of a recurrent ischemic event is high during the following 3–6 months. Many of these "new" events are probably caused by reactivation of the original culprit lesion (rethrombosis), but both postmortem and clinical observations indicate that patients with ACS often have many ruptured and/or "active" plaques in their coronary arteries, indicating widespread disease activity [26]. The role of active nonculprit lesion (vulnerable plaques) for subsequent ischemic events is unknown.

Coronary thrombosis caused by plaque rupture

A worldwide search revealed 18 autopsy studies in which 1460 coronary thrombi were identified and studied carefully with the purpose to characterize the surface of the underlying atherosclerotic plaque (Table 2.2). Plaque rupture was the major cause of coronary thrombosis, being responsible for approximately 76% of the fatal thrombotic events worldwide, regardless of clinical presentation (myocardial infarction or sudden death). Plaque rupture is a more frequent cause of coronary thrombosis in males (81%) than in females (59%). It is rare in one extremely small subgroup of patients, namely premenopausal females, who constitute less than 1% of heart attack victims. A few studies have reported that diabetes (predominantly Type II), smoking, and hyperlipidemia tend to favor a particular type of thrombosis but, except for sex and menopause, no particular risk factor has consistently been related with a particular type of plaque or mechanism of thrombosis [1]. Even in China, where the average plasma cholesterol level is low, rupture of a lipid-rich plaque is the major cause of coronary thrombosis [42].

Coronary thrombosis not caused by plaque rupture

The term plaque erosion has gained popularity for the minority of thrombi not induced by plaque rupture (~20% in males and ~40% in females) [23]. It refers to a heterogenous group of atherothrombotic plaques where no deep injury is present to explain the overlying thrombus, only the endothelium is missing at the plaque–thrombus interface.

Table 2.2 Worldwide, 1114 (76%) of 1460 fatal coronary thrombi were precipitated by plaque rupture.

Patients		Age[a], y	n	Rupture	Study
Hospital,	—	—	19	19 = 100%	Chapman [27]
Hospital,	—	—	17	17 = 100%	Constantinides [28]
Hospital,	AMI + SCD	58	40	39 = 98%	Friedman et al. [29]
Hospital,	AMI	62	88	71 = 81%	Bouch et al. [30]
Hospital,	AMI	66	91	68 = 75%	Sinapius [31]
Coroner,	SCD	53	20	19 = 95%	Friedman et al. [32]
Hospital,	AMI	67	76	69 = 91%	Horie et al. [33]
Hospital,	AMI	67	49	40 = 82%	Falk [34]
Coroner,	SCD	<65	32	26 = 81%	Tracy et al. [35]
Med. exam,	SCD	<70	61	39 = 64%	el Fawal et al. [36]
Hospital,	AMI	—	83	52 = 63%	Yutani et al. [37]
Coroner,	—	—	85	71 = 84%	Richardson et al. [38]
Hospital,	AMI	63	20	12 = 60%	van der Wal et al. [39]
Coroner,	SCD	—	202	143 = 71%	Davies[b] [40]
Hospital,	AMI	69	291	218 = 75%	Arbustini et al. [41]
Hospital,	AMI	61	61	56 = 92%	Shi et al. [42]
Hospital,	AMI	69	100	81 = 81%	Kojima et al. [43]
Med. exam,	SCD	48	125	74 = 59%	Virmani et al.[b] [23]
AMI + SCD			**1460**	**1114 = 76%**	**Worldwide**

— = Not reported; AMI = acute myocardial infarction; SCD = sudden coronary death. [a]Mean. [b]Davies (Ref. 40) and Virmani et al. (Ref. 23) are updated summaries, including previously published data.

The precise mechanisms of thrombosis superimposed to eroded plaques are not known but probably reflect the heterogeneity of these plaques. It is conceivable that systemic thrombogenic factors, such as platelet hyper-aggregability, hypercoagulability, circulating tissue factor, and/or depressed fibrinolysis, play a major role in thrombosis over plaques that are only eroded (versus ruptured) [12]. Recent studies have suggested that activated circulating leukocytes may transfer active tissue factor by shedding microparticles and transferring them onto adherent platelets [20,44,45]. Accordingly, such circulating sources of tissue factor rather than plaque-derived tissue factor can contribute to thrombosis at sites of endothelial denudation as seen in plaque erosion.

Thrombotic response

Rupture of the plaque surface occurs frequently during plaque growth [46]. Most frequently, only a small "resealing" mural thrombus forms at the rupture site, and only occasionally does a major and life-threatening luminal thrombosis evolve. There are three major determinants of the thrombotic response to plaque rupture (or the amount of thrombosis formed on top of an eroded plaque): the local thrombogenic substrate, local flow disturbances, and the systemic thrombotic propensity.

Local thrombogenic substrate

Ongoing inflammation, in particular macrophage infiltration and activation, and lipid accumulation not only destabilize plaques making them vulnerable to rupture, but these plaque components also appear to be highly thrombogenic when exposed to the flowing blood after plaque rupture [47,48]. Activated macrophages express tissue factor and the lipid-rich atheromatous core contains high amounts of active tissue factor, probably originating from dead macrophages [20]. Culprit lesions responsible for ACSs contain more tissue factor than plaques responsible for stable angina [49]. Oxidized lipids in the lipid-rich core may also directly stimulate platelet aggregation.

Local flow disturbances

In contrast to venous thrombosis, rapid flow and high shear forces promote arterial thrombosis, probably via shear-induced platelet activation [50]. A platelet-rich thrombus may indeed form and grow within a severe stenosis, where the blood velocity and shear forces are highest. Irregularities of the exposed surface also increase the platelet-mediated thrombus formation.

Systemic thrombotic propensity

The state (activation) of platelets, coagulation, and fibrinolysis are critical for the outcome of plaque rupture, documented by the protective effect of antiplatelet agents and anticoagulant treatment in patients at risk of coronary thrombosis. Tissue factor probably plays an important prothrombotic role, both locally (expressed by macrophages in the culprit lesion) and systemically (expressed by activated leukocytes in the peripheral blood) [20,44,45,49].

Platelets, fibrin, and thrombotic burden

In coronary thrombosis, the initial flow obstruction is usually caused by platelet aggregation, but fibrin is important for the subsequent stabilization of the early and fragile platelet thrombus. Thus, both platelets and fibrin are involved in the evolution of a stable and persisting coronary thrombus.

If the platelet-rich thrombus (macroscopically white) at the site of plaque disruption occludes the lumen totally – as it is usually the case in myocardial infarction with ST-elevation myocardial infarction (STEMI) – the blood proximal and distal to the occlusion will stagnate and may coagulate, giving rise to a secondarily formed venous-type stagnation thrombosis (macroscopically red). Stagnation thrombosis may contribute significantly to the overall thrombotic burden, particularly in occluded vein grafts (no side branches), and thus hamper recanalization. Clinical observations indicate that it is indeed very dif-ficult to recanalize an occluded vein graft rapidly by intravenous thrombolytic therapy alone.

Dynamic thrombosis and microembolization

The thrombotic response to plaque rupture is dynamic: thrombosis and thrombolysis, often associated with vasospasm, tend to occur simultaneously, causing intermittent flow obstruction and distal embolization (1). The latter leads to microvascular obstruction that may prevent myocardial reperfusion despite a "successfully" recanalized infarct-related artery [51].

The purpose of coronary recanalization is, of course, to provide oxygenated blood to the ischemic myocardium, and "successful" recanalization (a patent culprit artery with brisk flow angiographically) is assumed to improve the perfusion at the tissue level. However, mechanical crushing and fragmenta-tion of atherothrombotic lesion during percutaneous coronary intervention (PCI) has emerged as a major cause of intracoronary (micro) embolization leading to downstream microvascular occlusion and thus preventing optimal reperfusion of the ischemic myocardium despite "successful" recanalization of the infarct-related artery [51]. Both spontaneous as well as iatrogenic coron-ary microembolization appear to be associated with an unfavorable long-term prognosis.

Development of myocardial infarction

Myocardial infarction (i.e. irreversible injury) caused by complete coron-ary artery occlusion begins to develop after 15–20 min of severe ischemia (no forward or collateral flow). Within the perfusion area of the occluded artery, flow deprivation and myocardial ischemia are usually most severe in the subendocardium (apart from the innermost ~10 cell layers nour-ished from the cavity) and, at least in dogs, cell death progresses from the subendocardium to the subepicardium in a time-dependent fashion, the *wave-front phenomenon* [52]. Although the susceptibility to ischemic necrosis differs significantly among patients (related to, e.g. variability in preconditioning and oxygen demand/consumption), there are two well-characterized major determinants of the ultimate extent of infarction:

- Location of the occlusion, defining the "area at risk" (amount of jeopard-ized myocardium).
- Severity and duration of myocardial ischemia (residual flow and rapidity of recanalization).

The speed and completeness of infarct development and, subsequently, the potential for myocardial salvage by reperfusion therapy is difficult to assess in the individual patient presenting with an evolving acute myocardial infarction (AMI). The amount of residual or spontaneously restored forward flow and collateral flow differ substantially among AMI patients. Rapid recruitment of collateral flow at the time of coronary occlusion (via preexisting collaterals) does not exist in some patients with MI as they do not have such protective collaterals. They develop a transmural AMI rapidly (like rabbits and pigs that lack collaterals), whereas other MI patients have collaterals, probably because of the presence of a severe collateral-promoting atherosclerotic stenoses prior to the acute occlusion (e.g. they develop a relatively small MI slowly, possibly none at all, like cats and guinea pigs that possess native collaterals).

Collaterals

The available collateral flow, at the time of occlusion, may limit or even avert the development of MI. In unstable angina with pain at rest, about 10% of patients have an occluded culprit artery at the time of presentation, but no definite infarction evolves because of well-developed collateral circulation [1]. In infarction without Q-wave development, about 25% of patients have an occluded culprit artery at early angiographic examination, increasing to 40% in the subsequent few days, but a significant amount of myocardium is salvaged because of parallel development of collateral vessels. Conversely, in STEMI, nearly all patients initially have an occluded culprit artery. Unless recanalization occurs rapidly, these patients usually develop extensive transmural infarction with Q waves on the ECG because of poor collateral circulation. Thus, collaterals may save myocardium at risk, and improve clinical outcome.

Reperfusion and no-reflow

Timely, complete, and sustained reperfusion may save myocardium at risk of undergoing necrosis in patients with evolving STEMI. Such infarcts nearly always remain anemic and pale if not reperfused. Therapeutic reperfusion is, however, associated with extravasation of erythrocytes in the ischemic tissues that already have passed the point of no return, giving rise to a hemorrhagic red infarct acutely. In addition, reperfusion is not homogeneous and, in particular, "no-reflow" may be a cause and/or a consequence of infarction [51].

   No-reflow in human AMI is more complex than that seen after ligation of a normal coronary artery in animals (classical no-reflow model), because the clinical setting involves an atherothrombotic dynamic occlusion with its innate risk of distal embolization, or when crushed or fragmented mechanically during PCI [51]. Thus, coronary no-reflow and myocardial hypoperfusion, after otherwise successful recanalization of infarct-related arteries, does not simply represent nonreperfusion confined to myocardium that is already dead. No-reflow may also result from PCI-induced (micro)vascular obstruction caused by distal (micro)embolization and/or microvascular spasm. Because emboli necessarily stream preferentially to well-perfused and viable myocardium, potentially salvageable myocardium may vanish. PCI-induced (micro)embolization may, in fact, not only prevent optimal reperfusion, it may worsen the ischemia if distal branches receiving collateral flow are occluded. Thus, the vital question is, of course: how much of the coronary no-reflow and myocardial hypoperfusion seen after primary PCI reflects the classical no-reflow phenomenon caused by necrosis, and how much reflects PCI-induced distal microembolization (and microvascular spasm?) causing more necrosis? The thrombotic burden may prove to be critical.

Clinical implications

Coronary atherosclerosis with ruptured and eroded plaques is common and clinically silent for long periods of time. However, acute thrombosis (±vasospasm) may cause sudden flow obstruction, giving rise to an ACS. The culprit lesion is frequently "dynamic," causing intermittent flow obstruction, and the clinical presentation and the outcome depend on the location of the obstruction and the severity and duration of myocardial ischemia. A nonocclusive or transiently occlusive thrombus – overall modified by vascular tone and collateral flow – most frequently underlies ACS without ST-segment elevation, whereas a more stable and occlusive thrombus prevails in STEMI. A critical thrombotic component is also frequent in culprit lesions responsible for out-of-hospital cardiac arrest and sudden coronary death.

For the prevention and treatment of the ACS, it is important to keep in mind that they are the result of an interaction between two distinct processes: atherosclerosis and thrombosis. *Atherosclerosis* is a chronic and fixed process that sets the limit for what is achievable by antithrombotic and thrombolytic therapy. Atherosclerosis persists after thrombolysis and may, if severe, prevent optimal and durable reperfusion. The atherosclerotic obstruction may, however, be eliminated by mechanical intervention or bypass surgery. In contrast, *thrombosis* is an acute and dynamic process that is highly susceptible to treatment with drugs. Thrombosis may appear and disappear rapidly, either spontaneously or accelerated by treatment. Vasospasm and thrombosis often coexist. Overall, drug therapy and mechanical intervention may complement each other in the treatment of the ACS, to obtain *rapid, complete*, and *sustained reperfusion*.

An invasive approach (PCI) may be needed to obtain rapid, complete, and sustained reperfusion of infarct-related arteries or to "passivate" one or a few complex lesions with a particularly high short-term risk in ACS, but a target lesion-based approach alone will not eliminate the threat posed by all the other existing coronary plaques, and their overall risk determines the prognosis at long term. Therefore, life-long systemic therapy is important in patients with diseases caused by atherosclerosis.

References

1. Falk E, Shah PK, Fuster V. Atherothrombosis and thrombosis-prone plaques. In: Fuster V, Alexander RW, O'Rourke RA *et al.*, eds. *Hurst's the Heart*. McGraw-Hill, New York, 2004.
2. Davies MJ. The pathophysiology of acute coronary syndromes. *Heart* 2000; **83**: 361–366.
3. Libby P. Current concepts of the pathogenesis of the acute coronary syndromes. *Circulation* 2001; **104**: 365–372.
4. Lucis AEJ. Atherosclerosis. *Nature* 2000; **47**: 233–241.
5. Glass CK, Witztum JL. Atherosclerosis: the road ahead. *Cell* 2001; **104**: 503–516.
6. Libby P. Inflammation in atherosclerosis. *Nature* 2002; **420**: 868–874.
7. Burke AP, Virmani R, Galis Z, Haudenschild CC, Muller JE. 34th Bethesda Conference: task force #2 – what is the pathologic basis for new atherosclerosis imaging techniques? *J Am Coll Cardiol* 2003; **41**: 1874–1886.
8. Hoffmann U, Brady TJ, Muller J. Cardiology patient page. Use of new imaging techniques to screen for coronary artery disease. *Circulation* 2003; **108**: e50–e53.
9. Bogaty P, Hackett D, Davies G, Maseri A. Vasoreactivity of the culprit lesion in unstable angina. *Circulation* 1994; **90**: 5–11.
10. Naghavi M, Libby P, Falk E *et al.* From vulnerable plaque to vulnerable patient: a call for new definitions and risk assessment strategies. Part I. *Circulation* 2003; **108**: 1664–1672.
11. Schaar JA, Muller JE, Falk E *et al.* Terminology for high-risk and vulnerable coronary artery plaques. Report of a meeting on the vulnerable plaque, June 17 and 18, 2003, Santorini, Greece. *Eur Heart J* 2004; **25**: 1077–1082.
12. Naghavi M, Libby P, Falk E *et al.* From vulnerable plaque to vulnerable patient: a call for new definitions and risk assessment strategies. Part II. *Circulation* 2003; **108**: 1772–1778.
13. Guyton JR. Phospholipid hydrolytic enzymes in a "cesspool" of arterial intimal lipoproteins: a mechanism for atherogenic lipid accumulation. *Arterioscler Thromb Vasc Biol* 2001; **21**: 884–886.
14. Geng YJ, Libby P. Progression of atheroma: a struggle between death and procreation. *Arterioscler Thromb Vasc Biol* 2002; **22**: 1370–1380.
15. Naruko T, Ueda M, Haze K *et al.* Neutrophil infiltration of culprit lesions in acute coronary syndromes. *Circulation* 2002; **106**: 2894–2900.
16. Kaartinen M, van der Wal AC, van der Loos CM *et al.* Mast cell infiltration in acute coronary syndromes: implications for plaque rupture. *J Am Coll Cardiol* 1998; **32**: 606–612.
17. Kolodgie FD, Gold HK, Burke AP *et al.* Intraplaque hemorrhage and progression of coronary atheroma. *N Engl J Med* 2003; **349**: 2316–2325.
18. Schwartz SM, Virmani R, Rosenfeld ME. The good smooth muscle cells in atherosclerosis. *Curr Atheroscler Rep* 2000; **2**: 422–429.
19. Varnava AM, Mills PG, Davies MJ. Relationship between coronary artery remodeling and plaque vulnerability. *Circulation* 2002; **105**: 939–943.
20. Tedgui A, Mallat Z. Apoptosis as a determinant of atherothrombosis. *Thromb Haemost* 2001; **86**: 420–426.

21. Beckman JA, Ganz J, Creager MA, Ganz P, Kinlay S. Relationship of clinical presentation and calcification of culprit coronary artery stenoses. *Arterioscler Thromb Vasc Biol* 2001; **21**: 1618–1622.

22. Sangiorgi G, Rumberger JA, Severson A *et al.* Arterial calcification and not lumen stenosis is highly correlated with atherosclerotic plaque burden in humans: a histologic study of 723 coronary artery segments using nondecalcifying methodology. *J Am Coll Cardiol* 1998; **31**: 126–133.

23. Virmani R, Kolodgie FD, Burke AP, Farb A, Schwartz SM. Lessons from sudden coronary death: a comprehensive morphological classification scheme for atherosclerotic lesions. *Arterioscler Thromb Vasc Biol* 2000; **20**: 1262–1275.

24. Vink A, Schoneveld AH, Richard W *et al.* Plaque burden, arterial remodeling and plaque vulnerability: determined by systemic factors? *J Am Coll Cardiol* 2001; **38**: 718–723.

25. Servoss SJ, Januzzi JL, Muller JE. Triggers of acute coronary syndromes. *Prog Cardiovasc Dis* 2002; **44**: 369–380.

26. Falk E. Widespread targets for friendly fire in acute coronary syndromes. *Circulation* 2004; **110**: 4–6.

27. Chapman I. Morphogenesis of occluding coronary artery thrombosis. *Arch Pathol* 1965; **80**: 256–261.

28. Constantinides P. Plaque fissures in human coronary thrombosis. *J Atheroscler Res* 1966; **6**: 1–17.

29. Friedman M, van den Bovenkamp GJ. The pathogenesis of a coronary thrombus. *Am J Pathol* 1966; **48**: 19–44.

30. Bouch DC, Montgomery GL. Cardiac lesions in fatal cases of recent myocardial ischemia from a coronary care unit. *Br Heart J.* 1970; **32**: 795–803.

31. Sinapius D. Beziehungen zwischen Koronarthrombosen und Myokardinfarkten. *Dtsch Med Wochenschr* 1972; **97**: 443–448.

32. Friedman M, Manwaring JH, Rosenman RH, Donlon G, Ortega P, Grube SM. Instantaneous and sudden deaths. Clinical and pathological differentiation in coronary artery disease. *JAMA* 1973; **225**: 1319–1328.

33. Horie T, Sekiguchi M, Hirosawa K. Coronary thrombosis in pathogenesis of acute myocardial infarction. Histopathological study of coronary arteries in 108 necropsied cases using serial section. *Br Heart J* 1978; **40**: 153–161.

34. Falk E. Plaque rupture with severe pre-existing stenosis precipitating coronary thrombosis. Characteristics of coronary atherosclerotic plaques underlying fatal occlusive thrombi. *Br Heart J* 1983; **50**: 127–134.

35. Tracy RE, Devaney K, Kissling G. Characteristics of the plaque under a coronary thrombus. *Virchows Arch A Pathol Anat Histopathol* 1985; **405**: 411–427.

36. el Fawal MA, Berg GA, Wheatley DJ, Harland WA. Sudden coronary death in Glasgow: nature and frequency of acute coronary lesions. *Br Heart J* 1987; **57**: 329–335.

37. Yutani C, Ishibashi-Ueda H, Konishi M, Shibata J, Arita M. Histopathological study of acute myocardial infarction and pathoetiology of coronary thrombosis: a comparative study in four districts in Japan. *Jpn Circ J* 1987; **51**: 352–361.

38. Richardson PD, Davies MJ, Born GV. Influence of plaque configuration and stress distribution on fissuring of coronary atherosclerotic plaques. *Lancet* 1989; **2**: 941–944.

39. van der Wal AC, Becker AE, van der Loos CM, Das PK. Site of intimal rupture or erosion of thrombosed coronary atherosclerotic plaques is characterized by an

inflammatory process irrespective of the dominant plaque morphology. *Circulation* 1994; **89**: 36–44.

40. Davies MJ. The composition of coronary-artery plaques. *N Engl J Med* 1997; **336**: 1312–1314 (Editorial).
41. Arbustini E, Dal Bello B, Morbini P *et al*. Plaque erosion is a major substrate for coronary thrombosis in acute myocardial infarction. *Heart* 1999; **82**: 269–272.
42. Shi H, Wei L, Yang T, Wang S, Li X, You L. Morphometric and histological study of coronary plaques in stable angina and acute myocardial infarctions. *Chin Med J* 1999; **112**: 1040–1043.
43. Kojima S, Nonogi H, Miyao Y *et al*. Is preinfarction angina related to the presence or absence of coronary plaque rupture? *Heart* 2000; **83**: 64–68.
44. Mallat Z, Benamer H, Hugel B *et al*. Elevated levels of shed membrane microparticles with procoagulant potential in the peripheral circulating blood of patients with acute coronary syndromes. *Circulation* 2000; **101**: 841–843.
45. Bogdanov VY, Balasubramanian V, Hathcock J, Vele O, Lieb M, Nemerson Y. Alternatively spliced human tissue factor: a circulating, soluble, thrombogenic protein. *Nat Med* 2003; **9**: 458–462.
46. Mann J, Davies MJ. Mechanisms of progression in native coronary artery disease: role of healed plaque disruption. *Heart* 1999; **82**: 265–268.
47. Fernandez-Ortiz A, Badimon JJ, Falk E *et al*. Characterization of the relative thrombogenicity of atherosclerotic plaque components: implications for consequences of plaque rupture. *J Am Coll Cardiol* 1994; **23**: 1562–1569.
48. Corti R, Hutter R, Badimon JJ, Fuster V. Evolving concepts in the triad of atherosclerosis, inflammation and thrombosis. *J Thromb Thrombolysis* 2004; **17**: 35–44. (Review).
49. Ardissino D, Merlini PA, Ariens R, Coppola R, Bramucci E, Mannucci PM. Tissue-factor antigen and activity in human coronary atherosclerotic plaques. *Lancet* 1997; **349**: 769–771.
50. Ruggeri ZM. Platelets in atherothrombosis. *Nat Med* 2002; **8**: 1227–1234.
51. Falk E, Thuesen L. Pathology of coronary microembolisation and no reflow. *Heart* 2003; **89**: 983–985.
52. Reimer KA, Jennings RB. The "wavefront phenomenon" of myocardial ischemic cell death. II. Transmural progression of necrosis within the framework of ischemic bed size (myocardium at risk) and collateral flow. *Lab Invest* 1979; **40**: 633–644.

CHAPTER 3
Vascular biology of acute coronary syndromes

Lina Badimon

Introduction

Thrombus formation in a coronary artery with obstruction of coronary blood flow and reduction in oxygen supply to the myocardium produces the acute coronary syndromes (ACSs). These thrombotic episodes largely occur in response to atherosclerotic lesions that have progressed to a high risk-inflammatory/prothrombotic stage. Although apparently distinct, the atherosclerotic and thrombotic processes appear to be closely interrelated as the causal presentation of ACS through a complex multifactorial process named atherothrombosis. ACS represents a spectrum of ischemic myocardial events that share similar pathophysiology and include unstable angina, non-Q-wave myocardial infarction, Q-wave myocardial infarction, and sudden death.

Atherosclerosis is a chronic systemic disease involving the intima of large- and medium-sized arteries including the aorta, carotids, coronaries, and peripheral arteries, which is characterized by intimal thickening due to cellular- and lipid-accumulation [1]. Endothelial dysfunction and inflammation are the major facilitators of atherosclerotic disease progression. Lipid accumulation results from an imbalance between mechanisms responsible for lipid influx and efflux. Secondary changes may occur in the underlying media and adventitia, particularly in advanced disease stages. Indeed, fibroblasts from the adventitia have been shown to have an important partnership with the medial smooth muscle cells (SMCs), resulting in neointima formation and compensatory vascular enlargement (remodeling). The early atherosclerotic lesions might progress without compromising the lumen due to this remodeling [2]. When fatty streaks progress to fibroatheroma, they develop a cap of SMCs and collagen, and when this plaque is disrupted, the subsequent thrombus formation is the first step of ACS and strokes. Importantly, the culprit lesions leading to ACS are usually mildly stenotic and therefore are poorly detected by angiography [3]. The composition of the plaque, rather than the stenosis, appears to be the main determinant of risk of plaque rupture and following thrombogenicity. High-risk rupture-prone lesions usually have a large lipid core, a thin fibrous cap, high density of inflammatory cells (particularly at the shoulders of the plaque where disruptions most often occur) and a high tissue factor (TF) content [4,5]. Inflammatory processes also contribute markedly to atherosclerosis and its acute thrombotic complications, as is shown by the fact that many inflammatory mediators can augment TF gene expression by vascular cells, thus triggering the coagulation cascade [6]. Due to the baffling heterogeneity in the composition of atherothrombotic plaques even within the same individual, a reliable, noninvasive imaging tool able to detect early atherosclerotic disease and characterize lesion composition would be clinically relevant. Indeed, it would improve our understanding of the pathophysiological mechanisms of atherothrombosis and help in patient risk stratification [7]. The variety of lesion types is shown by the fact that two-thirds of ACSs take place after the disruption of a high-risk atherothrombotic plaque with superimposed thrombus formation, but, on the other hand, in one-third of the cases there is no plaque rupture but a superficial erosion of a markedly stenotic and fibrotic lesion [8]. In the latter, thrombosis may be triggered by a hyperthrombogenicity due to systemic factors [9].

Growing thrombi on atherosclerotic vessels may locally occlude the lumen, or embolize and be washed away by the blood flow to occlude distal vessels. However, thrombi may be physiologically and spontaneously lysed by mechanisms that block thrombus propagation. Thrombus size, location, and composition are regulated by (1) hemodynamic forces (mechanical effects); (2) thrombogenicity of exposed substrate (local molecular effects), which are strongly related to the degree of plaque disruption or substrate exposure, relative concentration of fluid phase, and cellular blood components (local cellular effects); and the (3) efficiency of the physiologic mechanisms to control the system, mainly fibrinolysis [10].

Cellular and molecular mechanisms in atherogenesis

Role of lipids and lipoproteins

Cholesterol is transported into the vessel wall as a component of the lipoproteins. Low-density lipoprotein (LDL) is considered the most atherogenic lipoproteins since they accumulate in the intima and carry large amounts of plasmatic cholesterol (up to 70%).

High levels of circulating LDL are predictive markers for cardiovascular disease. It appears that discrete LDL subclasses carry different levels of atherogenicity. The "atherogenic lipoprotein phenotype" describes a combination of moderate hypertriglyceridemia, low high-density lipoprotein (HDL) – cholesterol, and a predominance of small, dense LDL particles. This dyslipemia is prevalent in patients with the metabolic syndrome, in those with Type II diabetes, and in postmenopausal women.

Dietary fats and oils differ in the chain lengths of their constituent fatty acids and the number and geometry of their double bonds. These differences markedly affect concentrations of lipids in plasma and differences in the amount and type of fat from the diet can induce differences of 30–40% in serum LDL concentrations. When saturated fatty acids are replaced by unsaturated fats, total plasma cholesterol is lowered. A review of metabolic studies, prospective cohort studies, and clinical trials indicates that there are multiple mechanisms by which diet potentially influences risk of congenital heart disease (CHD), and there are dietary strategies effective in preventing CHD. As such, the substitution of nonhydrogenated unsaturated fats for saturated and trans-fats, the increase in the consumption of omega-3 fatty acids from fish, fish oil supplements, or plant sources, and the consumption of a diet high in fruits, vegetables, nuts, and whole grains and low in refined grain products are good strategies to prevent CHD [11].

Extracellular accumulation of lipids in the arterial intima occurs very early in response to increased plasma lipoproteins levels. Proteoglycan (PG) and protein-bound lipoprotein particles, perhaps, in a microenvironment shielded from plasma antioxidants, can undergo modifications. Such modifications include oxidation, aggregation, enzymatic, and nonenzymatic modifications of LDL. Modified forms of LDL are associated with increased atherogenicity because the physicochemical properties of the lipoprotein become altered. This may change the biological properties of the LDL and also increase the susceptibility of the LDL to other types of modifications.

Endothelial dysfunction
Hypercholesterolemia induces an increase of leukocyte recruitment by an increased expression of adhesion molecules per se and those induced by cytokines, a decrease in endothelium-dependent vasodilatation, and alterations in the thrombosis/fibrinolysis balance. Recently, our group has demonstrated that hypercholesterolemia can induce endothelial dysfunction by altering the expression of genes that are regulated through the downregulation of sterol regulatory element binding proteins (SREBPs) in endothelial cells [12].

Synthesis and degradation of extracellular matrix
Modified LDL can modulate the synthesis of PGs in different cell types. The increase of PG synthesis induced by LDL might have important consequences for the intimal LDL retention. Additionally, the exposure of endothelial cells to apoE-containing HDL has also shown to stimulate the production of heparan sulfate proteoglycans (HS-PGs) that have increased sulfation [13].

Lipoproteins also modulate the expression of matrix metalloproteinases (MMPs), enzymes that are able to digest various connective tissue components. An increase in the expression and activity of metalloproteinases is associated with the disruption of the fibrous cap of lesions and plaque rupture. Additionally, the breakdown products of the extracellular matrix (ECM) may be biologically active and might increase processes that are fundamental for the pathogenesis of the atherosclerosis.

Foam cell formation

Modified lipoproteins are taken up through mechanisms not regulated by cholesterol, leading to high intracellular cholesteryl ester accumulation and foam cell formation. The accumulation of lipid-laden foam cells is one of the earliest steps in the progression of the atherosclerotic plaque. In macrophages, the scavenger receptors (SRs) are mainly responsible for modified LDL uptake. We have recently described a main role for low density lipoprotein receptor-related protein (LRP) in the uptake of agLDL by vascular smooth muscle cells (VSMCs) [14]. SR and the LRP have been detected in human atherosclerotic lesions and could, therefore, play an important role in foam cell formation in the arterial intima. Several modified lipoproteins have demonstrated to upregulate their own receptors, for example, oxLDL increase the expression of several SRs, such as CD36, SR-A, and LOX-1, in different cell types. In addition, agLDL upregulate the expression of their receptor LRP in VSMCs [15]. Most of the modified lipoproteins could lead to a progressive cholesteryl ester accumulation not only by being taken up through non-downregulated receptors, but also by upregulating their own receptors.

Lipoproteins and the metabolic syndrome

The metabolic syndrome has recently been defined by the National Institutes of Health (2001) [16] as a cluster of disorders including abdominal obesity, insulin resistance, diabetes, endothelial dysfunction, blood pressure, and impaired fibrinolysis. The risk factors that constitute the metabolic syndrome consist of atherogenic dyslipemia, elevated blood pressure, elevated plasma glucose, and a prothrombotic state [17]. The metabolic syndrome is closely linked to the metabolic derangement called insulin resistance. This condition is characterized by a generalized defect in the insulin-signaling pathway [18]. Because insulin induces a myriad of metabolic responses, a defect in insulin-signaling results in several metabolic changes. The presence of insulin resistance predisposes to the development of Type II diabetes. There are four major causes of insulin resistance: genetics, obesity, lack of exercise, and diet composition. Insulin resistance and metabolic syndrome are related to the atherogenic dyslipemia also called "atherogenic lipoprotein phenotype" characterized by increased triglyceride-rich lipoproteins, increased small LDL particles, and reduced levels of HDL [19]. These changes in lipoprotein and fatty acid profile observed in insulin resistance may influence different proatherosclerotic mechanisms such as membrane lipid composition, metabolism or signal-transduction pathways [20].

Role of inflammation

Different constituents of the modified lipoproteins trigger the production of mediators of innate immunity. There are also nonlipid mediators involved in inflammation, such as homocystein, angiotensin II, and microbial products that can induce the synthesis of cytokines in atheroma-associated cells.

Under normal circumstances, the endothelial monolayer in contact with flowing blood is inert to the adhesion of leukocytes. The situation changes in dysfunctional endothelium. One of the endothelial–leukocyte adhesion molecules mainly involved in the early adhesion of mononuclear leukocytes to arterial endothelium is VCAM-1, which binds particularly those classes of leukocytes found in nascent atheroma: the monocyte and the T-lymphocyte. In addition to VCAM-1, P- and E-selectin, and ICAM-1 also seem to contribute to leukocyte recruitment. After leukocyte adhesion to the endothelium, the cells enter into the intima by diapedesis, a process that is facilitated by different chemokines, such as MCP-1, IL-8, and a trio of CXC chemokines induced by interferon-γ. Once in the intima, monocytes acquire characteristics of macrophage by expressing certain scavenger receptors, such as scavenger receptor A (SRAI and II) and CD36, that internalize modified lipoproteins leading to foam cell formation (as previously described).

One of the most important clinical markers of inflammation is C-reactive protein (CRP), which has been shown in multiple epidemiological studies to predict incidence of myocardial infarction, stroke, peripheral arterial disease, and sudden cardiac death. In terms of clinical application, some data indicate that CRP seems to be a strong predictor of cardiovascular events and it adds prognostic information at all levels of calculated Framingham risk and at all levels of metabolic syndrome [21]. The feature that distinguishes CRP from LDL cholesterol is the fact that inflammation (but not elevated cholesterol LDL) plays a major role in almost all processes associated with the metabolic syndrome.

Role of the different components of the vascular wall
Extracellular matrix
The ECM of the arterial intima is a relatively large compartment made of collagen, elastin, complex PGs, and hyaluronate and multidomain proteins such as fibronectin, laminin, and tenascin [13]. ECM occupies 60% of the arterial intima and regulates numerous cellular functions. The main PGs structuring the ECM are chondroitin sulfate proteoglycans CS-PGs, such as versican or biglycan, which have the longest negatively charged glycosaminoglycan (GAG) chains and are mainly synthesized by VSMC. HS-PGs, such as perlecan, are constituents of the basement membrane and are mainly synthesized by endothelial cells and VSMCs. In addition, other HS-PGs, such as syndecans and glypicans, are found in the cell membranes of the vascular cells. While CS-PGs play a major role for LDL retention in the arterial intima, cell-surface HS-PGs are dynamic molecules that mediate ligand catabolism [22]. Collagens play a central role not only in maintaining the integrity and stability of the wall, but also in many cellular functions.

Cellular components

Endothelium

Normally, vascular endothelium forms a multifunctional interface between circulating blood and the various tissues and organs in the body. It constitutes a selectively permeable barrier for macromolecules, as well as a nonthrombogenic surface that actively maintains the fluidity of blood. Endothelial dysfunction, as well as a breach of the endothelial integrity, triggers a series of biochemical and molecular reactions aimed at arresting blood flow and vessel wall repair. One of its main traits is the reduction of the availability of vasodilators, especially nitric oxide (NO), and an increase in endothelium-derived contracting factors leading to vasoconstriction, such as angiotensin II (AGII).

These vasoactive substances mediate vascular tone, structure, and function influencing VSMC growth, apoptosis, platelet aggregation, monocyte and leukocyte adhesion, and thrombosis. The homeostasis of vasoactive substances is disrupted by endothelial dysfunction, leading to changes in vascular structure and function. Hypertension and other risk factors for cardiovascular disease are associated with endothelial dysfunction and vascular remodeling. Elevated AGII activity, which is strongly correlated with hypertension, is a major trigger of endothelial dysfunction in hypertensive patients. AGII stimulates NADPH/NADH oxidase in endothelium, VSMC, and adventitia of blood vessels to generate reactive oxygen species, leading to endothelial dysfunction, cell growth, and inflammation [23]. These changes result in upregulation of endothelin-1, adhesion molecules, NF-kb, and other inflammatory mediators, as well as increased breakdown of nitric oxide and uncoupling of nitric oxide synthase. The balance of vasoconstriction and vasodilatation is thus disrupted, leading to vascular remodeling and injury. Physiopathological stimuli especially relevant to atherogenesis include cytokines and bacterial endotoxins, infection by viruses, advanced glycosylation end products that are generated in diabetes and with aging, hyperhomocysteinemia, and hypercholesterolemia, and oxidized LDL. In addition to these humoral stimuli, it is also clear that biochemical forces generated by flowing blood can also influence endothelial cell structure and function, modulating the expression of relevant genes. Hemodynamic effects on endothelium are supported by the long-standing observation that the earliest lesions develop in a nonrandom pattern, the geometry of which correlates with branch points and other regions of altered blood flow. A variety of changes in the metabolic and synthetic activities of endothelial cells in response to defined biomechanical forces have been reported. These include the production of arachidonate metabolites, growth factors, coagulation and fibrinolytic factors, ECM components, and vasoactive mediators. Certain of the most acute shear-induced changes appear to involve regulation at the level of rate-limiting enzymes and/or substrate availability. However, especially in the case of delayed responses, in which *de novo* synthesis occurs, upregulation of gene expression appears to occur as a direct consequence of exposure to fluid mechanical forces. There are genes such as *PDGF-B, MCP-1,*

VCAM-1, and *endothelin-1* that have a "shear stress response element" in their promoter.

Monocyte/macrophages

The state and function of the macrophages in the atherosclerotic lesions may be critical for the development of atherosclerosis. Macrophages play an important role in innate immune responses, cellular adhesion, phagocytosis of apoptotic cells, and lipid uptake. Most of these macrophage functions are mediated by SRs. Since the cloning of the first two macrophage SR (now called SR-A Type I and Type II), the broad SR family has grown considerably. On the basis of functional studies and expression in the arterial intima, only some of the SRs are good candidates to contribute to atherosclerotic foam cell formation. Besides its role in lipid accumulation, macrophages may also contribute to atherosclerosis through secretory inflammatory products. Activated lymphocytes and macrophages with a wide expression of Class II histocompatibility antigen have been found at every stage of atherosclerotic lesions indicating that macrophages may participate in local immune responses.

Vascular smooth muscle cells

Vascular smooth muscle cells represent an average of 50% of the cellular component in advanced atherosclerotic plaque and may reach 90–95% in early lesions. In response to multiple stimuli, VSMC from the arterial tunica media are activated and migrate to the intima where they proliferate. These seem to be early steps at the onset of the atherosclerotic process. The proliferation and migration of VSMC from the media to the intima is one of the key events in early atherosclerosis. The understanding of the molecular mechanisms involved in VSMC activation and differentiation requires an accurate mapping of the cascade of transcription factors induced by atherogenic stimuli. Recently, different nuclear receptors including PPARs, retinoid receptors, retinoid X receptors (RXRs), retinoic acid receptors (RARs), and retinoid-related orphan receptors (RORs) have been identified in VSMC activation/proliferation, and consequently have been involved in atherogenesis [24,25]. Recently our group has identified neuron-derived organ receptor-1 (*NOR-1*) as a new early response gene in VSMCs [26]. *NOR-1* is strongly induced by growth factors and thrombin, and is overexpressed in atherosclerotic lesions from patients with coronary artery disease (CAD). It is transiently induced by PTCA in porcine coronary arteries. It is also induced by high cholesterol levels [27]. These results suggest that *NOR-1* may play a role in the molecular mechanisms underlying both spontaneous and accelerated atherosclerosis.

Vascular smooth muscle cells also contribute to the lesion by synthesizing ECM. In fact, proliferative VSMCs have a high capacity to synthesize sulfated-PGs, and it is well established that PGs in the arterial wall are involved in the focal deposition of cholesterol-rich particles in the early phases of atherogenesis.

Finally, VSMCs also have a great importance in foam cell formation. We demonstrated that agLDL can cause high intracellular cholesteryl ester accumulation in VSMCs [14,15,28]. We showed, for the first time, that in VSMCs, LRP mediates the binding and internalization of agLDL and that in absence of LRP function, VSMCs are unable to accumulate cholesterol. Additionally, this receptor is expressed in atherosclerotic plaques [29] and it is upregulated by agLDL uptake, leading to intracellular lipid accumulation.

Cellular and molecular mechanisms in thrombus formation

The endothelium is an active organ system playing a crucial role in maintaining vascular homeostasis via regulation of hemostatic, inflammatory, and reparative responses to local injury, and it has many antithrombotic and fibrinolytic properties. Vasoconstriction and platelet adhesion at the place of vascular injury cooperate to form a hemostatic aggregate, as the first step in vessel wall repair and the prevention of excessive blood loss. A few scattered platelets may interact with subtly injured, dysfunctional endothelium, and contribute by the release of growth factors to intimal hyperplasia. In contrast, from a monolayer to a few layers of platelets may deposit on the lesion with mild injury that may or may not evolve to a mural thrombus. The release of platelet growth factors may contribute significantly to an accelerated intimal hyperplasia, as it occurs in the coronary vein grafts within the first postoperative year. In severe injury, with exposure of components of deeper layers of the vessel, as in spontaneous plaque rupture or in angioplasty, marked platelet aggregation with mural thrombus formation follows. Vascular injury of this magnitude also stimulates thrombin formation through both the intrinsic (surface-activated) and extrinsic (tissue-factor dependent) coagulation pathways, in which the platelet membrane facilitates interactions between clotting factors.

Platelets

After plaque rupture, some of the atherosclerotic plaque components exhibit a potent activating effect on platelets and coagulation [30–32]. Exposed matrix from the vessel wall and thrombin generated by the activation of the coagulation cascade as well as epinephrine and ADP are powerful platelet agonists. Each agonist stimulates the discharge of calcium and promotes the subsequent release of its granule content. Although platelets are classically relegated to this passive role as a responder to thrombotic stimuli, they are also increasingly evincing importance as a source of inflammatory mediators. For example, they can both produce and respond to chemoattractant cytokines [33], or express CD154 (CD40 ligand), the molecule which regulates TF gene expression in the macrophage and SMCs [34]. Platelet-related ADP and 5HT stimulate adjacent platelets, further enhancing the process of platelet aggregation. Arachidonate, which is released from the platelet membrane by the stimulatory effect of collagen, thrombin, ADP, and 5HT, promotes the synthesis of thromboxane A_2 by the sequential effects of cyclooxygenase and thromboxane synthetase. Thromboxane A_2 not only promotes further platelet aggregation, but is also a potent vasoconstrictor.

The initial recognition of damaged vessel wall by platelets involves (1) adhesion, activation, and adherence to recognition sites on the thromboactive substrate [ECM proteins e.g. von Willebrand factor (vWF), collagen, fibronectin, vitronectin, laminin]; (2) spreading of the platelet on the surface; and (3) aggregation of platelets with each other to form a platelet plug or white thrombus. The efficiency of the platelet recruitment will depend on the underlying substrate and the local geometry (local factors). A final step of recruitment of other blood cells also occurs; erythrocytes, neutrophils, and occasionally monocytes are found on evolving mixed thrombus.

Platelet function depends on adhesive interactions and most of the glycoproteins on the platelet membrane surface are receptors for adhesive proteins. Many of these receptors have been identified, cloned, sequenced, and classified within large gene families that mediate a variety of cellular interactions [35]. The most abundant is the integrin family, which includes GPIIIbIIa, GPIaIIa, GPIcIIa, the fibronectin receptor, and the vitronectin receptor, in decreasing order of magnitude. Another gene family present in the platelet membrane glycocalyx is the leucine-rich glycoprotein family represented by the GPIbIX complex, receptor for vWF on unstimulated platelets that mediates adhesion to subendothelium and GPV. Other gene families include the selectins (such as GMP-140) and the immunoglobulin domain protein (HLA Class I antigen and platelet/endothelial cell adhesion molecule-1, PECAM-1). Unrelated to any other gene family is the GPIV (IIIa).

Another recently discovered receptor on platelets is P-selectin. P-selectin is a transmembrane protein present in the alpha granules of platelets, from where it quickly moves to the platelet surface after activation. It interacts with the P-selectin glycoprotein ligand-1 on leukocytes, forming aggregates and upregulating TF formation. It also enforces platelet aggregates through interaction with platelet sulfatides. This might explain why P-selectin expression in platelets has been linked to arterial thrombosis and coronary artery disease [36]. P-selectin is also present on activated endothelial cells, where it helps in the recruitment of leukocytes [37]. Indeed, selectins are specialized in lymphocyte homing and involved in inflammation processes.

Thrombin plays an important role in the pathogenesis of arterial thrombosis. It is one of the most potent known agonists for platelet activation and recruitment. The thrombin receptor has 425 amino acids with 7 transmembrane domains and a large NH_2-terminal extracellular extension that is cleaved by thrombin to produce a "tethered" ligand that activates the receptor to initiate signal transduction [38]. Thrombin is a critical enzyme in early thrombus formation, cleaving fibrinopeptides A and B from fibrinogen to yield insoluble fibrin, which effectively anchors the evolving thrombus. Both free and fibrin-bound fibrin thrombin are able to convert fibrinogen to fibrin, allowing propagation of thrombus at the site of injury.

Therefore, platelet activation triggers intracellular signaling and expression of platelet membrane receptors for adhesion and initiation of cell contractile processes that induce shape change and secretion of the granular contents. The expression of the integrin IIb/IIa (αIIbβ_3) receptors for adhesive glycoprotein ligands (mainly fibrinogen and vWF) in the circulation initiates platelet-to-platelet interaction. The process becomes perpetuated by the arrival of platelets brought by the circulation. Most of the glycoproteins in the platelet membrane surface are receptors for adhesive proteins or mediate cellular interactions. vWF has been shown to bind to platelet membrane glycoproteins in both adhesion (platelet–substrate interaction) and aggregation (platelet–platelet interaction), leading to thrombus formation in perfusion studies conducted at high shear rates [35]. Ligand binding to the different membrane receptors triggers platelet activation with different relative potencies. A lot of interest has been recently generated on the platelet ADP-receptors (P2Y$_{AC}$, P2y1R, P2X$_{1R}$) because of available pharmacological inhibitors.

Activation of the coagulation system

During plaque rupture, in addition to platelet deposition in the injured area, the clotting mechanism is activated by the exposure of the plaque contents. The activation of the coagulation leads to the generation of thrombin, which is a powerful platelet agonist in addition to an enzyme that catalyzes the formation and polymerization of fibrin. Fibrin is essential in the stabilization of the platelet thrombus and its withstanding to removal forces by flow, shear, and high intravascular pressure. The efficacy of fibrinolytic agents pointedly demonstrates the importance of fibrin in thrombosis associated with myocardial infarction.

The blood coagulation system involves a sequence of reactions integrating zymogens – proteins susceptible to be activated to enzymes (via limited proteolysis) and cofactors (nonproteolytic enzyme activators) in three groups: (1) the contact activation (generation of factor XIa via the Hageman factor); (2) the conversion of factor X to factor Xa in a complex reaction requiring the participation of factors IX and VIII; and (3) the conversion of prothrombin to thrombin and fibrin formation [35,39].

Glycosaminoglycans and sulfatides have been suggested to be the triggering surfaces for *in vivo* initiation of contact activation; however, the physiologic role of coagulation contact activation is unclear, since the absence of Hageman factor, prekallikrein, or high-molecular-weight kininogen does not induce a clinically apparent pathology. On the contrary, factor XI deficiency is associated with abnormal bleeding. Activated factor XI induces the activation of factor IX in the presence of Ca^{2+}. Factor IXa forms a catalytic complex with factor VIII on a membrane surface and efficiently activates factor X in the presence of Ca^{2+}. Factor IX is a vitamin K-dependent enzyme, as are factor VII, factor X, prothrombin, and protein C.

The TF pathway, previously known as extrinsic coagulation pathway, through TF factor VIIa complex in the presence of Ca^{2+} induces the formation of Xa. A second TF-dependent reaction catalyzes the transformation of IX into IXa. TF is an integral membrane protein that serves to initiate the activation of factors IX and X and localize the reaction to cells on which TF is expressed. Other cofactors include factor VIIIa, which binds to platelets and forms the binding site for IXa, thereby forming the machinery for the activation of X, and factor Va, which binds to platelets and provides a binding site for Xa. The human genes for these cofactors have been cloned and sequenced. In physiologic conditions, no cells in contact with blood contain active TF, although cells such as monocytes and polymorphonuclear leukocytes can be induced to synthesize and express TF [39].

Activated Xa converts prothrombin into thrombin. The complex, which catalyzes the formation of thrombin, consists of factors Xa and Va in a 1 : 1 complex. The activation results in the cleavage of fragment 1.2 and formation of thrombin from fragment 2. The interaction of the four components of the "prothrombinase complex" (Xa, Va, phospholipid, and Ca^{2+}) yields a more efficient reaction [40].

Activated platelets provide procoagulant surface for the assembly and expression of both intrinsic Xase and prothrombinase enzymatic complexes. These complexes, respectively, catalyze the activation of factor X to factor Xa and prothrombin to thrombin. The expression of activity is associated with the binding of both the proteases, factor IXa and factor Xa, and the cofactors, VIIIa and Va, to procoagulant surfaces. The binding of IXa and Xa is promoted by VIIIa and Va, respectively, such that Va and VIIIa is likely to provide the equivalent of receptors for the proteolytic enzymes. The surface of the platelet expresses the procoagulant phospholipids that bind coagulation factors and contribute to the procoagulant activity of the cell [40].

Thrombin acts on multiple substrates, including fibrinogen, factor XIII, factors V and VIII, and protein C, in addition to its effects on platelets. It plays a central role in hemostasis and thrombosis. The catalytic transformation of fibrinogen into fibrin is essential in the formation of the hemostatic plug and in the formation of arterial thrombi. It binds to the fibrinogen central domain and cleaves fibrinopeptides A and B, resulting in fibrin monomer and polymer formation. The fibrin mesh holds the platelets together and contributes to the attachment of the thrombus to the vessel wall. Thrombin makes sure the coagulation cascade is activated and stimulates platelet aggregation, thus becoming pivotal to the stability of the mural thrombus, which forms over the plaque and releases growth factors and platelet vasoconstrictors, favoring the onset of ischemic events.

Spontaneous anticoagulation and fibrinolysis

The control of the coagulation reactions occurs by diverse mechanisms, such as hemodilution and flow effects, proteolytic feedback by thrombin, inhibition by plasma proteins (such as antithrombin III [ATIII]) and endothelial cell-localized activation of an inhibitory enzyme (protein C), and fibrinolysis. Although ATIII readily inactivates thrombin in solution, its catalytic site is inaccessible while bound to fibrin, and it may still cleave fibrinopeptides even in the presence of heparin. Thrombin has a specific receptor in endothelial cell surfaces, thrombomodulin, that triggers a physiologic anticoagulative system. The thrombin–thrombomodulin complex serves as a receptor for the vitamin K-dependent protein C which is activated and released from the endothelial cell surface. Activated protein C, in the presence of protein S, inactivates factors Va and VIIIa and limits thrombin effects. Thrombin generated at the site of injury binds to thrombomodulin, an endothelial surface membrane protein, initiating activation of protein C, which in turn (in the presence of protein S) inactivates factors Va and VIIIa. Loss of Va decreases the role of thrombin formation to negligible levels [40]. Thrombin stimulates successive release of both tissue plasminogen activator (tPA) and plasminogen-activator inhibitor type 1 from endothelial cells, thus initiating endogenous lysis through plasmin generation from plasminogen by tPA with subsequent modulation through plasminogen-activator inhibitor type 1. Thrombin therefore plays a pivotal role in maintaining the complex balance of initial prothrombotic reparative events and subsequent endogenous anticoagulant and fibrinolytic pathways. Endogenous fibrinolysis (repair mechanism) involves catalytic activation of zymogens, positive and negative feedback control, and inhibitor blockade.

Blood clotting is blocked at the level of the prothrombinase complex by the physiologic anticoagulant-activated protein C and oral anticoagulants. Oral anticoagulants prevent posttranslational synthesis of γ-carboxyglutamic acid groups on the vitamin K-dependent clotting factors, preventing binding of prothrombin and Xa to the membrane surface. Activated protein C cleaves factor Va to render it functionally inactive. Endothelial loss, contributes to the high thrombogenicity of atherosclerotic plaques. Overall, it is likely that when injury to the vessel wall is mild, the thrombogenic stimulus is relatively limited, and the resulting thrombotic occlusion is transient, as occurs in unstable angina. On the other hand, deep vessel injury secondary to plaque rupture or ulceration results in exposure of collagen, TF, and other elements of the vessel matrix, leading to relatively persistent thrombotic occlusion and myocardial infarction [1].

It is likely that the nature of the substrate exposed after spontaneous or angioplasty-induced plaque rupture determines whether an unstable plaque proceeds rapidly to an occlusive thrombus or persists as nonocclusive mural thrombus. The analysis of the relative contribution of different components of human atherosclerotic plaques (fatty streaks, sclerotic plaques, fibrolipid plaques, atheromatous plaques, hyperplasic cellular plaque, and normal intima) to acute thrombus formation showed that the atheromatous core was up to sixfold more active than the other substrates, in triggering thrombosis [4]. The atheromatous core, together with the residual mural thrombus

[41], remained the most thrombogenic substrate when the substrates were normalized by the degree of irregularity as defined by the roughness index. Therefore ruptured plaques with a large atheromatous core are at high risk to lead to ACS, and this core shows the most intense TF staining compared with other components [4,5]. As proof of concept, we showed that local tissue blockade of TF, by treatment with TFPI, significantly reduces thrombosis [42]. Recently, the use of active site inhibited recombinant FVIIa (FF-rFVIIa) has shown to significantly reduce thrombus growth on damaged vessels without TF, indicating the efficacy of blocking blood-borne TF [43].

Monocyte/macrophage are key to the development of vulnerable plaques [44]. The vulnerable plaques (AHA Type IV and Va), commonly composed of an abundant lipid core separated from the lumen by a thin fibrotic cap, are particularly soft and prone to disruption [45]. A high density of activated inflammatory cells has been detected in the disrupted areas of atherectomy specimens from patients with acute coronary syndromes [46]. These cells are capable of degrading ECM by secreting proteolytic enzymes, such as MMPs [47], among which some can further promote thrombogenicity through the activation of platelet aggregation, as MMP-2 does [48]. In addition, T-cells isolated from rupture prone sites can stimulate macrophages to produce metalloproteinases and may predispose lesions disruption by weakening their fibrous cap. Recently, LDLs have shown to downregulate the expression of lysil-oxidase (LOX) in vascular wall cells [49]. LOX is an enzyme that contributes to the maturation of the elastin and collagen fibrils of the ECM. Its decrease is associated to an increased permeability of the vascular wall and hence may contribute to plaque destabilization. Cell apoptosis and microparticles with procoagulant activity and postulated apoptotic origin have also been linked to inflammation and thrombosis [50,51]. Finally, it merits mentioning that atherosclerotic plaques often demonstrate increased adventitial and intimal neovascularization, especially at the lesions responsible for ACSs [52,53]. These new vessels may provide a way to recruit inflammatory cells into the plaque, and due to their thin walls easily rupture and hemorrhage, with the consequent secondary plaque expansion or rupture [54,55].

Summary

The formation of a thrombus within a coronary artery with obstruction of coronary blood flow and reduction in oxygen supply to the myocardium produce ACSs. These thrombotic episodes largely occur in response to atherosclerotic lesions that have progressed to a high risk-inflammatory/prothrombotic stage by a process modulated by local and systemic factors. Although distinct from one another, the atherosclerotic and thrombotic processes appear to be closely interrelated as the cause of ACS through a complex multifactorial process named atherothrombosis. The cellular and molecular mechanisms at play in atherothrombosis are subject of extensive investigation. The identification of dangerous lesions by angiography is often rendered impossible because, due to remodeling, their stenosis is mild. Advances in noninvasive imaging techniques will help recognize subclinical pathology, identify plaques at risk, and reduce the clinical impact of atherothrombosis, enabling us to better risk stratify the disease and perhaps to customize the treatment and directly monitor its effect.

References

1. Fuster V, Badimon L, Badimon JJ *et al.* The pathogenesis of coronary artery disease and the acute coronary syndromes: (Part I) and (Part II). *New Engl J Med* 1992; **326**, 242–250.
2. Glagov S, Weisenberg E, Zarins CK *et al.* Compensatory enlargement of human atherosclerotic coronary arteries. *New Engl J Med* 1987; **316**: 1371–1375.
3. Ambrose JA, Weinrauch M. Thrombosis in ischemic heart disease. *Arch Intern Med* 1996; **156**: 1382–1394.
4. Fernández-Ortiz A, Badimon JJ, Falk E, Fuster V *et al.* Characterization of the relative thrombogenicity of atherosclerotic plaque components: implications for consequences of plaque rupture. *J Am Coll Cardiol* 1994; **23**: 1562–1569.
5. Toschi V, Gallo R, Lettino M *et al.* Tissue factor modulates the thrombogenicity of human atherosclerotic plaques. *Circulation* 1997; **95**: 594–599.
6. Libby P and Simon DI. Inflammation and thrombosis: the clot thickens. *Circulation* 2001; **103**: 1718–1720.
7. Corti R, Fuster V, Badimon JJ *et al.* New understanding of atherosclerosis (clinically and experimentally) with evolving MRI technology *in vivo*. *Ann N Y Acad Sci* 2001; **947**: 181–195; discussion 195–198.
8. Virmani R, Kolodgie FD, Burke AP *et al.* Lessons from sudden coronary death: a comprehensive morphological classification scheme for atherosclerotic lesions. *Arterioscler Thromb Vasc Biol* 2000; **20**: 1262 1275.
9. Rauch U, Osende JI, Fuster V *et al.* Thrombus formation on atherosclerotic plaques: pathogenesis and clinical consequences. *Ann Intern Med* 2001; **134**: 224–238.
10. Badimon L, Chesebro JH, Badimon JJ. Thrombus formation on ruptured atherosclerotic plaques and rethrombosis on evolving thrombi. *Circulation* 1992; **86**: III-74–III-85.
11. Hu FB, Willett WC. Optimal diets for prevention of coronary heart disease. *JAMA* 2002; **288**(20): 2569–2578.
12. Rodriguez C, Martínez-González J, Sánchez-Gómez S, Badimon L. LDL downregulates CYP51 in porcine vascular endothelial cells and in the arterial wall through a sterol regulatory element binding protein-2-dependent mechanism. *Circ Res* 2001; **88**: 268–274.
13. Newby AC. Dual role of matrix metalloproteinases (matrixins) in intimal thickening and atherosclerotic plaque rupture. *Physiol Rev* 2005; **85**: 1–31.
14. Llorente-Cortés V, Martínez-González J, Badimon L. LDL receptor-related protein mediates uptake of aggregated LDL in human vascular smooth muscle cells. *Arterioscler Thromb Vasc Biol* 2000; **20**: 1572–1579.
15. Llorente-Cortés V, Otero-Viñas M, Sanchez S, Rodríguez C, Badimon L. Low density lipoprotein upregulates low-density lipoprotein receptor-related protein expression in vascular smooth muscle cells. *Circulation* 2002; **106**: 3104–3110.

16. Grundy SM, D'Agostino Sr RB, Mosca L *et al.* Cardiovascular risk assessment based on US cohort studies: findings from a National Heart, Lung, and Blood institute workshop. *Circulation* 2001; **104**(4): 491–496.

17. Grundy SM. Hypertriglyceridemia, atherogenic dylipemia, and the metabolic syndrome. *Am J Cardiol* 1998; **81**: 18B–25B.

18. DeFronzo RA, Ferrannini E. Insulin resistance: a multifactorial syndrome responsible for NIDDM, obesity, hypertension, dyslipidemia and atherosclerotic cardiovascular disease. *Diabetes Care* 1991; **14**: 173–194.

19. Grundy SM, Abate N, Chandalia M. Diet composition and the metabolic syndrome: what is the optimal fat intake. *Am J Med* 2002; **113**(9B): 25S–29S.

20. Wessby B. Dietary fat, fatty acid composition in plasma and the metabolic syndrome. *Curr Opin Lipidol* 2003; **14**: 15–19.

21. Ridker PM. Clinical application of C-reactive protein for cardiovascular disease detection and prevention. *Circulation* 2003; **107**: 363–369.

22. Williams KJ. Arterial wall chondroitin sulfate proteoglycans: diverse molecules with distint roles in lipoprotein retention and atherogenesis. *Curr Opin Lipidol* 2001; **12**: 477–487.

23. Schiffrin EL. Beyond blood pressure: the endothelium and atherosclerosis progression. *Am J Hypertens* 2002; **15**: 115S–122S.

24. Marx N, Schonbeck V, Lazar MA, Libby P, Plutzky J. Peroxisome proliferator-activated receptor activators inhibit gene expression and migration in human vascular smooth muscle cells. *Circ Res* 1998; **83**: 1097–1103.

25. Staels B, Koening W, Habbib A *et al.* Activation of human aortic smooth-muscle cells is inhibited by PPARα but not by PPARβ activator. *Nature* 1998; **393**: 790–793.

26. Martínez-González J, Rius J, Castelló A, Cases-Langhoff C, Badimon L. Neuron-derived orphan receptor-1 (NOR-1) modulates vascular smooth muscle cell proliferation. *Circ Res* 2003; **92**: 96–103.

27. Rius J, Martinez-Gonzalez J, Crespo J, Badimon L. Involvement of neuron-derived orphan receptor-1 (NOR-1) in LDL-induced mitogenic stimulus in vascular smooth muscle cells: role of CREB. *Arterioscler Thromb Vasc Biol* 2004; **24**(4): 697–702.

28. Llorente-Cortés V, Otero-Viñas M, Camino-López S, Llampayas O, Badimon L. Aggregated low-density lipoprotein uptake induces membrane tissue factor procoagulant activity and microparticle release in human vascular smooth muscle cells. *Circulation* 2004; **110**: 452–459.

29. Llorente-Cortés V, Otero-Viñas M, Berrozpe M, Badimon L. Intracellular lipid accumulation, low density lipoprotein receptor-related protein expression, and cell survival in vascular smooth muscle cells derived from normal and atherosclerotic human coronaries. *Eur J Clin Inves* 2004; **34**(3): 182–190.

30. Badimon L, Fuster V, Badimon JJ. (2004). Interaction of platelet activation and thrombosis. In: Fuster V, Topol EJ, & Nabel EG, eds. *Atherosclerosis and Coronary Artery Disease*, 2nd edn. Lippincott-Raven Publishers, Philadelphia, PA, 2004: 583–597, chapter 41.

31. Badimon JJ, Fuster V, Chesebro JH, Badimon L. Coronary atherosclerosis. *Circulation* 1993; **87**: II-3–II-16.

32. Marcus A, Safier LB. Thromboregulation: multicellular modulation of platelet reactivity in hemostasis and thrombosis. *FASEB J* 1993; **7**: 516–522.

33. Abi-Younes S, Sauty A, Mach F *et al.* The stromal cell-derived factor-1 chemokine is a potent platelet agonist highly expressed in atherosclerotic plaques. *Circ Res* 2000; **86**: 131–138.

34. Henn V, Slupsy JR, Grafe M *et al.* CD40 ligand on activated platelets triggers an inflammatory reaction of endothelial cells. *Nature* 1998; **391**: 591–594.
35. Badimon L, Fuster V, Corti R, Badimon JJ. Coronary thrombosis: local and systemic factors. In: Fuster V, ed. *Hurst's the Heart,* 11th edn. McGraw-Hill, New York, 2004: 1141–1151.
36. Merten M, Thiagarajan P. P-selectin in arterial thrombosis. *Z Kardiol* 2004; **93**: 855–863.
37. Vandedries ER, Furie BC, Furie B. Role of P-selectin and PSGL-1 in coagulation and thrombosis. *Thromb Haemost* 2004; **92**: 459–466.
38. Coughlin SR. Thrombin receptor structure and function. *Thromb Haemostasis* 1993; **70**: 184–187.
39. Nemerson Y. Mechanism of coagulation. In: Williams WJ, Beutler E, Erslev AJ, & Lichtman MA, eds. *Hematology.* McGraw-Hill, New York, 1990: 1295–1304.
40. Nemerson Y, Williams WJ. Biochemistry of plasma coagulation factors. In: Williams WJ, Beutler E, Erslev AJ & Lichtman MA, eds. *Hematology.* McGraw-Hill, New York, 1990: 1267–1284.
41. Meyer BJ, Badimon JJ, Mailhac A *et al.* Inhibition of growth of thrombus on fresh mural thrombus. Targeting optimal therapy. *Circulation* 1994; **90**: 2432–2438.
42. Badimon JJ, Lettino M, Toschi V *et al.* Local inhibition of tissue factor reduces the thrombogenicity of disrupted human atherosclerotic plaques. Effects of TFPI on plaque thrombogenicity under flow conditions. *Circulation* 1999; **99**: 1780–1787.
43. Sánchez-Gómez S, Casani L, Vilahur G *et al.* FFR-rFVIIa inhibits thrombosis triggered by ruptured and eroded vessel wall. *Thromb Haemostasis* 2001; (#OC999).
44. Ross R. Atherosclerosis: an inflammatory disease. *N Engl J Med* 1999; **340**: 115–126.
45. Davies MJ. Stability and instability: two faces of coronary atherosclerosis. (The Paul Dudley White Lecture 1995.) *Circulation* 1996; **94**: 2013–2020.
46. Moreno PR, Falk E, Palacios IF *et al.* Macrophage infiltration in acute coronary syndromes. Implications for plaque rupture. *Circulation* 1994; **90**: 775–778.
47. Galis ZS, Khatri JJ. Matrix metalloproteinases in vascular remodeling and atherogenesis: the good, the bad, and the ugly. *Circ Res* 2002; **90**: 251–262.
48. Sawicki G, Salas E, Murat J *et al.* Release of gelatinase A during platelet activation mediates aggregation. *Nature* 1997; **386**: 616–619.
49. Rodríguez C, Raposo B, Martínez-González J *et al.* Low density lipoproteins down-regulate lysyl oxidase in vascular endothelial cells and in the arterial wall. *Arterioscl Throm Vasc Biol* 2002; **22**: 1409–1414.
50. Mallat Z, Tedgui A. Current perspective on the role of apoptosis in atherothrombotic disease. *Circ Res* 2001; **88**: 998–1003.
51. Mallat Z, Hugel B, Ohan J *et al.* Shed membrane microparticles with procoagulant potential in human atherosclerotic plaques: a role for apoptosis in plaque thrombogenicity. *Circulation* 1999; **99**: 348–353.
52. Tenaglia AN, Peters KG, Sketch MH Jr. *et al.* Neovascularization in atherectomy speciments from patients with unstable angina: implications for pathogenesis of unstable angina. *Am Heart J* 1998; **135**: 10–14.
53. Juan-Babot JO, Martínez-González J, Berrozpe M, Badimon L. Neovascularización en arterias coronarias humanas con distintos grados de lesión. *Rev Esp Cardiol* 2003; **56**(10): 978–986.
54. Shah PK. Mechanisms of plaque vulnerability and rupture. *J Am Coll Cardiol* 2003; **41**(4 suppl S): 15S–22S.
55. Kolodgie FD, Gold HK, Burke AP *et al.* Intraplaque hemorrhage and progression of coronary atheroma. *N Engl J Med* 2003; **349**: 2316–2325.

Section three:
Clinical aspects of ACS

CHAPTER 4

Clinical aspects of acute coronary syndromes

Eugene McFadden

The term acute coronary syndrome (ACS) is widely used to describe any clinical presentation suggestive of acute myocardial ischemia. Faced with such a patient, the initial priority for the clinician is to identify immediately life-threatening conditions such as ST-segment elevation myocardial infarction (STEMI) or aortic dissection. Patients with STEMI should receive, when indicated, immediate reperfusion therapy. The appropriate diagnostic and therapeutic pathways in the subgroup of patients with STEMI is comprehensively addressed in the European Society of Cardiology guidelines for the management of STEMI [1].

The remaining patients with an initial diagnosis of suspected ACS constitute a heterogeneous group. In some, a diagnosis of acute myocardial ischemia will be confirmed. They will be ultimately classified as having non-ST-segment elevation myocardial infarction (NSTEMI), if ischemia has resulted in myocardial damage or unstable angina (UA), if no myocardial necrosis has occurred [2,3]. As this classification can only be made retrospectively, and because both conditions are presumed to share a common underlying pathophysiology, the term suspected UA/NSTEMI is commonly used to describe patients with ACS in whom STEMI has been ruled out at initial presentation but who are judged to require further diagnostic workup. Other potential diagnoses include specific noncoronary cardiac causes (such as pericarditis) and specific noncardiac causes (such as esophageal spasm). Finally, many patients will be classified as having a noncardiac, but undefined, cause for their symptoms.

The initial evaluation of patients with suspected ACS should address two issues; first, the likelihood that the clinical presentation represents ACS due to underlying coronary artery disease (CAD); second, the likelihood that the patient will experience an adverse outcome (e.g. death, myocardial infarction). The history, the baseline electrocardiogram (ECG), and to a lesser extent the physical examination, have a central role in the diagnosis and further management of suspected UA/NSTEMI. They provide information that guides decisions regarding the drugs that should be administered, the environment in which the patient should be managed (coronary care unit, high dependency unit, etc.), and the further investigations (stress testing, angiography, etc.)

that are required. They also provide important elements that help assess the prognosis. This information is particularly relevant nowadays because the benefit of many of the more recently introduced therapies for UA/NSTEMI is greatest in those with the highest level of baseline risk. The diagnostic and prognostic information they provide will subsequently be refined in the light of the results of markers of myocardial damage (see Chapter 5). However, the history and baseline ECG still form the cornerstone of clinical assessment in this situation; first, they are immediately available; second, highly suspicious clinical or ECG findings should always guide clinical judgment, irrespective of other apparently reassuring information.

The European guidelines differ slightly in their approach to the classification of patients with suspected ACS from the American guidelines. The former adopt a pragmatic approach in defining high- and low-risk patient groups. The latter include an extra intermediate level of risk [2,3]. Where there are significant differences between the two sets of guidelines, they will be alluded to in the text.

History: role in diagnosis and risk stratification

Patients who present with suspected ACS fall into two categories depending on whether or not they have previously documented CAD. While a prior history of CAD correctly increases the initial index of clinical suspicion, the most important aspect of the history is the nature of the current symptoms. The presence of a history of CAD, sex, age, and the number of traditional risk factors are the other aspects of the history that help define the likelihood that the current presentation is due to myocardial ischemia [4–6].

Diagnostic value of symptoms at presentation: angina, anginal equivalents, and atypical presentations

While the most frequent presenting symptom of UA/NSTEMI is typical anginal chest pain, there are well-recognized, more subtle, presentations that should be regarded as "anginal equivalents." Equally, there are symptoms that render the diagnosis of UA/NSTEMI much less likely, while not entirely excluding it. Classically, angina is defined as chest discomfort, often radiating into the left arm, which is provoked by exertion or by emotional stress, and is relieved by rest [4]. Prompt (<5 min) relief of pain by sublingual nitrates supports the diagnosis. The Canadian Cardiovascular Society classification of angina, initially proposed by Campeau, provides the basis for the current classification of chest pain in UA/NSTEMI patients. In the Canadian classification, symptoms were graded into four classes: Class I – where angina does not occur during normal activity, Class II – where angina leads to a limitation of normal activities, Class III – where angina leads to marked limitation of normal activity, and Class IV – where angina precludes any normal activity and may occur at rest [7].

In UA/NSTEMI, three principal patterns of angina have been described: prolonged (>20 min) anginal pain at rest, new onset severe (Class III) angina, or recent destabilization of previously stable angina (crescendo angina) with at least CCS III (Canadian Cardiovascular Society Class III) angina characteristics [8]. The presence of any of these typical symptom patterns substantially increases the likelihood that the patient has acute ischemia related to underlying CAD.

Occasionally, chest pain may be less prominent and the predominant localization may be in the arms, the epigastium, the neck, or the jaws. If such symptoms are promptly (<5 min) relieved by sublingual nitrates, it is highly likely that they are ischemic in origin, and they should be regarded as "anginal equivalents." There are symptoms, other than chest pain, that may represent "anginal equivalents." The most frequent are new onset or sudden worsening of dyspnea, sweating, or nausea; such presentations, without chest pain, are more frequent in elderly patients and are particularly common in women.

Atypical presentations of ACS are not uncommon. They are often observed in younger (25–40 years) and older (>75 years) patients, in patients with diabetes mellitus, and in women. Such atypical presentations include pain that occurs predominantly at rest, epigastric pain, recent onset indigestion, stabbing chest pain, chest pain with some pleuritic features, or increasing dyspnea. In the Multicenter Chest Pain Study, acute myocardial ischemia was diagnosed in 22% of patients presenting to emergency departments with sharp or stabbing chest pain, 13% of those whose chest pain had some pleuritic features, and 7% of those whose chest pain was fully reproduced by palpation [9]. However, the presence of pain localized in the chest or radiating to the left arm and the description of the pain as a sensation of pressure are the presenting symptoms that are most consistently associated with the presence of acute ischemia [10,11].

Risk stratification: presenting symptoms and other aspects of the history

When patients present with angina, the tempo of the symptoms, the occurrence of pain at rest, the duration of the episodes, and their frequency in the preceding 24 h are prognostically important [12–14]. Some of these elements have been included in prognostic scores that also include information from the EGG and from the results of biomarkers and are discussed further below [15,16]. Other important indicators of risk are a history of previous myocardial infarction, older age (particularly >70 years), and if the sex is male. A prior history of myocardial infarction strongly suggests the presence of underlying multivessel coronary disease. Older patients have a greater likelihood of underlying coronary disease than younger patients and when this is present it is more likely to be multivessel disease and associated with significant left ventricular dysfunction. Furthermore, older patients are more likely to have significant comorbidity, such as renal impairment and diabetes mellitus.

Women who present with suggestive symptoms are much less likely to have obstructive coronary disease than men; furthermore, when CAD is present, it tends to be less severe. Overall, the outcome of women with proven UA is better that that of men and the outcome for proven NSTEMI is similar for both sexes [17].

Of the other traditional risk factors, smoking, hypercholesterolemia, and hypertension, are only very weak predictors of the likelihood of acute ischemia and their presence or absence should not influence early management decisions [11]. In patients with an established diagnosis of ACS, hypercholesterolemia, hypertension, and diabetes mellitus are associated with a worse prognosis due to the greater likelihood of both more extensive CAD and of underlying left ventricular dysfunction. Diabetes mellitus, however, does appear to have independent pejorative prognostic implications. Current smoking is associated with a lower risk of death probably because smokers develop ACS due to thrombosis at nonocclusive plaques at a younger age.

Physical examination: role in diagnosis and risk stratification

Physical examination is most often normal, including chest examination, auscultation, and measurement of heart rate and blood pressure. The purpose of the examination is to identify potential precipitating extracardiac factors (such as thyroid disease, anemia, and severe hypertension) and to exclude noncardiac causes of chest pain (such as dissecting aneurysm or pneumothorax) and nonischemic cardiac disorders (such as pericarditis) that cause chest pain. The physical examination can also identify significant peripheral vascular disease, which raises the likelihood of coexisting CAD. Finally, it will identify signs of potential hemodynamic instability and of left ventricular dysfunction. Patients with ACS who have evidence of left heart failure or of new onset, presumably ischemic, mitral regurgitation are a very high-risk group.

ECG: role in diagnosis and risk stratification

Diagnostic value of the resting ECG

The resting ECG is a key tool in the assessment of patients with suspected ACSs. It is a useful screening tool in patients with atypical presentations and it may provide evidence of alternative diagnoses such as pericarditis, pulmonary embolism, or cardiomyopathy. Ideally, a tracing should be obtained when the patient is symptomatic and compared with a tracing obtained when symptoms have resolved. Comparison with a previous ECG, if available, is extremely valuable, particularly in patients with coexisting cardiac pathology such as left ventricular hypertrophy or a previous myocardial infarction. Significant Q-waves, consistent with previous myocardial infarction, are highly suggestive of the presence of significant coronary atherosclerosis, but do not necessarily imply current instability.

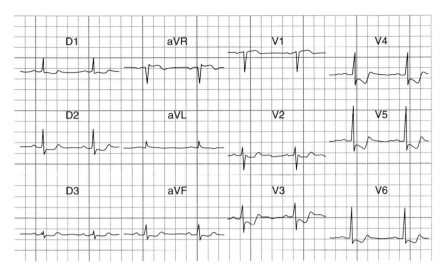

Figure 4.1 ST-segment depression in anterior leads.

ST-segment shift (Figure 4.1) and T-wave changes (Figure 4.2) are the most reliable electrocardiographic indicators of unstable coronary disease [18–20]. The European and American guidelines differ in their definition of significant ST-shift: the American guidelines consider ST-segment depression greater than 0.05 mV as significant whereas the European guidelines consider ST-segment depression greater than 0.1 mV as significant [2,3]. In both situations, the presence of significant ST-segment depression in two or more contiguous leads, in the appropriate clinical context, is considered highly suggestive for the presence of acute ischemia. Inverted T-waves (>1 mm) in leads with predominant R-waves are also highly suggestive, although the latter finding is less specific. Deep symmetrical inversion of the T-waves in the anterior chest leads is often related to significant proximal left anterior descending coronary artery stenosis [21]. Nonspecific ST-segment shift and T-wave changes (>1 mm) are less specific. Indeed, in the Multicenter Chest Pain Study, such nonspecific changes were often noted in patients in whom UA was ultimately ruled out. Transient episodes of bundle branch block occasionally occur during ischemic attacks. It should be appreciated that a completely normal ECG in patients presenting with suspicious symptoms does not exclude the possibility of an ACS. In several studies, around 5% of patients with normal ECGs who were discharged from the emergency department were ultimately found to have either an acute myocardial infarction or ACS [10,22,23]. However, a completely normal ECG recorded during an episode of significant chest pain should direct attention to other possible causes for the presenting symptoms.

ST-segment elevation indicates transmural ischemia due to epicardial coronary occlusion. New-onset, persistent, ST-segment elevation characterizes evolving myocardial infarction and is an indication for immediate reperfusion

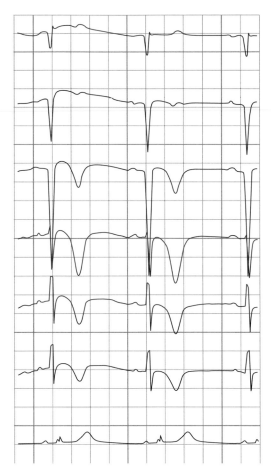

Figure 4.2 Negative T-waves in anterior leads.

therapy. Episodes of transient ST-segment elevation in conjunction with episodes of ST-segment depression may also be observed in patients who will be ultimately classified as having UA/NSTEMI. One condition that forms part of the spectrum of ACS is variant angina. The classic clinical presentation with recurrent episodes of chest pain, predominantly at rest and often occurring in the early morning, is well known. However, if there is not a high index of clinical suspicion, the diagnosis may be missed when the patient presents for the first time. In this situation, an ECG recorded during pain that demonstrates ST-segment elevation, which resolves spontaneously, or after nitrates, establishes the diagnosis [24]. In all patients with suspected ACS, it is extremely useful to institute multilead ST-segment monitoring during the initial evaluation or subsequent hospitalization, in order to detect or to rule out ST-segment changes during chest pain or to detect silent ischemia [25].

Risk stratification based on the ECG

Electrocardiographic findings provide important prognostic information. Several studies have demonstrated that a gradient of risk for death or other major adverse cardiac events can be determined based on the type of changes on the baseline ECG. Patients who present with an ACS and who have bundle branch block, are pacemaker dependent, or have ECG signs of left ventricular hypertrophy are at the highest risk of death. Among those with no confounding features on the baseline ECG, patients with significant ST-segment shift (ST-depression and or transient ST-segment elevation) are at highest risk, followed by those with isolated T-wave inversion, and those with a normal ECG [20,26–28]. The risk does not seem to differ significantly between the latter two categories. These prognostic elements on the ECG remain significant when clinical and biomarker data are taken into account [27–30].

Integration of clinical and ECG data into risk stratification algorithms

Diagnostic aids for risk stratification have been developed based on data obtained in large clinical trials. These risk scores incorporate clinical variables, ECG findings, and the result of cardiac biomarkers. While they cannot replace clinical judgment, they may be useful as a checklist, especially in situations where patients are first evaluated in an environment such as the emergency department where they do not have immediate access to an experienced cardiologist.

Conclusions

Despite the increasing sophistication of modern medicine, the initial management of patients with suspected ACS still relics on a careful clinical history that focuses on the presenting symptoms. It is critical that the physician who first encounters the patient rapidly excludes potentially life-threatening alternative diagnoses, such as aortic dissection. Furthermore, he should be able to recognize presentations that are at first sight atypical as "anginal equivalent" symptoms. The ECG, albeit, imperfect is a powerful adjunct to clinical judgment. It allows immediate recognition of STEMI, and helps rapidly stratify risk in the remaining patients. Finally, integration of the results of biomarkers of cardiac myocyte necrosis with clinical and ECG variables into decision-making algorithms are invaluable guides to management, particularly when patients are first encountered in settings where the initial evaluation is performed by physicians who are not experienced cardiologists [15,16].

References

1. Van de Werf F, Ardissino D, Betriu A *et al.* Management of acute myocardial infarction in patients presenting with ST-segment elevation. The Task Force on the

Management of Acute Myocardial Infarction of the European Society of Cardiology. *Eur Heart J* 2003; **24**: 28–66.

2. Braunwald E, Antman EM, Beasley JW *et al*. ACC/AHA guideline update for the management of patients with unstable angina and non-ST-segment elevation myocardial infarction – 2002: summary article. A report of the American College of Cardiology/American Heart Association Task Force on Practice Guidelines (Committee on the Management of Patients with Unstable Angina). *Circulation* 2002; **106**: 1893–1900.

3. Bertrand ME, Simoons ML, Fox KA *et al*. Management of acute coronary syndromes in patients presenting without persistent ST-segment elevation. *Eur Heart J* 2002; **23**: 1809–1840.

4. Gibbons RJ, Chatterjee K, Daley J *et al*. ACC/AHA/ACP-ASIM guidelines for the management of patients with chronic stable angina: a report of the American College of Cardiology/American Heart Association Task Force on Practice Guidelines (Committee on Management of Patients with Chronic Stable Angina). *J Am Coll Cardiol* 1999; **33**: 2092–2197.

5. Pryor DB, Harrell FE, Jr, Lee KL, Califf RM, Rosati RA. Estimating the likelihood of significant coronary artery disease. *Am J Med* 1983; **75**: 771–780.

6. Chaitman BR, Bourassa MG, Davis K *et al*. Angiographic prevalence of high-risk coronary artery disease in patient subsets (CASS). *Circulation* 1981; **64**: 360–367.

7. Campeau L. Letter: grading of angina pectoris. *Circulation* 1976; **54**: 522–523.

8. Braunwald E. Unstable angina. A classification. *Circulation* 1989; **80**: 410–414.

9. Lee TH, Cook EF, Weisberg M, Sargent RK, Wilson C, Goldman L. Acute chest pain in the emergency room. Identification and examination of low-risk patients. *Arch Intern Med* 1985; **145**: 65–69.

10. Pozen MW, D'Agostino RB, Selker HP, Sytkowski PA, Hood WB, Jr. A predictive instrument to improve coronary-care-unit admission practices in acute ischemic heart disease. A prospective multicenter clinical trial. *N Engl J Med* 1984; **310**: 1273–1278.

11. Selker HP, Griffith JL, D'Agostino RB. A tool for judging coronary care unit admission appropriateness, valid for both real-time and retrospective use. A time-insensitive predictive instrument (TIPI) for acute cardiac ischemia: a multicenter study. *Med Care* 1991; **29**: 610–627.

12. Califf RM, Mark DB, Harrell FE, Jr *et al*. Importance of clinical measures of ischemia in the prognosis of patients with documented coronary artery disease. *J Am Coll Cardiol* 1988; **11**: 20–26.

13. Califf RM, Phillips HR, III, Hindman MC *et al*. Prognostic value of a coronary artery jeopardy score. *J Am Coll Cardiol* 1985; **5**: 1055–1063.

14. White LD, Lee TH, Cook EF *et al*. Comparison of the natural history of new onset and exacerbated chronic ischemic heart disease. The Chest Pain Study Group. *J Am Coll Cardiol* 1990; **16**: 304–310.

15. Antman EM, Cohen M, Bernink PJ *et al*. The TIMI risk score for unstable angina/non-ST elevation MI: a method for prognostication and therapeutic decision making. *JAMA* 2000; **284**: 835–842.

16. Boersma E, Pieper KS, Steyerberg EW *et al*. Predictors of outcome in patients with acute coronary syndromes without persistent ST-segment elevation. Results from an international trial of 9461 patients. The PURSUIT Investigators. *Circulation* 2000; **101**: 2557–2567.

17. Hochman JS, Tamis JE, Thompson TD *et al.* Sex, clinical presentation, and outcome in patients with acute coronary syndromes. Global Use of Strategies to Open Occluded Coronary Arteries in Acute Coronary Syndromes IIb Investigators. *N Engl J Med* 1999; **341**: 226–232.

18. Selker HP, Zalenski RJ, Antman EM *et al.* An evaluation of technologies for identifying acute cardiac ischemia in the emergency department: a report from a National Heart Attack Alert Program Working Group. *Ann Emerg Med* 1997; **29**: 13–87.

19. Selker HP, Zalenski RJ, Antman EM *et al.* An evaluation of technologies for identifying acute cardiac ischemia in the emergency department: executive summary of a National Heart Attack Alert Program Working Group Report. *Ann Emerg Med* 1997; **29**: 1–12.

20. Savonitto S, Ardissino D, Granger CB *et al.* Prognostic value of the admission electrocardiogram in acute coronary syndromes. *JAMA* 1999; **281**: 707–713.

21. de Zwaan C, Bar FW, Janssen JH *et al.* Angiographic and clinical characteristics of patients with unstable angina showing an ECG pattern indicating critical narrowing of the proximal LAD coronary artery. *Am Heart J* 1989; **117**: 657–665.

22. Rouan GW, Lee TH, Cook EF, Brand DA, Weisberg MC, Goldman L. Clinical characteristics and outcome of acute myocardial infarction in patients with initially normal or nonspecific electrocardiograms (a report from the Multicenter Chest Pain Study). *Am J Cardiol* 1989; **64**: 1087–1092.

23. McCarthy BD, Wong JB, Selker HP. Detecting acute cardiac ischemia in the emergency department: a review of the literature. *J Gen Intern Med* 1990; **5**: 365–373.

24. Maseri A, Pesola A, Marzilli M *et al.* Coronary vasospasm in angina pectoris. *Lancet* 1977; **1**: 713–717.

25. Cohn PF. The value of continuous ST segment monitoring in patients with unstable angina. *Eur Heart J* 2001; **22**: 1972–1973.

26. Zaacks SM, Liebson PR, Calvin JE, Parrillo JE, Klein LW. Unstable angina and non-Q wave myocardial infarction: does the clinical diagnosis have therapeutic implications? *J Am Coll Cardiol* 1999; **33**: 107–118.

27. Cannon CP, McCabe CH, Stone PH *et al.* The electrocardiogram predicts one-year outcome of patients with unstable angina and non-Q wave myocardial infarction: results of the TIMI III Registry ECG Ancillary Study. Thrombolysis in Myocardial Ischemia. *J Am Coll Cardiol* 1997; **30**: 133–140.

28. Ohman EM, Armstrong PW, Christenson RH *et al.* Cardiac troponin T levels for risk stratification in acute myocardial ischemia. GUSTO IIA Investigators. *N Engl J Med* 1996; **335**: 1333–1341.

29. Antman EM, Tanasijevic MJ, Thompson B *et al.* Cardiac-specific troponin I levels to predict the risk of mortality in patients with acute coronary syndromes. *N Engl J Med* 1996; **335**: 1342–1349.

30. Hyde TA, French JK, Wong CK, Straznicky IT, Whitlock RM, White HD. Four-year survival of patients with acute coronary syndromes without ST-segment elevation and prognostic significance of 0.5-mm ST-segment depression. *Am J Cardiol* 1999; **84**: 379–385.

CHAPTER 5

Circulating biomarkers for risk stratification

Christopher Heeschen

Introduction

For several decades, circulating biomarkers have been used to assess myocardial injury in patients with suspected non-ST-elevation acute coronary syndromes (NSTE-ACSs). However, the purpose of biochemical marker determination in cardiovascular disease has shifted from the exclusive detection of myocardial injury to risk stratification and guidance of treatment in patients with ACS [1–3]. A substantial number of studies supports the use of cardiac troponins for diagnostic and therapeutic risk stratification. Data for concurrent measurement of markers of general inflammation (e.g. high-sensitivity C-reactive protein – CRP), as well as markers of vascular inflammation (e.g. placental growth factor – PlGF), platelet activation (e.g. soluble CD40 ligand), or neurohumoral activation (e.g. brain natriuretic peptide), are currently emerging and may prove that a multimarker approach will provide additional information. Although limitations inherent to markers that are not specific for the coronary arteries and/or myocardium remain, these novel markers may represent important tools for diagnostic and therapeutic stratification of patients with ACS.

Cardiac troponins as specific markers of cardiac necrosis (and thrombosis)

Angioscopic studies have revealed that the thrombus responsible for the clinical manifestation of unstable angina is more commonly white (platelet rich) and less likely red (fibrin rich), whereas the latter tends to be more prominent in acute myocardial infarction [4]. Pathological studies in patients with unstable angina who died suddenly have demonstrated that the fatal event is often preceded by repetitive embolization of thrombi from an unstable atheroma [5,6]. This determines focal myocardial necrosis that is too small to be detected by an increase in creatine kinase or CK-MB but can be detected by troponin measurements. Indeed, it has been shown that troponin T elevation in patients with ACS was significantly linked to visibility of thrombus formation even after prolonged treatment with heparin and morphological complexity of the target lesion [7]. Failed resolution of thrombus and complex lesion characteristics provided important prognostic information. In a multivariable analysis, however, troponin T represented the only independent and most powerful marker for the prediction of cardiac risk in patients with ACS. The angiographic findings of this study, related to the troponin status, are in full agreement with the concept that troponin T release is related to coronary thrombosis and consecutive embolization leading to minor myocardial damage. Thus, even a small increase in troponin levels in patients with ACS is related to "minor myocardial injury" and should be interpreted as an indicator for microembolization from liable thrombus formation.

Subsequently, numerous studies provide convincing evidence that the troponin blood level is a powerful indicator of the risk of patients with NSTE-ACS [8–18], whereas creatine kinase-MB (CK-MB) and myoglobin are less powerful predictors [8]. A metaanalysis of 14 trials showed that troponins are highly predictive for the risk of death or acute myocardial infarction. During 30-day follow-up, the relative risk was 2.7 (95% CI = 2.1–3.4) in patients with unstable angina and elevated troponin T. Respective values for troponin I were 4.2 (95% CI = 2.7–6.4) [19]. This predictive capacity of the troponins is independent of important clinical risk factors including age, ST-segment deviations, and presence of heart failure. Another metaanalysis calculated a more than ninefold increase in the risk for death or myocardial infarctions in patients with elevated troponins [20].

Based on pathophysiological considerations, the increased cardiac risk of troponin-T-positive patients may be less related to minor myocardial damage itself rather than to a more complex coronary morphology and thrombus formation in the culprit lesion.

The acute phase reactant CRP as a marker of general inflammation

Elevated levels of circulating cardiac troponin are found in about one-third of the patients with NSTE ACS. Although the absolute short-term risk of troponin-negative patients is significantly lower as compared to troponin-positive patients, the large number of patients without troponin elevation remains clinically challenging with respect to risk assessment and therapeutic management. Specifically, the 6-month risk of death or nonfatal myocardial infarction in troponin-negative patients was 8.4% in the CAPTURE (C7E3 Fab Antiplatelet Therapy in Unstable Refractory Angina) trial [21]. Therefore, the availability of a sensitive marker of plaque instability, whose levels become elevated before or even in the absence of myocardial necrosis, should improve diagnostic and therapeutic decision-making. Over the past decade, CRP, as a prototypic, but nonspecific, acute-phase reactant has emerged as a powerful predictor of cardiovascular events. There is compelling epidemiological evidence that CRP is a sensitive marker of inflammation and/or metabolic processes associated with atherogenesis and cardiovascular events (e.g. death, myocardial infarction, or stroke).

Although CRP has been shown to be useful for risk assessment in different populations [22–24] including patients with ACS [25–27], the controversial debate about whether CRP is indeed a clinically useful biomarker continues. Indeed, Danesh *et al.* [24] found in the Reykjavik prospective cohort study, which included 2459 patients with stable coronary heart disease and 3969 selected controls, that the predictive value of a single baseline measurement of CRP for the 20-year incidence of cardiovascular events was much less impressive than previously reported [28,29]. Surprisingly, they found that CRP adds little to the predictive value provided by the assessment of traditional risk factors, including LDL whereas Ridker *et al.* had previously reported that CRP could even be more predictive than LDL [30]. Since the Reykjavik study included by far the largest number of events (albeit during a follow-up of 20 years) that have been studied in such analyses, these new findings emphasize the need for more research to clarify the use of CRP as a marker of cardiovascular risk in clinical practice.

Only very recently, however, two studies, one by Nissen *et al.* [31] and one by Ridker *et al.* [32], confirmed that reducing the inflammatory component of cardiovascular disease through the use of statin therapy improves the clinical outcome independently of the reduction in serum cholesterol levels. In the REVERSAL trial (Reversing Atherosclerosis with Aggressive Lipid Lowering), including 502 patients with angiographically documented stable coronary disease, the reduced rate of progression of atherosclerosis associated with intensive statin treatment (80 mg atorvastatin), as compared with moderate statin treatment (40 mg pravastatin), was significantly related to greater reductions in the levels of both atherogenic lipoproteins and CRP [31]. In the PROVE IT-TIMI 22 study (Pravastatin or Atorvastatin Evaluation and Infection Therapy), including 3745 patients with ACS, atorvastatin (80 mg) was more likely than pravastatin (40 mg) to result in low levels of LDL cholesterol and CRP [32]. However, meeting these targets was more important in determining the patients' outcome than was the specific choice of therapy. Patients who had low CRP levels after statin therapy had better clinical outcomes than those with higher CRP levels, regardless of the resultant level of LDL cholesterol.

It should be noted that the exact source of elevated CRP levels among patients with ACS remains unclear to date. Given that myocardial damage is also a major inflammatory stimulus, it is important to notice that in a recent combined analysis of FRISC II (FRISC II – Fragmin and Fast Revascularization during Instability in Coronary artery disease) and GUSTO-IV (GUSTO – Global Utilization of Strategies To Open Occluded Arteries), CRP elevation over a period of up to 120 h after onset of symptoms was found only in patients with elevated troponin levels [33]. Consistently, in CAPTURE patients, CRP levels were significantly higher in troponin-positive patients [27] suggesting that an acute inflammatory process induced by myocardial damage is superimposed on a chronic inflammatory condition. Thus, current research activities have shifted to the identification of more upstream markers of the inflammatory cascade that may be more representative of vascular inflammation (Figure 5.1).

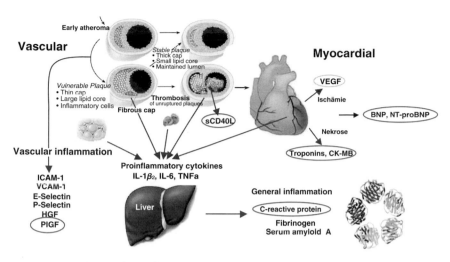

Figure 5.1 Earlier markers of vascular inflammatory and thromboinflammatory activation, respectively, may precede the development of myocardial injury (troponin release) or neurohumoral activation (BNP or NT-proBNP release) in patients with ACS.

PlGF as a primary vascular inflammatory instigator

Placental growth factor, a member of the vascular endothelial growth factor (VEGF) family, was recently shown to be profoundly upregulated in early and advanced atherosclerotic lesions [34]. PlGF, originally identified in the placenta [35], stimulates vascular smooth muscle growth, recruits macrophages into atherosclerotic lesions, upregulates the TNF-α and MCP-1 production by macrophages, enhances production of tissue factor, and stimulates pathological angiogenesis [34,36]. All these processes are known contributors to plaque progression and destabilization. Most importantly, however, inhibition of the PlGF effects by blocking its receptor Flt-1 was experimentally shown to suppress both atherosclerotic plaque growth and vulnerability via inhibition of inflammatory cell infiltration [34]. These data suggest that PlGF may act as a primary inflammatory instigator of atherosclerotic plaque instability.

Indeed, PlGF blood levels are markedly upregulated in patients with ACS independent of the presence of myocardial injury [37]. Moreover, data from the CAPTURE trial established PlGF blood levels as a novel, powerful, and independent prognostic determinant of clinical outcome in patients with ACS [37]. Measuring PlGF levels significantly extends the predictive and prognostic information gained from traditional inflammatory markers in ACS. The predictive value of PlGF levels was independent of myocardial necrosis as evidenced by elevated troponin levels [38], as well as platelet activation as evidenced by elevation of soluble CD40 ligand [39]. Intriguingly, elevated PlGF levels enabled identification of not only those patients with acute chest pain, who developed ACS, but also those patients who suffered from an increased risk of recurrent instability after discharge from initial ACS. Thus, measuring PlGF levels may not only represent a reliable and powerful clinical tool for identifying patients with high-risk lesion formation, but also with ongoing vascular inflammation of the coronary circulation.

The role of PlGF as a primary inflammatory instigator of atherosclerotic lesion instability can be well rationalized by its well-documented proinflammatory effects in animal models of atherosclerosis or arthritis [34]. Although PlGF belongs to the family of VEGF, its etiopathogenetical role appears to be more related to vascular inflammation than to angiogenesis [34]. Indeed, whereas VEGF is activated by hypoxia, and elevation of VEGF levels is regarded as an early adaptation of the myocardium to deprivation of blood flow [40], PlGF is not affected or even downregulated by hypoxia [41,42]. In line with these data, the analysis of the CAPTURE data did not reveal any correlation between PlGF levels and VEGF levels as a marker of myocardial ischemia or between PlGF levels and troponin levels as a marker of myocardial necrosis. Thus, PlGF levels do not appear to be confounded by myocardial necrosis, whereas VEGF levels are linked to troponin elevation, impaired TIMI flow, and clinical evidence of myocardial ischemia [43]. Most notably, however, since the proinflammatory effects of PlGF can be specifically inhibited by blocking its receptor Flt-1, these findings may also provide a rationale for a novel antiinflammatory therapeutic target in patients with coronary artery disease [44].

Soluble CD40 ligand as a marker for platelet activation

Troponins are surrogate markers for unstable thrombus formation [7] but more immediate biochemical markers of platelet activation may prove to be helpful for identifying patients that are in a prothrombotic state, even before myocardial necrosis occurs. In this respect, increasing evidence suggests that CD40 ligand is associated with platelet activation [45]. Soluble CD40 ligand is actively released following platelet stimulation (Figure 5.2) [46,47]. Circulating soluble CD40 ligand can activate CD40 on endothelial cells and, thereby, induce a proinflammatory cascade in the vessel wall. Moreover, soluble CD40 ligand can activate CD40 that is also expressed on inflammatory cells, such as monocytes and T cells. The subsequent activation of these inflammatory cells and their invasion into the ruptured or eroded plaque results in a further inflammatory perturbation of the vessel wall. In patients with coronary heart disease, soluble CD40 ligand is primarily released from activated platelets. Subsequently, elevated levels have been reported for patients with ACS [48,49]. Moreover, it has been shown that soluble CD40 ligand is a powerful biochemical marker of thrombotic inflammatory activation in patients with ACS, supporting the close relationship between inflammation, thrombotic activation, and ACS [39,50]. Furthermore, the latter two studies have clearly demonstrated that combining this new marker with classical

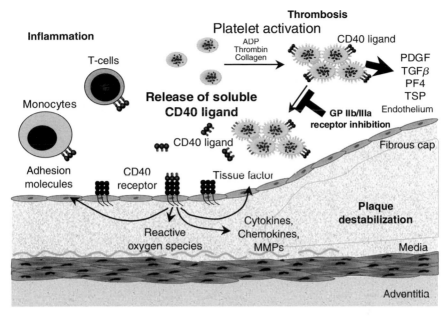

Figure 5.2 The pathophysiological role of soluble CD40 ligand in plaque destabilization and thrombosis of patients with ACS.

markers of necrosis (troponins) can help us to identify patients at the highest risk for subsequent cardiovascular events.

Natriuretic peptides as markers of neurohumoral activation of the heart

After the description of elevated levels of the neurohormone B-type natriuretic peptide (BNP) and the N-terminal fragment of the BNP prohormone, NT-proBNP, respectively, in patients with congestive heart failure, several investigations focused on the prognostic value of neurohumoral activation in the setting of AMI. More recently, however, the prognostic implications of BNP and NT-proBNP, respectively, have also been extended to patients with unstable angina and non-ST-elevation myocardial infarction (NSCTE-ACS). In a first small case–control study of patients with NSCTE-ACS, NT-proBNP levels were higher among patients who died than those who survived [51]. This pilot study was followed by a post hoc analysis of the *O*rbofiban in *P*atients with *U*nstable coronary *S*yndromes (OPUS)-TIMI 16 trial including 2525 patients in which BNP was measured approximately 40 h after onset of symptoms [52]. Rates of death and heart failure during 10 months of follow-up increased with higher baseline levels of BNP that was consistent across the spectrum of ACS. More recently, in a consecutive series of patients with chest pain and non-ST-segment elevation, Jernberg and colleagues also found that NT-proBNP levels measured at the time of arrival in the emergency room are strongly associated with long-term mortality, again independent of the index diagnosis (myocardial infarction versus unstable angina) [53]. Moreover, a more recent study in patients with stable coronary heart disease demonstrated that elevated levels of BNP are independently associated with inducible ischemia and therefore provide the rationale for the hypothesis that NT-proBNP levels in patients with ACS may also reflect ischemia-induced left ventricular dysfunction even in the absence of myocardial necrosis [54].

In a heterogeneous population of patients with a NSCTE-ACS enrolled in the PRISM trial, it was demonstrated that serial measurements of NT-proBNP, significantly enhance the predictive value as compared with a single baseline NT-proBNP measurement [55]. In addition to the baseline NT-proBNP sample, a second blood sample, drawn 72 h after the onset of symptoms, provided important information about the further clinical course of the patients. A rapid decline in NT-proBNP levels may indicate responsiveness to the therapeutic regimen that was chosen for the individual patient and, thus, may explain the reduced event rates observed in patients with declining NT-proBNP levels during the first days after onset of symptoms. Intriguingly, none of the other investigated biomarkers (troponin T and CRP) demonstrated a similar pattern during clinical stabilization of the patients. These data suggest for the first time that serial measurements of NT-proBNP in patients with ACS can be used for dynamic risk assessment and may be helpful for rapidly identifying patients that are suitable for early discharge or that may need more intensive therapy.

Summary

The electrocardiogram still remains the most useful and cost-effective first line tool in the evaluation of patients with chest pain. After exclusion of the presence of ST-segment elevations, repeat quantitative or qualitative troponin measurements provide valuable diagnostic tools for improving efficacy and safety in decision-making in patients suspected of having an ACS. Increasing evidence suggests that the combined use of biomarkers reflecting distinct pathophysiological features, such as myocardial necrosis, vascular inflammation, oxidative stress, and neurohumoral activation, may significantly add to our ability to correctly identify patients who are at high risk for short-term and long-term cardiovascular events and subsequently tailor medical treatment to improve their adverse outcome.

References

1. Hamm CW, Bertrand M, Braunwald E. Acute coronary syndrome without ST elevation: implementation of new guidelines. *Lancet* 2001; **358**: 1533–1538.
2. Hamm CW, Braunwald E. A classification of unstable angina revisited. *Circulation* 2000; **102**: 118–122.

3. Klootwijk P, Hamm C. Acute coronary syndromes: diagnosis. *Lancet* 1999; **353**: SII10–15.

4. Mizuno K, Satomura K, Miyamoto A *et al.* Angioscopic evaluation of coronary-artery thrombi in acute coronary syndromes. *N Engl J Med* 1992; **326**: 287–291.

5. Davies MJ, Thomas AC, Knapman PA, Hangartner JR. Intramyocardial platelet aggregation in patients with unstable angina suffering sudden ischemic cardiac death. *Circulation* 1986; **73**: 418–427.

6. Falk E. Unstable angina with fatal outcome: dynamic coronary thrombosis leading to infarction and/or sudden death. Autopsy evidence of recurrent mural thrombosis with peripheral embolization culminating in total vascular occlusion. *Circulation* 1985; **71**: 699–708.

7. Heeschen C, van Den Brand MJ, Hamm CW, Simoons ML. Angiographic findings in patients with refractory unstable angina according to troponin T status. *Circulation* 1999; **100**: 1509–1514.

8. Hamm CW, Goldmann BU, Heeschen C, Kreymann G, Berger J, Meinertz T. Emergency room triage of patients with acute chest pain by means of rapid testing for cardiac troponin T or troponin I. *N Engl J Med* 1997; **337**: 1648–1653.

9. Hamm CW, Ravkilde J, Gerhardt W *et al.* The prognostic value of serum troponin T in unstable angina. *N Engl J Med* 1992; **327**: 146–150.

10. Ravkilde J, Horder M, Gerhardt W *et al.* Diagnostic performance and prognostic value of serum troponin T in suspected acute myocardial infarction. *Scand J Clin Lab Invest* 1993; **53**: 677–685.

11. Wu AH, Abbas SA, Green S *et al.* Prognostic value of cardiac troponin T in unstable angina pectoris. *Am J Cardiol* 1995; **76**: 970–972.

12. Ohman EM, Armstrong PW, Christenson RH *et al.* Cardiac troponin T levels for risk stratification in acute myocardial ischemia. GUSTO IIA Investigators. *N Engl J Med* 1996; **335**: 1333–1341.

13. Lindahl B, Venge P, Wallentin L. Relation between troponin T and the risk of subsequent cardiac events in unstable coronary artery disease. The FRISC study group. *Circulation* 1996; **93**: 1651–1657.

14. Heeschen C, Goldmann BU, Moeller RH, Hamm CW. Analytical performance and clinical application of a new rapid bedside assay for the detection of serum cardiac troponin I. *Clin Chem* 1998; **44**: 1925–1930.

15. Heeschen C, Goldmann BU, Langenbrink L, Matschuck G, Hamm CW. Evaluation of a rapid whole blood ELISA for quantification of troponin I in patients with acute chest pain. *Clin Chem* 1999; **45**: 1789–1796.

16. Antman EM, Tanasijevic MJ, Thompson B *et al.* Cardiac-specific troponin I levels to predict the risk of mortality in patients with acute coronary syndromes. *N Engl J Med* 1996; **335**: 1342–1349.

17. Galvani M, Ottani F, Ferrini D *et al.* Prognostic influence of elevated values of cardiac troponin I in patients with unstable angina. *Circulation* 1997; **95**: 2053–2059.

18. Luscher MS, Thygesen K, Ravkilde J, Heickendorff L. Applicability of cardiac troponin T and I for early risk stratification in unstable coronary artery disease. TRIM Study Group. Thrombin inhibition in myocardial ischemia. *Circulation* 1997; **96**: 2578–2585.

19. Olatidoye AG, Wu AH, Feng YJ, Waters D. Prognostic role of troponin T versus troponin I in unstable angina pectoris for cardiac events with meta-analysis comparing published studies. *Am J Cardiol* 1998; **81**: 1405–1410.

20. Ottani F, Galvani M, Nicolini FA *et al.* Elevated cardiac troponin levels predict the risk of adverse outcome in patients with acute coronary syndromes. *Am Heart J* 2000; **140**: 917–927.

21. Hamm CW, Heeschen C, Goldmann B *et al.* Benefit of abciximab in patients with refractory unstable angina in relation to serum troponin T levels. c7E3 Fab Anti-platelet Therapy in Unstable Refractory Angina (CAPTURE) Study Investigators. *N Engl J Med* 1999; **340**: 1623–1629.

22. Ridker PM. Clinical application of C-reactive protein for cardiovascular disease detection and prevention. *Circulation* 2003; **107**: 363–369.

23. Koenig W, Lowel H, Baumert J, Meisinger C. C-reactive protein modulates risk prediction based on the Framingham score: implications for future risk assessment: results from a large cohort study in southern Germany. *Circulation* 2004; **109**: 1349–1353.

24. Danesh J, Wheeler JG, Hirschfield GM *et al.* C-reactive protein and other circulating markers of inflammation in the prediction of coronary heart disease. *N Engl J Med* 2004; **350**: 1387–1397.

25. Liuzzo G, Biasucci LM, Gallimore JR *et al.* The prognostic value of C-reactive protein and serum amyloid a protein in severe unstable angina. *N Engl J Med* 1994; **331**: 417–424.

26. Morrow DA, Rifai N, Antman EM *et al.* C-reactive protein is a potent predictor of mortality independently of and in combination with troponin T in acute coronary syndromes: a TIMI 11A substudy. Thrombolysis in myocardial infarction. *J Am Coll Cardiol* 1998; **31**: 1460–1465.

27. Heeschen C, Hamm CW, Bruemmer J, Simoons ML. Predictive value of C-reactive protein and troponin T in patients with unstable angina: a comparative analysis. CAPTURE Investigators. Chimeric c7E3 Antiplatelet Therapy in Unstable Angina Refractory to standard treatment trial. *J Am Coll Cardiol* 2000; **35**: 1535–1542.

28. Danesh J, Whincup P, Walker M *et al.* Low grade inflammation and coronary heart disease: prospective study and updated meta-analyses. *BMJ* 2000; **321**: 199–204.

29. Koenig W. Update on C-reactive protein as a risk marker in cardiovascular disease. *Kidney Int Suppl* 2003; **84**: S58–S61.

30. Ridker PM, Rifai N, Rose L, Buring JE, Cook NR. Comparison of C-Reactive protein and low-density lipoprotein cholesterol levels in the prediction of first cardiovascular events. *N Engl J Med* 2002; **347**: 1557–1565.

31. Nissen SE, Tuzcu EM, Schoenhagen P *et al.* Statin therapy, LDL cholesterol, C-reactive protein, and coronary artery disease. *N Engl J Med* 2005; **352**: 29–38.

32. Ridker PM, Cannon CP, Morrow D *et al.* C-reactive protein levels and outcomes after statin therapy. *N Engl J Med* 2005; **352**: 20–28.

33. James SK, Lindahl B, Siegbahn A *et al.* N-terminal pro-brain natriuretic peptide and other risk markers for the separate prediction of mortality and subsequent myocardial infarction in patients with unstable coronary artery disease: a Global Utilization of Strategies To Open Occluded Arteries (GUSTO)-IV substudy. *Circulation* 2003; **108**: 275–281.

34. Luttun A, Tjwa M, Moons L *et al.* Revascularization of ischemic tissues by PlGF treatment, and inhibition of tumor angiogenesis, arthritis and atherosclerosis by anti-Flt1. *Nat Med* 2002; **8**: 831–840.

35. Maglione D, Guerriero V, Viglietto G, Delli-Bovi P, Persico MG. Isolation of a human placenta cDNA coding for a protein related to the vascular permeability factor. *Proc Natl Acad Sci USA* 1991; **88**: 9267–9271.

36. Autiero M, Luttun A, Tjwa M, Carmeliet P. Placental growth factor and its receptor, vascular endothelial growth factor receptor-1: novel targets for stimulation of ischemic tissue revascularization and inhibition of angiogenic and inflammatory disorders. *J Thromb Haemost* 2003; **1**: 1356–1370.

37. Heeschen C, Dimmeler S, Fichtlscherer S *et al.* Prognostic value of placental growth factor in patients with acute chest pain. *JAMA* 2004; **291**: 435–441.

38. Heeschen C, Hamm CW, Goldmann B, Deu A, Langenbrink L, White HD. Troponin concentrations for stratification of patients with acute coronary syndromes in relation to therapeutic efficacy of tirofiban. PRISM Study Investigators. Platelet receptor inhibition in ischemic syndrome management. *Lancet* 1999; **354**: 1757–1762.

39. Heeschen C, Dimmeler S, Hamm CW *et al.* Soluble CD40 ligand in acute coronary syndromes. *N Engl J Med* 2003; **348**: 1104–1111.

40. Lee SH, Wolf PL, Escudero R, Deutsch R, Jamieson SW, Thistlethwaite PA. Early expression of angiogenesis factors in acute myocardial ischemia and infarction. *N Engl J Med* 2000; **342**: 626–633.

41. Khaliq A, Dunk C, Jiang J *et al.* Hypoxia down-regulates placenta growth factor, whereas fetal growth restriction up-regulates placenta growth factor expression: molecular evidence for "placental hyperoxia" in intrauterine growth restriction. *Lab Invest* 1999; **79**: 151–170.

42. Cao Y, Linden P, Shima D, Browne F, Folkman J. *In vivo* angiogenic activity and hypoxia induction of heterodimers of placenta growth factor/vascular endothelial growth factor. *J Clin Invest* 1996; **98**: 2507–2511.

43. Heeschen C, Dimmeler S, Hamm CW, Boersma E, Zeiher AM, Simoons ML. Prognostic significance of angiogenic growth factor serum levels in patients with acute coronary syndromes. *Circulation* 2003; **107**: 524–530.

44. Luttun A, Tjwa M, Carmeliet P. Placental growth factor (PlGF) and its receptor Flt-1 (VEGFR-1): novel therapeutic targets for angiogenic disorders. *Ann N Y Acad Sci* 2002; **979**: 80–93.

45. Cipollone F, Mezzetti A, Porreca E *et al.* Association between enhanced soluble CD40L and prothrombotic state in hypercholesterolemia – effects of statin therapy. *Circulation* 2002; **106**: 399–402.

46. Henn V, Steinbach S, Buchner K, Presek P, Kroczek RA. The inflammatory action of CD40 ligand (CD154) expressed on activated human platelets is temporally limited by coexpressed CD40. *Blood* 2001; **98**: 1047–1054.

47. Lee Y, Lee WH, Lee SC *et al.* CD40L activation in circulating platelets in patients with acute coronary syndrome. *Cardiology* 1999; **92**: 11–16.

48. Garlichs CD, Eskafi S, Raaz D *et al.* Patients with acute coronary syndromes express enhanced CD40 ligand/CD154 on platelets. *Heart* 2001; **86**: 649–655.

49. Prasad KS, Andre P, Yan Y, Phillips DR. The platelet CD40L/GP IIb–IIIa axis in atherothrombotic disease. *Curr Opin Hematol* 2003; **10**: 356–361.

50. Varo N, de Lemos JA, Libby P *et al.* Soluble CD40L: risk prediction after acute coronary syndromes. *Circulation* 2003; **108**: 1049–1052.

51. Omland T, de Lemos JA, Morrow DA *et al.* Prognostic value of N-terminal pro-atrial and pro-brain natriuretic peptide in patients with acute coronary syndromes. *Am J Cardiol* 2002; **89**: 463–465.

52. de Lemos JA, Morrow DA, Bentley JH *et al.* The prognostic value of B-type natriuretic peptide in patients with acute coronary syndromes. *N Engl J Med* 2001; **345**: 1014–1021.

53. Jernberg T, Stridsberg M, Venge P, Lindahl B. N-terminal pro brain natriuretic peptide on admission for early risk stratification of patients with chest pain and no ST-segment elevation. *J Am Coll Cardiol* 2002; **40**: 437–445.
54. Bibbins-Domingo K, Ansari M, Schiller NB, Massie B, Whooley MA. B-type natriuretic peptide and ischemia in patients with stable coronary disease: data from the Heart and Soul study. *Circulation* 2003; **108**: 2987–2992.
55. Heeschen C, Hamm CW, Mitrovic V, Lantelme NH, White HD. N-terminal pro-B-type natriuretic peptide levels for dynamic risk stratification of patients with acute coronary syndromes. *Circulation* 2004; **110**: 3206–3212.

Section four:
Investigation in ACS

CHAPTER 6

Coronary angiography, angioscopy, and intravascular ultrasound in non-ST-segment elevation acute coronary syndromes

Eric Van Belle, Christophe Bauters, François Schiele, and Michel E. Bertrand

The development of invasive imaging techniques of the coronary tree (angiography, angioscopy, and intravascular ultrasound, IVUS) has been very useful to describe the natural history and to validate concepts in the setting of acute coronary syndromes (ACSs). Coronary angiography, historically the "gold standard," illustrates luminal narrowing but does not provide direct information on the changes within the vessel wall necessary to detect vulnerable plaque [1]. This limitation has promoted interest in alternate, invasive catheter-based techniques, such as angioscopy or IVUS, to directly visualize the blood stream–arterial wall interface, and to characterize plaque composition.

Validation of invasive imaging techniques

Angiography

The X-ray coronary angiogram reflects luminal diameter and provides a measure of stenosis with excellent resolution of irregular luminal surface implying the presence of atherosclerotic disease. But this method does not provide an image of the vessel wall or provide information about the composition of the atherosclerotic plaque. The phenomenon of remodeling makes angiography a poor technique for assessing the true atherosclerotic burden (Table 6.1). The shadows of the coronary lumen, seen on angiography, only provide indirect and incomplete information concerning the extent of the atherosclerotic process in the arterial wall [2,3].

Angioscopy

Although, historically, attempts have been made to visualize intracardiac structures, it was not until the development and application of fiber optics that

Table 6.1 Comparison of invasive methods for detection of individual characteristics of vulnerable plaque.

Imaging modality	Resolution (μm)	Penetration	Vessel size	Plaque burden	Calcium	Fibrous cap	Lipid core	Inflammation	Intimal disruption	Thrombus
Angiography	200	Excellent	++	++	++	−	−	−	+	++
IVUS	100	Good	++++	++++	++++	+	+	−	+	+
Angioscopy	50	Poor	−	−	−	+	+++	−	+++	++++

Notes −, no detection; + to + + ++, from poor to excellent ability to detect the individual characteristics.

direct visualization of coronary arteries could be achieved. Coronary angioscopy complements angiography by characterizing plaque composition and illuminating the presence of thrombus or endoluminal irregularities, such as ulcerations, fissures, or tears. The normal artery appears angioscopically as glistening white, whereas atherosclerotic plaque can be categorized on the basis of its angioscopic color as yellow or white [4,5]. Histologic correlation has demonstrated high concentrations of cholesterol-laden crystals seen through a thin, fibrous cap in yellow plaque and a thick, fibrous cap in smooth white plaques [4]. Platelet-rich thrombus at the site of plaque rupture is characterized as white granular material, and fibrin/erythrocyte-rich thrombus, as an irregular, red structure protruding into the lumen [5].

The interrogative capabilities of angioscopy are confined to the intraluminal space and surrounding endoluminal surface. It represents the only diagnostic technique capable of providing information on true color. Angioscopy is especially suitable to detect surface plaque color, intimal tears and flap, and intraluminal/parietal thrombi (Table 6.1). Inter- and intraobserver variability are good [6].

The anatomopathological significance of the plaque color was validated *in vivo* using atherectomy specimen. It was demonstrated, in particular, that yellow plaque color by angioscopy is closely related to degenerated plaque or atheroma [7]. Similarly, the sensitivity to detect thrombus is excellent ($\approx$100%, Table 6.1) [8].

Intravascular ultrasound

Intravascular ultrasound is a technology that allows *in vivo* visualization of variations in arterial geometry and atherosclerotic plaque by utilizing a miniature transducer at the end of a flexible catheter. IVUS provides a two-dimensional cross-sectional image of the arterial wall and can accurately assess the plaque burden (Table 6.1) [9].

Intravascular ultrasound has provided insight into the extent and distribution of atherosclerotic plaque, allowing characterization of vessel wall and plaque morphology [10]. IVUS is capable of characterizing the plaque core, although with less sensitivity for lipid-rich than calcified lesions. Plaque morphology can be described by ultrasound as echoreflective, corresponding to calcified plaque; hyperechoic, representing fibrous plaque; and hypoechoic, indicating a lipid-rich core [11]. Plaque characterization is reliable in distinguishing fibrous and calcified plaque but not soft or lipid-rich plaque, owing in part to variable concentrations of cholesterol crystals and calcospherites that form the heterogeneous components of the cholesterol core [12]. In terms of macrocalcification, IVUS yields a three-fold higher detection rate compared with angiography, with a sensitivity and specificity of 89% and 97%, respectively. However, the echoreflective properties of calcium result in acoustic shadows that preclude accurate quantification and obscure imaging of adjacent structures [13,14].

The two-dimensional IVUS image, derived from ultrasound frequencies in the range of 20–40 MHz, results in an axial resolution of 100–200 μm and a lateral resolution of 250 μm [11]. These properties, though beneficial for visualizing deep structures, limit imaging of microstructures, yielding a sensitivity of only 37% for the detection of plaque rupture with IVUS [15]. Although three-dimensional image reconstruction improves border definition, it has not yet been tested for detection of vulnerable plaque or plaque disruption.

Histopathological studies mostly report low sensitivity for IVUS in detecting lipid-rich lesions [16,17] and the axial resolution remains too low for measuring cap thickness. The sensitivity of IVUS to detect thrombi is relatively low (57%) due to false-negative interpretation of laminar clots and an inability to distinguish disrupted atheroma from intraluminal thrombus [8]. Indeed, thrombus possesses an acoustic density that differs only slightly from nearby normal and abnormal tissues, making a positive identification particularly difficult [18].

Description of the culprit lesion at the time of acute coronary syndrome

Pathologic studies [19] in patients whose death was due to infarction or was sudden have shown that a thrombus is usually superimposed on a ruptured atherosclerotic plaque. Angiography and angioscopy were very useful to confirm these findings *in vivo*.

Indeed, Ambrose *et al.* reported that an eccentric stenosis with a narrow neck due to one or more overhanging edges or irregular borders, or both, (Ambrose's Type II eccentric) was found by angiography in the majority of patients with unstable angina (54%) or a recent myocardial infarction (MI) (66%) [20,21]. Comparison with angioscopy confirmed that Ambrose's Type II eccentric stenoses and complex lesions were strongly associated with disrupted plaques and/or thrombus [22]. More specifically, angioscopic studies demonstrated that a disrupted yellow plaque was observed in 50–70% of patients with unstable angina or non-Q-wave MI [23,24] and in 70–95% of patients with an acute myocardial infraction (AMI) (Figure 6.1) [25–27]. While an intraluminal thrombus was observed in only 20% of patients with unstable angina or non-Q-wave MI by angiography [28,29], it was found in 40–75% of patients by angioscopy [23,28]. Finally, angioscopy confirmed that in patients with AMI, a thrombus is present in the culprit lesion in almost every case (95–100%, Figure 6.1) [25,26,30], and that in more than 80% of cases it is a platelet-rich, white, or a mixed (red–white) thrombus [5,25,26].

Angioscopy was also very helpful in demonstrating that diabetic patients with unstable angina were more likely to have an ulcerated plaque with thrombus than nondiabetic patients (94% versus 55%) [31], and that rise in troponin in patients with non-ST-elevation ACS was more frequently associated with thrombus at the culprit site (86% versus 34%) [32].

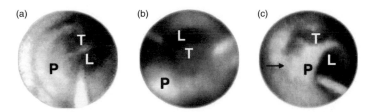

Figure 6.1 Coronary angioscopic findings in patients with ACS. (a) Yellow plaque (P) with a lining thrombus (T). (b) Yellow plaque (P) with a large protruding thrombus (T). (c) Predominantly white plaque (P) with a localized yellow area (arrow) and an adjacent lining thrombus (T). L indicates lumen. From Ref. 39.

By contrast, the sensitivity of IVUS to describe plaque rupture was disappointing. Indeed, in patients with AMI or unstable angina, IVUS evidence of a disrupted plaque – described as a plaque with an echolucent zone communicating with the lumen – is only found in about one-third of culprit lesions [26,33,34] (Figure 6.2). As discussed above, this lack of sensibility of IVUS is probably related to the inability of current IVUS technology to distinguish the fresh thrombus from the soft plaque. However, IVUS studies provided additional interesting information. In particular, they demonstrated that the site of plaque rupture is usually associated with local vessel enlargement [35–37] and less calcification of the vessel wall [38], suggesting that a "positive" coronary remodeling could be a marker of increased plaque "vulnerability."

Healing and natural history of the culprit lesion

Most information in this area has been obtained using serial angioscopy investigations in patients with an AMI [5,25,26,39,40]. After investigating AMI patients initially treated with thrombolysis or medical conservative therapy, we reported that a complex plaque morphology – a yellow plaque and a mural or protruding thrombus – was present for at least 1 month in the majority of cases (≈80%) [39]. The use of mechanical reperfusion (balloon angioplasty or stent implantation) was associated with an immediate reduction in thrombus burden [25] and with a significant reduction in the prevalence and burden of thrombus by 1 month, without significant impact on plaque morphology and color [25,26]. By 6 months, mechanical reperfusion was associated with an almost complete plaque stabilization, described as a white plaque with a smooth shape and no thrombus [5,25,26,40].

Overall, these findings demonstrate that plaque healing takes several weeks after the occurrence of ACS. The persistence of plaque instability, even in the absence of symptoms, provides a possible explanation for the previously described higher rates of restenosis and reocclusion when angioplasty is performed at recent infarct-related lesions [41,42], as well as the high rate of late vessel occlusion after successful thrombolysis [43]. It also provides an

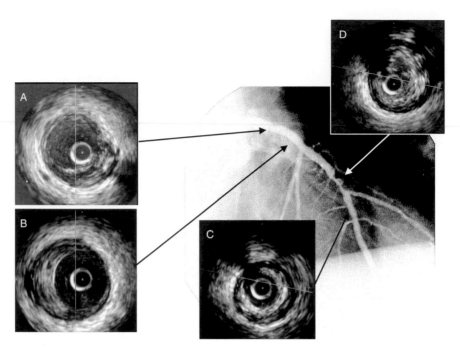

Figure 6.2 IVUS findings in patients with ACS. An eccentric plaque is observed in the proximal (a,b) and distal (c) left anterior descending artery. A plaque with an echolucent zone communicating with the lumen (d) is observed in the culprit lesion. This typical aspect of plaque rupture is observed in only one-third of culprit lesions [26,33,34].

explanation for the clinical benefits associated with the use of coronary stenting and for the powerful and prolonged antiplatelet therapies in patients suffering from ACS.

Predictive value

The prediction of outcome based on coronary imaging of the culprit lesion in patients with ACS

In patients with ACS, lesion complexity by angiography [44,45] and angiographic evidence of thrombus at the culprit lesion site [44–46] are predictors of poor outcome after percutaneous coronary revascularization. However, the ability to predict outcome for lesion complexity and thrombus is relatively low. Of these criteria, the angiographic presence of an intraluminal thrombus has been associated most consistently with an increased risk of early adverse outcome [45,46].

In patients with unstable angina and non-Q-wave infarction, angioscopic features of disruption, yellow color, or thrombus at the culprit lesion site can identify patients at high risk of early adverse outcome after percutaneous transluminal coronary angioplasty (PTCA) [23,28,47]. Similarly, Fukuda *et al.* reported that the presence of an intracoronary mobile mass, detected by IVUS, in patients with ACS is more frequently associated with distal embolization following PTCA [48]; while Tanaka *et al.* reported that large vessels with lipid pool-like image, as detected by IVUS, are at high risk for no-reflow following primary PTCA for an AMI [49].

Finally, comparative studies have demonstrated that the predictive value of angioscopy was superior to angiography [23,28,47] and IVUS [47], this being mainly related to the superiority of angioscopy to detect intraluminal thrombus [28,47].

The prediction of ACS based on coronary imaging: the detection of the vulnerable plaque

Plaque rupture or endothelial damage and subsequent occlusive thrombi and bleeding in the plaque are considered to be a pathognomonic mechanism of AMI [50,51]. Preexisting stenosis of the infarct-related coronary segments has been reported to be mostly mild, and their morphology is smooth on the basis of coronary angiograms that were mostly performed 1 year or even 3 months before the onset of AMI [52–54]. However, coronary angiographies performed within 1 week (3±3 days) before an AMI, reported that an Ambrose Type II eccentric lesion with multiple irregularities and a significant stenosis was common at the infarct-related vessel [55]. These data suggest that the onset of plaque rupture and/or thrombi occurs usually a few days before the onset of AMI.

Retrospective IVUS studies of culprit lesions in patients with ACS demon strate that a "positive" remodeling was one of the characteristic features of such lesions [35–37]. This observation has recently been confirmed by a prospective study. In this study, Yamagishi *et al.* reported that large eccentric plaques containing an echolucent zone by IVUS were at risk for instability during the following 2 years [56]. These findings support recent pathologic studies in which a close link between positive vessel remodeling and histopathologic characteristics of plaque vulnerability, such as size of the lipid-rich core and the degree of plaque inflammation, was found [57,58].

Xanthomatous yellow plaques by angioscopy indicate a high concentration of cholesterol-laden crystals seen through a thin fibrous cap whereas white plaques have a thick fibrous cap. Studies comparing IVUS and angioscopic features of atherosclerotic plaques have also demonstrated that compensatory enlargement occurs more frequently with yellow plaques than with white plaques [59]. Based on retrospective analysis, it has been shown that yellow plaques were more frequently observed at the culprit lesion in patients with ACS while white plaques were more frequently observed in patients with stable angina [4,7,59]. This relationship was confirmed by Uchida *et al.* in a prospective study in which yellow plaques were associated with a higher risk of ACS at 1 year than white plaques (28% versus 3%) [60].

Unstable/vulnerable plaques: a pancoronary process?

Recent studies using various clinical imaging modalities found evidence of ruptured plaques that were distant from the culprit lesion in patients with acute cardiovascular events.

Goldstein *et al.* [61] reported the presence of additional complex angiographic lesions in 21% of patients presenting with MI. Using IVUS, Schoenhagen *et al.* [62] reported the presence of a ruptured plaque distant from the culprit site in 10/105 (10%) patients presenting with an AMI and in 2/95 (2%) patients with stable/unstable angina. Rioufol *et al.* reported a plaque rupture distant from the culprit site in 19/24 patients (79%) with an ACS [33]. By contrast angioscopic studies identified additional ruptured/thrombotic plaques in only 5–10% of cases [60,63].

The apparent discrepancy between the results observed by angioscopy and by IVUS is probably related to the inability of IVUS to detect mural thrombus and therefore to distinguish chronic "healed" from fresh "thrombotic" ulcers, while angioscopy can only detect fresh ulcers. Therefore, the presence of a plaque that has already ruptured, as detected by IVUS, does not necessarily imply that this site is still biologically active.

While these studies examined plaques that had already ruptured, another issue is to detect additional vulnerable plaque before rupture in patients with ACS. In an angioscopic study, Uchida *et al.* found that approximately 20% of patients with ACS had a second "vulnerable yellow" plaque [60], while Asakura *et al.* [63] reported the presence of "vulnerable yellow" coronary plaques distant from the culprit lesion in all patients ($n = 20$) with ACS. Schoenhagen *et al.* [62], in an IVUS study analyzing morphology of plaques distant from the culprit/angioplasty site reported no difference in plaque morphology between patients with ACS compared to patients with stable angina. The authors interpreted the finding as a limitation of current IVUS methodology in detecting characteristics of plaque vulnerability.

Overall, these results have important implications for the morphological assessment of plaque rupture and vulnerability with *in vivo* imaging modalities. Recent histological studies suggest that episodes of plaque destabilization and rupture are common and most frequently not associated with clinical symptoms [64–66]. Presumably, after an episode of rupture, the local balance between thrombosis and spontaneous thrombolysis prevents the occlusion in most vessel segments. However, at the time of an AMI, the systemic inflammatory and procoagulant milieu seems to promote multifocal plaque instability, increasing the probability of additional atheroma disruption at multiple sites other than the culprit lesion [67–69]. Plaque vulnerability therefore describes a temporary biochemical stage of plaque activation with increased risk to rupture [57,58,70,71].

Conclusion

Over the last 30 years, the development of intravascular imaging, such as coronary angiography, angioscopy, and IVUS; has led to a better understanding of the physiopathology of ACS. *In vivo* validation of very important concepts, including the concept of ACS secondary to plaque rupture and thrombus formation or the concept of plaque vulnerability, were made possible by the development of such imaging modalities. These techniques were also very helpful in understanding the natural healing process of the disrupted plaque. Such findings had a tremendous impact on the nature and efficacy of the medical care provided to patients suffering an ACS and are providing the rationale for the development of new imaging modalities.

References

1. Falk E, Shah PK, Fuster V. Coronary plaque disruption. *Circulation* 1995; **92**: 657–671.
2. Arnett EN, Isner JM, Redwood DR *et al.* Coronary artery narrowing in coronary heart disease: comparison of cineangiographic and necropsy findings. *Ann Intern Med* 1979; **91**: 350–356.
3. Roberts WC, Jones AA. Quantitation of coronary arterial narrowing at necropsy in sudden coronary death: analysis of 31 patients and comparison with 25 control subjects. *Am J Cardiol* 1979; **44**: 39–45.
4. Mizuno K, Miyamoto A, Satomura K *et al.* Angioscopic coronary macromorphology in patients with acute coronary disorders. *Lancet* 1991; **337**: 809–812.
5. Ueda Y, Asakura M, Hirayama A, Komamura K, Hori M, Kodama K. Intracoronary morphology of culprit lesions after reperfusion in acute myocardial infarction: serial angioscopic observations. *J Am Coll Cardiol* 1996; **27**: 606–610.
6. den Heijer P, Foley DP, Hillege HL *et al.* The "Ermenonville" classification of observations at coronary angioscopy. Evaluation of intra- and inter-observer agreement. *Eur Heart J* 1994; **15**: 815–822.
7. Thieme T, Wernecke KD, Meyer R *et al.* Angioscopic evaluation of atherosclerotic plaques: validation by histomorphologic analysis and association with stable and unstable coronary syndromes. *J Am Coll Cardiol* 1996; **28**: 1–6.
8. Siegel R, Ariani M, Fishbein M *et al.* Histopathologic validation of angioscopy and intravascular ultrasound. *Circulation* 1991; **84**: 109–117.
9. Gussenhoven EJ, Essed CE, Lancee CT *et al.* Arterial wall characteristics determined by intravascular ultrasound imaging: an *in vitro* study. *J Am Coll Cardiol* 1989; **14**: 947–952.
10. Regar E, Serruys PW. Ten years after introduction of intravascular ultrasound in the catheterization laboratory: tool or toy? *Z Kardiol* 2002; **91**(Suppl. 3): 89–97.
11. Nissen SE, Yock P. Intravascular ultrasound: novel pathophysiological insights and current clinical applications. *Circulation* 2001; **103**: 604–616.
12. Hiro T, Leung CY, De Guzman S *et al.* Are soft echoes really soft? Intravascular ultrasound assessment of mechanical properties in human atherosclerotic tissue. *Am Heart J* 1997; **133**: 1–7.

13. Kostamaa H, Donovan J, Kasaoka S, Tobis J, Fitzpatrick L. Calcified plaque cross-sectional area in human arteries: correlation between intravascular ultrasound and undecalcified histology. *Am Heart J* 1999; **137**: 482–488.
14. Tuzcu EM, Berkalp B, De Franco AC *et al.* The dilemma of diagnosing coronary calcification: angiography versus intravascular ultrasound. *J Am Coll Cardiol* 1996; **27**: 832–838.
15. van der Lugt A, Gussenhoven EJ, Stijnen T *et al.* Comparison of intravascular ultrasonic findings after coronary balloon angioplasty evaluated *in vitro* with histology. *Am J Cardiol* 1995; **76**: 661–666.
16. Peters RJ, Kok WE, Havenith MG, Rijsterborgh H, van der Wal AC, Visser CA. Histopathologic validation of intracoronary ultrasound imaging. *J Am Soc Echocardiogr* 1994; **7**: 230–241.
17. Komiyama N, Berry GJ, Kolz ML *et al.* Tissue characterization of atherosclerotic plaques by intravascular ultrasound radiofrequency signal analysis: an *in vitro* study of human coronary arteries. *Am Heart J* 2000; **140**: 565–574.
18. Frimerman A, Miller HI, Hallman M, Laniado S, Keren G. Intravascular ultrasound characterization of thrombi of different composition. *Am J Cardiol* 1994; **73**: 1053–1057.
19. Davies MJ. A macro and micro view of coronary vascular insult in ischemic heart disease. *Circulation* 1990; **82**(Suppl. II): II-38–II-46.
20. Ambrose J, Winters S, Stern A *et al.* Angiographic morphology and the pathogenesis of unstable angina. *J Am Coll Cardiol* 1985; **5**: 609–616.
21. Ambrose J, Winters S, Arora R *et al.* Coronary angiographic morphology in myocardial infarction: a link between the pathogenesis of unstable angina and myocardial infarction. *J Am Coll Cardiol* 1985; **6**: 1233–1238.
22. Waxman S, Mittleman MA, Zarich SW *et al.* Plaque disruption and thrombus in Ambrose's angiographic coronary lesion types. *Am J Cardiol* 2003; **92**: 16–20.
23. Waxman S, Sassower MA, Mittleman MA *et al.* Angioscopic predictors of early adverse outcome after coronary angioplasty in patients with unstable angina and non-Q-wave myocardial infarction. *Circulation* 1996; **93**: 2106–2113.
24. Nesto RW, Waxman S, Mittleman MA *et al.* Angioscopy of culprit coronary lesions in unstable angina pectoris and correlation of clinical presentation with plaque morphology. *Am J Cardiol* 1998; **81**: 225–228.
25. Sakai S, Mizuno K, Yokoyama S *et al.* Morphologic changes in infarct-related plaque after coronary stent placement: a serial angioscopy study. *J Am Coll Cardiol* 2003; **42**: 1558–1565.
26. Ueda Y, Asakura M, Yamaguchi O, Hirayama A, Hori M, Kodama K. The healing process of infarct-related plaques. Insights from 18 months of serial angioscopic follow-up. *J Am Coll Cardiol* 2001; **38**: 1916–1922.
27. Arakawa K, Mizuno K, Shibuya T *et al.* Angioscopic coronary macromorphology after thrombolysis in acute myocardial infarction. *Am J Cardiol* 1997; **79**: 197–202.
28. White C, Ramee S, Collins T *et al.* Coronary thrombi increase PTCA risk. Angioscopy as a clinical tool. *Circulation* 1996; **93**: 253–258.
29. Dangas G, Mehran R, Wallenstein S *et al.* Correlation of angiographic morphology and clinical presentation in unstable angina. *J Am Coll Cardiol* 1997; **29**: 519–525.
30. Mizuno K, Satomura K, Miyamoto A *et al.* Angioscopic evaluation of coronary-artery thrombi in acute coronary syndromes. *N Engl J Med* 1992; **326**: 287–291.

31. Silva JA, Escobar A, Collins TJ, Ramee SR, White CJ. Unstable angina. A comparison of angioscopic findings between diabetic and nondiabetic patients. *Circulation* 1995; **92**: 1731–1736.

32. Okamatsu K, Takano M, Sakai S *et al.* Elevated troponin T levels and lesion characteristics in non-ST-elevation acute coronary syndromes. *Circulation* 2004; **109**: 465 470.

33. Rioufol G, Finet G, Ginon I *et al.* Multiple atherosclerotic plaque rupture in acute coronary syndrome: a three-vessel intravascular ultrasound study. *Circulation* 2002; **106**: 804–808.

34. Fukuda D, Kawarabayashi T, Tanaka A *et al.* Lesion characteristics of acute myocardial infarction: an investigation with intravascular ultrasound. *Heart* 2001; **85**: 402–406.

35. Schoenhagen P, Ziada KM, Kapadia SR, Crowe TD, Nissen SE, Tuzcu EM. Extent and direction of arterial remodeling in stable versus unstable coronary syndromes: an intravascular ultrasound study. *Circulation* 2000; **101**: 598–603.

36. Nakamura M, Nishikawa H, Mukai S *et al.* Impact of coronary artery remodeling on clinical presentation of coronary artery disease: an intravascular ultrasound study. *J Am Coll Cardiol* 2001; **37**: 63–69.

37. von Birgelen C, Klinkhart W, Mintz GS *et al.* Plaque distribution and vascular remodeling of ruptured and nonruptured coronary plaques in the same vessel: an intravascular ultrasound study *in vivo. J Am Coll Cardiol* 2001; **37**: 1864–1870.

38. Beckman JA, Ganz J, Creager MA, Ganz P, Kinlay S. Relationship of clinical presentation and calcification of culprit coronary artery stenoses. *Arterioscler Thromb Vasc Biol* 2001; **21**: 1618–1622.

39. Van Belle E, Lablanche JM, Bauters C, Renaud N, McFadden EP, Bertrand ME. Coronary angioscopic findings in the infarct-related vessel within 1 month of acute myocardial infarction: natural history and the effect of thrombolysis [see comments]. *Circulation* 1998; **97**: 26–33.

40. Bauters C, Lablanche JM, Renaud N, McFadden EP, Hamon M, Bertrand ME. Morphological changes after percutaneous transluminal coronary angioplasty of unstable plaques. Insight from serial angioscopic follow-up. *Eur Heart J* 1996; **17**: 1554–1559.

41. Bauters C, Khanoyan P, McFadden EP, Quandalle P, Lablanche JM, Bertrand ME. Restenosis after delayed coronary angioplasty of the culprit vessel in patients with a recent myocardial infarction treated by thrombolysis. *Circulation* 1995; **91**: 1410–1418.

42. Bauters C, Delomez M, Van Belle E, McFadden EP, Lablanche JM, Bertrand ME. Angiographically documented late reocclusion after successful coronary angioplasty of an infarct-related lesion is a powerful predictor of long-term mortality. *Circulation* 1999; **99**: 2243–2250.

43. Veen G, Meyer A, Verheugt FWA *et al.* Culprit lesion morphology and stenosis severity in the prediction of reocclusion after coronary thrombolysis: angiographic results of the APRICOT study. *J Am Coll Cardiol* 1993; **22**: 1755–1762.

44. Ellis SG, Vandormael MG, Cowley MJ *et al.* Coronary morphologic and clinical determinants of procedural outcome with multivessel coronary artery disease. Implications for patient selection. *Circulation* 1990; **82**: 1193–1202.

45. Smith SC, Jr., Dove JT, Jacobs AK *et al.* ACC/AHA guidelines for percutaneous coronary intervention (revision of the 1993 PTCA guidelines) – executive summary: a report of the American College of Cardiology/American Heart Association

task force on practice guidelines (committee to revise the 1993 guidelines for percutaneous transluminal coronary angioplasty) endorsed by the Society for Cardiac Angiography and Interventions. *Circulation* 2001; **103**: 3019–3041.

46. Myler RK, Shaw RE, Stertzer SH *et al.* Lesion morphology and coronary angioplasty: current experience and analysis. *J Am Coll Cardiol* 1992; **19**: 1641–1652.
47. Feld S, Ganim M, Carell MZ *et al.* Comparison of angioscopy, intravascular ultrasound imaging and quantitative coronary angiography in predicting clinical outcome after coronary intervention in high risk patients. *J Am Coll Cardiol* 1996; **28**: 97–105.
48. Fukuda D, Tanaka A, Shimada K, Nishida Y, Kawarabayashi T, Yoshikawa J. Predicting angiographic distal embolization following percutaneous coronary intervention in patients with acute myocardial infarction. *Am J Cardiol* 2003; **91**: 403–407.
49. Tanaka A, Kawarabayashi T, Nishibori Y *et al.* No-reflow phenomenon and lesion morphology in patients with acute myocardial infarction. *Circulation* 2002; **105**: 2148–2152.
50. Falk E. Plaque rupture with severe pre-existing precipitating coronary thrombosis: characteristics of coronary atherosclerotic plaques underlying fatal occlusive thrombi. *Br Heart J* 1983; **50**: 127–134.
51. Davies MJ, Thomas AC. Plaque fissuring: the cause of acute myocardial infarction, sudden ischemia death, and crescendo angina. *Br Heart J* 1985; **53**: 363–373.
52. Little WC, Constantinescu M, Applegate RJ *et al.* Can coronary angiography predict the site of a subsequent myocardial infarction in patients with mild-to-moderate coronary artery disease? *Circulation* 1988; **78**: 1157–1166.
53. Ambrose JA, Tannenbaum MA, Alexopoulos D *et al.* Angiographic progression of coronary artery disease and the development of myocardial infarction. *J Am Coll Cardiol* 1988; **12**: 56–62.
54. Yokoya K, Takatsu H, Suzuki T *et al.* Process of progression of coronary artery lesions from mild or moderate stenosis to moderate or severe stenosis: a study based on four serial coronary arteriograms per year. *Circulation* 1999; **100**: 903–909.
55. Ojio S, Takatsu H, Tanaka T *et al.* Considerable time from the onset of plaque rupture and/or thrombi until the onset of acute myocardial infarction in humans: coronary angiographic findings within 1 week before the onset of infarction. *Circulation* 2000; **102**: 2063–2069.
56. Yamagishi M, Terashima M, Awano K *et al.* Morphology of vulnerable coronary plaque: insights from follow-up of patients examined by intravascular ultrasound before an acute coronary syndrome. *J Am Coll Cardiol* 2000; **35**: 106–111.
57. Burke AP, Kolodgie FD, Farb A, Weber D, Virmani R. Morphological predictors of arterial remodeling in coronary atherosclerosis. *Circulation* 2002; **105**: 297–303.
58. Varnava AM, Mills PG, Davies MJ. Relationship between coronary artery remodeling and plaque vulnerability. *Circulation* 2002; **105**: 939–943.
59. Takano M, Mizuno K, Okamatsu K, Yokoyama S, Ohba T, Sakai S. Mechanical and structural characteristics of vulnerable plaques: analysis by coronary angioscopy and intravascular ultrasound. *J Am Coll Cardiol* 2001; **38**: 99–104.
60. Uchida Y, Nakamura F, Tomaru T *et al.* Prediction of acute coronary syndromes by percutaneous coronary angioscopy in patients with stable angina. *Am Heart J* 1995; **130**: 195–203.

61. Goldstein JA, Demetriou D, Grines CL, Pica M, Shoukfeh M, O'Neill WW. Multiple complex coronary plaques in patients with acute myocardial infarction. *N Engl J Med* 2000; **343**: 915–922.

62. Schoenhagen P, Stone GW, Nissen SE *et al.* Coronary plaque morphology and frequency of ulceration distant from culprit lesions in patients with unstable and stable presentation. *Arterioscler Thromb Vasc Biol* 2003; **23**: 1895–1900.

63. Asakura M, Ueda Y, Yamaguchi O *et al.* Extensive development of vulnerable plaques as a pan-coronary process in patients with myocardial infarction: an angioscopic study. *J Am Coll Cardiol* 2001; **37**: 1284–1288.

64. Frink RJ. Chronic ulcerated plaques: new insights into the pathogenesis of acute coronary disease. *J Invasive Cardiol* 1994; **6**: 173–185.

65. Williams H, Johnson JL, Carson KG, Jackson CL. Characteristics of intact and ruptured atherosclerotic plaques in brachiocephalic arteries of apolipoprotein E knockout mice. *Arterioscler Thromb Vasc Biol* 2002; **22**: 788–792.

66. Burke AP, Kolodgie FD, Farb A *et al.* Healed plaque ruptures and sudden coronary death: evidence that subclinical rupture has a role in plaque progression. *Circulation* 2001; **103**: 934–940.

67. Libby P. Current concepts of the pathogenesis of the acute coronary syndromes. *Circulation* 2001; **104**: 365–372.

68. Mazzone A, De Servi S, Ricevuti G *et al.* Increased expression of neutrophil and monocyte adhesion molecules in unstable coronary artery disease. *Circulation* 1993; **88**: 358–363.

69. Buffon A, Biasucci LM, Liuzzo G, D'Onofrio G, Crea F, Maseri A. Widespread coronary inflammation in unstable angina. *N Engl J Med* 2002; **347**: 5–12.

70. Muller JE, Tofler GH, Stone PH. Circadian variation and triggers of onset of acute cardiovascular disease. *Circulation* 1989; **79**: 733–743.

71. Pasterkamp G, Schoneveld AH, van der Wal AC *et al.* Inflammation of the atherosclerotic cap and shoulder of the plaque is a common and locally observed feature in unruptured plaques of femoral and coronary arteries. *Arterioscler Thromb Vasc Biol* 1999; **19**: 54–58.

CHAPTER 7

New coronary imaging in acute coronary syndrome

Pim J. de Feyter, Evelyne Regar, and Nico R.A. Mollet

Introduction

Atherosclerosis begins early in life. Before the age of 20, half of asymptomatic individuals already have detectable coronary intimal lesions [1,2]. Coronary atherosclerosis progresses relentlessly over the years and accounts for more death and disability than any other disease entity in industrialized societies [3]. The progression from asymptomatic atherosclerosis to a high-risk (vulnerable) plaque and to a thrombosed plaque causing an acute coronary syndrome (ACS) has been unravelled to a large extent. The transition from a high-risk plaque to a thrombosed plaque is often caused by a rupture or erosion of the fibrous cap complicated by thrombosis extending into the coronary lumen [4–7]. The identification of a high-risk (vulnerable) plaque is of great clinical interest, but currently no widely accepted method is available to prospectively identify the vulnerable plaque. Many invasive and noninvasive imaging modalities have emerged that are now capable of identification of some, but not all, specific features of the vulnerable plaque [8]. In this chapter, we describe highly promising noninvasive diagnostic tools, such as Multislice computed tomography (MSCT), magnetic resonance imaging (MRI), and a few invasive intracoronary diagnostic tools that can be used in clinical practice, for example, optical coherence tomography (OCT), thermography, palpography, and intravascular MRI [9,10].

Definition of vulnerable plaque

Postmortem evaluation has shown that high-risk (vulnerable) plaques have several characteristics: a thin fibrous cap (<65 μm), a large, lipid-rich pool (>3 mm^3), often a non- or modestly stenotic plaque, and increased macrophage activity (inflammation) often associated with positive coronary wall remodeling [4–7]. It should be emphasized here that these histologic characteristics of the vulnerable plaque are "indirectly" and in retrospection obtained from plaques that show cap rupture or erosion with thrombus formation. The actual diagnosis of a vulnerable plaque, however, is a prospective diagnosis and implies the occurrence of a future adverse coronary event.

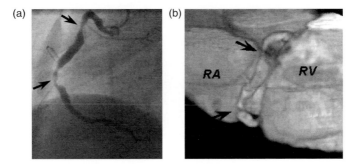

Figure 7.1 Noninvasive MR-coronary angiography of the right coronary artery
(RCA). (a) Diagnostic invasive coronary angiography of RCA demonstrating two
significant coronary stenoses (arrows). (b) Corresponding MR-coronary angiography.
RA: right atrium. RV: right ventricular.

Noninvasive imaging

Magnetic resonance imaging

Magnetic resonance imaging has emerged as a potential useful tool to image
coronary plaques. In the thoracic aorta or carotid arteries the composition
of the atherosclerotic plaque (lipid, fibrous, or calcium) can be assessed by
using a multiple contrast MRI imaging technique. Accurate measurements
of the carotid plaque size and fibrous cap thickness and visualization of the
ruptured cap are possible with MRI [11–15]. MRI coronary angiography can
detect coronary stenoses in the proximal and mid-coronary artery segments
but is limited by its inability to image distal epicardial coronary vessels and
approximately 15% of the proximal epicardial vessels cannot be assessed due
to motion artifacts [16–18] (Figure 7.1). Preliminary studies have shown that
MRI imaging of coronary plaques is possible, but so far it has remained limited
to measurements of the coronary wall (including the plaque) thickness [19,20]
(Figure 7.2).

Computed tomography (CT) – coronary calcium

Electron-beam computed tomography (EBCT) can accurately detect coronary
calcium (Figure 7.3). The coronary artery calcium score (CACS) is related to
the overall burden of coronary atherosclerosis [21,22] and can predict adverse
coronary events, as has been shown in several large-scale, long-term studies
(Table 7.1) [23–29]. These studies provide ample evidence that coronary calcium is a predictor of adverse coronary events. The greater the overall calcium
burden, which correlates with a greater overall coronary plaque burden, the
greater is the likelihood of an adverse event (Table 7.2) [28]. But calcification of an individual plaque is neither a marker for plaque vulnerability nor
for plaque stability. The absence of calcium does not exclude the presence of
coronary atherosclerosis but is associated with a low likelihood of advanced

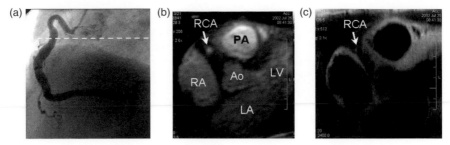

Figure 7.2 Noninvasive MR-coronary plaque imaging of diseased right coronary artery (RCA). (a) Diagnostic invasive coronary angiography. Dashed line indicated MR-cross-sectional images (b), (c). (b) MR-coronary angiography using bright blood imaging technique delineating the coronary lumen. (c) MR-coronary angiography using black blood imaging technique showing a thickened coronary wall. PA: pulmonary artery. RA: right atrium. Ao: aorta. LV: left ventricular. LA: left atrium.

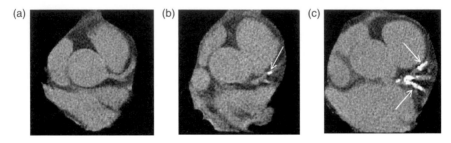

Figure 7.3 EBCT demonstrating (a) normal left coronary artery; (b) mild degree of calcium in left coronary artery; (c) high degree of calcium in left coronary artery.

coronary atherosclerosis and a very low likelihood of an adverse coronary event.

It would be important to establish that CACS assessment provides predictive information in addition to the predictive value of traditional risk factors or the Framingham risk score. Detrano *et al.* [25] showed that CACS offered no additional predictive value; but other studies showed that CACS results increased the risk prediction conveyed by traditional risk factors alone [27,29]. Furthermore, Kondos *et al.* [27] demonstrated in 5635 asymptomatic self-referred adults who responded to a questionnaire (only 65% of the initial group responded) that CACs provided incremental prognostic information in addition to age and risk factors. Greenland *et al.* [29] demonstrated that the Framingham score in combination with the CACS conveyed an increased risk compared with the Framingham score alone, and a CACS score greater than 300 was more predictive among various Framingham risk score categories.

Finally, Shaw *et al.* [28] showed in a large study of 10 377 asymptomatic individuals that coronary calcium provided independent incremental information

Table 7.1 Coronary calcium to predict adverse cardiac events.

Study	N	Mean age (years)	Gender (%male)	FUP (years)	Events (death/MI)	Calcium score cut-off	Risk ratio
Wong et al. [23]	926	54	79	3.3	28	>81–270	4.5*
Arad et al. [24]	1172	53	71	3.7	18	>271	8.8*
Detrano et al. [25]	1196	66	89	3.4	44	>44	2.3*
Raggi et al. [26]	676	52	51	2.7	30	>100	>4.1%**
Kondos et al. [27]	5635	51	74	3.1	222	≥0	Men = 10.5; women = 2.6
Shaw et al. [28]	10.377	53	60	5.0	249 (death)	>400–1000; >1000	6.15* 12.3*
Greenland et al. [29]	1029	65.7	90	7.0	84 (death, MI)	>300	3.9

*Compared with patients with 0 score.
**Annualized event rate.

Table 7.2 Coronary calcium score and risk adjusted mortality rate.

Coronary calcium score	Relative risk
11–100	1.64 (1.12 , 2.41)
101–400	1.74 (1.16 , 2.61)
401–1000	2.54 (1.62 , 3.99)
>1000	4.03 (2.52 , 6.40)

Source: From Ref. 28.

in addition to traditional risk factors in the prediction of all cause mortality (Table 7.2).

Thus CACS can modify the predicted risk obtained from traditional risk factors, especially among patients in the intermediate risk category in whom clinical decision-making is most uncertain [28]. Greenland et al. [30] suggested applying calcium quantification in patients with an intermediate risk, based on traditional risk factors. In these patients, the calcium score could determine whether they should be regarded as high risk and receive more intensive therapy, or regarded as low risk (no calcium present), where advice on the lifestyle might be sufficient [30].

Figure 7.4 CT-coronary plaque imaging. Maximum intensity projected CT image of the left main coronary artery. The arrowhead indicates the presence of a nonobstructive, predominantly noncalcified plaque located at the distal part of the left main and protruding in the circumflex coronary artery. A cross-sectional multiplanar reconstructed CT image (inlay) provides detailed information regarding the presence of noncalcified (low-density) plaque tissue adjacent to the contrast-enhanced coronary lumen.

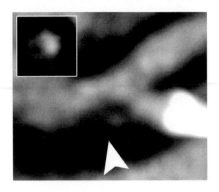

Figure 7.5 CT-coronary plaque imaging. Maximum intensity projected CT image of the left main coronary artery. The arrowhead indicates the presence of a calcified plaque extending along the entire left main coronary artery. A cross-sectional multiplanar reconstructed CT image (inlay) confirms the presence of calcified (high-density) plaque tissue adjacent to the contrast-enhanced coronary lumen.

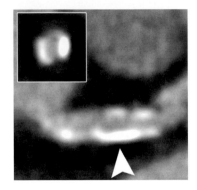

CT – coronary plaque imaging

Multislice computed tomography is able to detect obstructive and nonobstructive coronary plaques and may be useful in identifying the composition of the atherosclerotic plaque (Figures 7.4 and 7.5). Based on the differences in density measurements of various tissues, it is possible to differentiate among fibrous tissue, lipid, and calcium [31–36]. Lipid is a low-density structure, fibrous tissue is an intermediate-density structure, and calcium is a high-density structure. A very low-density obstruction in the setting of an ACS may represent a thrombotic occlusion.

Schroeder *et al.* [37] demonstrated that MSCT density measurements differed significantly among coronary plaques classified by Intravascular ultrasound (IVUS) as lipid (low echogenicity), fibrous (intermediate echogenicity), or calcified, thereby suggesting that MSCT was able to distinguish among lipid, fibrous tissue and calcium. These results were confirmed by the study of Leber *et al.* [38], who also compared IVUS, determined echogenicity values of plaques with CT-densities and showed that lipid and fibrous tissue could be distinguished by MSCT (Table 7.3), although there is some overlap between density values of lipid and fibrous tissue. Achenbach *et al.* [39] demonstrated that MSCT allowed the identification of positive and negative

Table 7.3 Plaque composition with contrast-enhanced CT coronary plaque imaging.

IVUS	MS CT	
	Schroeder HU ± SD (n = 17)	Leber HU ± SD (n = 37)
Hypoechoïc	14 ± 26	49 ± 22
Hyperechoïc	91 ± 21	91 ± 22
Calcified	419 ± 194	391 ± 156

Source: From Refs 37 and 38.

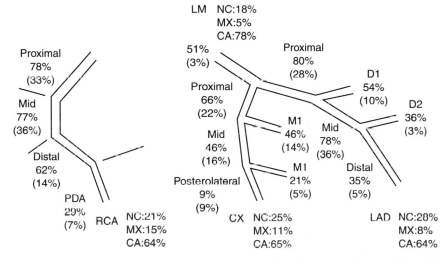

Figure 7.6 MSCT coronary plaque imaging. Extent, distribution, and composition of coronary plaques in the coronary tree. RCA: right coronary artery; Cx: circumflex artery; LAD: left anterior descending artery; LM: left main; NC: noncalcific plaque; MX: mixed plaque (calcific and noncalcific plaque); CA: calcific plaque.

coronary wall remodeling. The diagnostic accuracy of MSCT to detect coronary plaques compared with IVUS is reasonably good with a sensitivity of 82–86% and a specificity of 88–92% [38,39]. However, it appears that MSCT seriously underestimates the size of plaque by about 40% [40]. Mollet *et al.* [41] assessed the coronary plaque burden with MSCT, which was defined as the number of diseased coronary segments, location of disease, obstructive or nonobstructive plaque, and type of plaque (calcific or noncalcific). The results obtained in 41 patients are shown in Figure 7.6.

The role of MSCT to noninvasively detect a vulnerable plaque or to identify a vulnerable patient is currently being evaluated in many studies.

Table 7.4 Diagnostic performance of 16-slice MSCT.

	CT	β	NP (n)	D (%)	Excl. (%)	Sens. (%)	Spec. (%)	PPV (%)	NPV (%)
Nieman et al. [42]	12	+	58	50	—	95	86	80	97
Ropers et al. [43]	12	+	77	50	12	92	93	79	97
Kuettner et al. [44]	16	+	60	50	6	72	97	72	97
Mollet et al. [45]	16	+	128	50	—	92	95	79	98
Martuscelli et al. [46]	16	+	64	>50	16	94	97	91	98
Kuettner et al. [48]	16	+	72	>50	6.6	82	98	87	97
Mollet et al. [47]	16	+	51	>50	0	95	98	87	99

Notes: Use of β-blockers (β); diameter reduction considered significant (D); percentage of excluded segments or branches (Excl.); sensitivity (Sens.); specificity (Spec.); positive (PPV) and negative predictive value (NPV) regarding the assessable segments or branches; number of patients (NP).

Noninvasive imaging: CT – coronary stenosis

Over the past decade, great strides have been taken to detect coronary stenoses using CT. The most recent reports about the diagnostic performance concern the 16-MSCT scanner. The sensitivity and specificity to detect a significant coronary stenosis is high (Table 7.4), but one should bear in mind that only the larger coronary artery segments (>2 mm diameter) were analyzed and that in a few reports, 6–16% of the available segments were excluded from analysis in the majority due to motion artifacts or severe calcification obscuring the lumen [42–48]. In a recent report by Mollet et al. [47], patients with unstable angina were evaluated. It appeared that the diagnostic performance was equally high in patients with unstable and stable angina. Current limitations of MSCT are that patients with irregular heart rhythm cannot be evaluated, whereas the rather high radiation exposure with an effective dose ranging of 10–12 mSv is of great concern.

Invasive diagnostic tools

Thermography

Coronary atherosclerosis is considered a chronic inflammatory disease. One of the characteristics of a high-risk plaque is the presence of intense inflammatory reaction manifested by the local invasion of macrophages and lymphocytes. Based on these findings, a hypothesis was generated that these "activated" macrophages produce thermal energy, which might be detected on the surface of these atherosclerotic lesions. It appeared that the temperature heterogeneity is directly proportional to the degree of histologically detected inflammation [49,50]. Patients with an ACS had higher levels of coronary artery temperature heterogeneity, and in a follow-up study these thermographic findings were

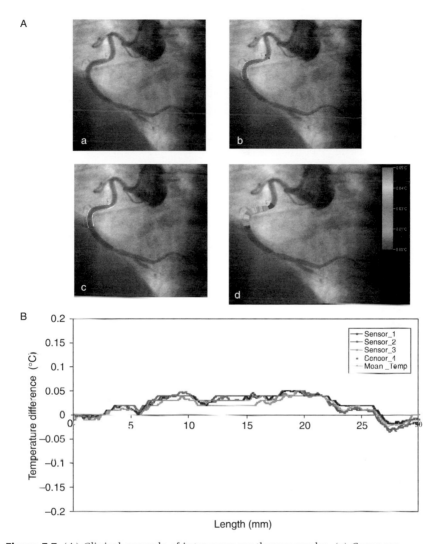

Figure 7.7 (A) Clinical example of intracoronary thermography. (a) Coronary angiogram of a mildly diseased right coronary artery with multiple lumen irregularities. (b) Automated delineation of the vessel wall; (c) plaque imaging and (d) collected temperature data on vessel anatomy. (B) Example for the display of intracoronary temperature measurements. The lines indicate the temperature differences between the reference temperature and the temperature measured at the coronary wall by each individual thermistor sensor over the length of the arterial segment.

predictive of an acute adverse coronary event [51,52]. An example of clinical thermography in a coronary artery is given in Figure 7.7. Further studies are needed to establish the capability of thermography to identify an individual vulnerable plaque in the coronary arteries. The impact of coronary blood flow

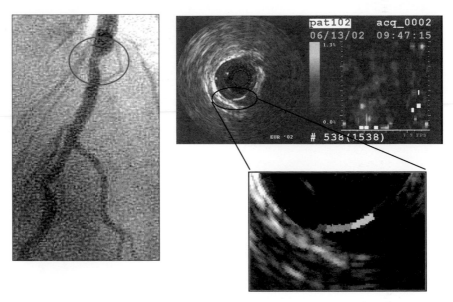

Figure 7.8 Clinical example of intracoronary palpography. Intravascular ultrasound palpography is assessing the local mechanical tissue properties of the luminal surface of the vessel wall. One strain value per angle lumen circumference is calculated and plotted as color-coded contour at the lumen vessel boundary.

on temperature, with the "cooling" effect of high blood flow, needs to be addressed [53].

Palpography

Features of the vulnerable plaque are the presence of a large lipid core covered by a rather thin fibrous cap that has different local mechanical properties, as is manifested more readily by a deformation of these plaques compared with adjacent coronary structures. Upon a defined mechanical excitation, soft tissue components will deform more (high strain) than hard components (low strain) [54]. The deformations of structures can be measured by ultrasound. It has been demonstrated in an animal study that the strain pattern is different for fibrous, fibro-fatty, and fatty plaques and that a high-strain value (a highly deformable structure) was associated with a fatty plaque and presence of macrophages [55]. The sensitivity and specificity of a high-strain spot to detect a vulnerable plaque, as assessed in postmortem human coronary arteries, was 88% and 89%, respectively [56]. *In vivo* intracoronary palpography is feasible and the finding of high-strain spots is highly reproducible [57,58] (Figure 7.8). In a recent study, it was shown that the number of high-strain spots in the coronary arteries was directly related to the magnitude of instability of patients with the highest number of high-strain spots in patients with an acute myocardial infarction, intermediate in unstable patients, and lowest in stable

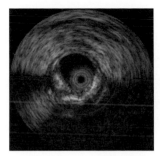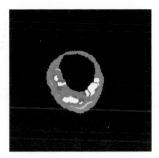

Figure 7.9 Virtual histology is based on backscatter analysis and mathematical modeling of the radiofrequency signals produced by the intravascular ultrasound unit. Data were used to develop classification schemes, which allow the differentiation between tissue types in regions of interest. Tissue types are assigned color values and overlaid on the tissue maps from IVUS (green = fibrous, yellow = lipid rich, red = lipid core, white = calcium tissue).

patients [59]. The acquisition of a palpogram can be obtained from a motorized catheter pullback using special IVUS catheters that are commercially available.

Virtual histology

More sophisticated tissue characterization by IVUS can be obtained by the use of radio-frequency signal analysis (Figure 7.9). Virtual histology is based on IVUS backscatter analysis and on the mathematical modeling of the radio-frequency signal. This allows to differentiate between tissue types: lipid, lipid-fibrous, calcified, and calcified necrotic, which has been validated by using *ex vivo* histology of human coronary arteries [60]. The data necessary for virtual histology are acquired during an IVUS catheter motorized pullback. Special IVUS catheters are commercially available. The data are displayed as a color map where the various tissue are represented by various colors. The clinical impact of the radiofrequency analysis of the ultrasound signal needs to be established and several prospective clinical trials are being initiated.

Optical coherence tomography

Optical coherence tomography is an imaging technique that allows for high-resolution (Figure 7.10) (axial resolution of 15 μm) imaging in biological systems. The high resolution capacity of OCT might allow for *in vivo* real-time visualization of a thin fibrous cap, which is present in high-risk (vulnerable) plaques. Postmortem studies demonstrated the accuracy of OCT in comparison to histology [61–63]. Intravascular application of OCT has proven feasible in the animal model. These studies showed that OCT can detect both normal and pathological artery structures. Recent experimental data suggest the possibility of detection of macrophages in atherosclerotic plaque *in vitro* [64]. The first clinical study proved the concept of *in vivo* intravascular OCT using

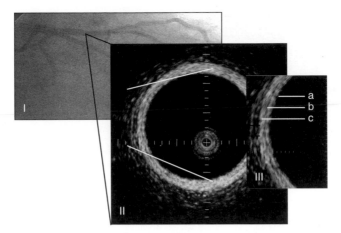

Figure 7.10 Clinical example of intravascular OCT imaging. (I) Coronary angiogram of a left descending coronary artery. (II) cross-sectional, optical coherence tomography of the coronary artery showing a normal coronary artery with clear demarcation between a highly reflective intimal layer (a), a low-reflective media (b), and a highly reflective adventitial layer (c).

a modified IVUS catheter. Ten patients scheduled for coronary stent implantation, with mild moderate coronary lesions, that were remote from the target stenosis, were investigated. Most coronary structures that were detected by IVUS could also be visualized with OCT. Intimal hyperplasia and echolucent regions, which may correspond to lipid pools, were identified more frequently by OCT than by IVUS [61,65].

We performed a pilot study using dedicated OCT imaging catheters in patients scheduled for percutaneous coronary intervention. OCT analysis of coronary artery wall was possible in all patients and the entire vessel circumference was visualized at all times (Figures 7.10 and 7.11). A wide spectrum of different plaque morphologies was seen. OCT allowed for differentiation of the normal artery wall for inhomogeneous, mixed plaques and thin cap fibroatheromas with inhomogeneous, low-reflecting necrotic cores, covered by highly reflecting fibrous caps with a thickness of approximately 50 μm. Prospective *in vivo* validation is pending.

Intravascular MRI
Intravascular MRI is another potential approach to determine plaque composition and locate potential "vulnerable plaques" within human coronary arteries. Hitherto, cardiac and respiratory motion has inhibited intravascular approaches but recent developments have allowed for the development of a self-contained intravascular MRI catheter unencumbered by cardiac motion.

Intravascular MRI can determine the presence of lipid within the arterial wall or, in combination with local delivery of contrast agents, determine the presence of specific cell types associated with plaque instability or thrombus.

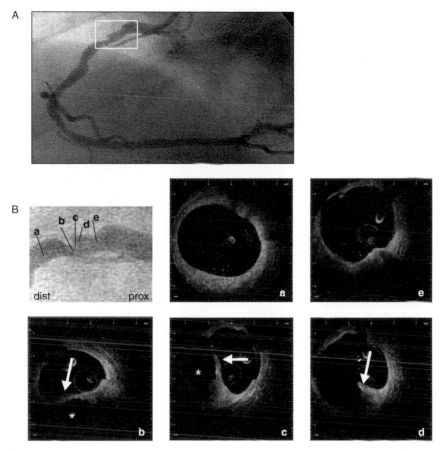

Figure 7.11 Clinical example of intravascular OCT imaging. (A) Angiogram of the right coronary artery showing an exulcerated plaque in the proximal segment. (B) Corresponding intravascular OCT image showing remnants of the ruptured fibrous cap. (a) Distal reference segment with circular lumen and eccentric, predominantly fibrous plaque, (b) distal portion of the lesion showing a fibrous cap that partially separates the true lumen from the neolumen (asterix), (c) mid-portion of the lesion: communication between the true lumen and the neolumen (asterix), (d) proximal portion of the lesion, (e) proximal reference showing circular lumen and eccentric fibro-fatty plaque.

The intravascular MRI system has been evaluated in nonatherosclerotic porcine coronary and femoral arteries to test proof of concept and device safety. *Ex vivo* human carotid tissue, aortic tissue, and coronary arteries were used to correlate MRI findings with histology. In *ex vivo* aortic studies, the MRI correctly predicted the histological results in 15 of 16 aortic cases (95% sensitivity, 100% specificity) and in *ex vivo* coronary arteries 16 of 18 lesions (89%) were correctly predicted, including the diagnosis of three thin cap fibroatheromas. Human safety studies have been initiated in Europe (Figure 7.12).

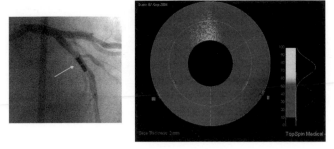

Figure 7.12 Clinical example of intracoronary MRI. Left: coronary angiogram showing the intravascular MRI catheter in the proximal left descending coronary artery. Right: corresponding intracoronary MRI. The vessel circumference is represented in three-color coded sectors of 120°. Blue color indicates the predominance of nonlipid tissue, yellow color indicates the predominance of lipid-rich tissue. In our patient, some lipid rich tissue signal (yellow) is visible in sector I, whereas the other sectors show nonlipid tissue (blue).

Conclusion

Noninvasive coronary plaque imaging with MRI and CT is feasible and have the potential to identify a vulnerable plaque but both techniques need substantial improvements before they can be accepted as clinically reliable tools. CT coronary calcium scoring is slowly emerging as an imaging technique that is able to identify high-risk individuals independent of the traditional risk factors. However, further studies are needed particularly in nonself referred individuals to establish the true predictive value of coronary calcium scoring.

To date, none of the described invasive techniques is validated on a broad basis *in vivo* and there is no gold standard available. However, these new modalities have the potential to provide new levels of anatomical detail and new dimensions of information for the diagnosis of coronary artery disease. In the future these technologies have to be validated. Their scientific, clinical, and prognostic value needs to be determined and the indications for clinical applications established.

References

1. Strong JP, Malcom GT, McMahan CA *et al*. Prevalence and extent of atherosclerosis in adolescents and young adults: implications for prevention from the pathobiological determinants of atherosclerosis in youth study. *JAMA* 1999; **281**(8): 727–735.
2. Tuzcu EM, Kapadia SR, Tutar E *et al*. High prevalence of coronary atherosclerosis in asymptomatic teenagers and young adults: evidence from intravascular ultrasound. *Circulation* 2001; **103**(22): 2705–2010.
3. Murray CJ, Lopez AD. Alternative projections of mortality and disability by cause 1990–2020: global burden of disease study. *Lancet* 1997; **349**(9064): 1498–1504.

4. Davies MJ, Thomas AC. Plaque fissuring – the cause of acute myocardial infarction, sudden ischaemic death, and crescendo angina. *Br Heart J* 1985; **53**(4): 363–373.

5. Falk E, Shah PK, Fuster V. Coronary plaque disruption. *Circulation* 1995; **92**(3): 657–671.

6. Virmani R, Kolodgie FD, Burke AP, Farb A, Schwartz SM. Lessons from sudden coronary death: a comprehensive morphological classification scheme for atherosclerotic lesions. *Arterioscler Thromb Vasc Biol* 2000; **20**(5): 1262–1275.

7. Libby P. Inflammation in atherosclerosis. *Nature* 2002; **420**(6917): 868–874.

8. Fayad ZA, Fuster V. Clinical imaging of the high-risk or vulnerable atherosclerotic plaque. *Circ Res* 2001; **89**(4): 305–316.

9. de Feyter PJ, Nieman K. New coronary imaging techniques: what to expect? *Heart* 2002; **87**(3): 195–197.

10. MacNeill BD, Lowe HC, Takano M, Fuster V, Jang IK. Intravascular modalities for detection of vulnerable plaque: current status. *Arterioscler Thromb Vasc Biol* 2003; **23**(8): 1333–1342. Epub Jun 12, 2003.

11. Fayad ZA, Nahar T, Fallon JT *et al. In vivo* magnetic resonance evaluation of atherosclerotic plaques in the human thoracic aorta: a comparison with transesophageal echocardiography. *Circulation* 2000; **101**(21): 2503–2509.

12. Yuan C, Mitsumori LM, Beach KW, Maravilla KR. Carotid atherosclerotic plaque: noninvasive MR characterization and identification of vulnerable lesions. *Radiology* 2001; **221**(2): 285–299.

13. Toussaint JF, LaMuraglia GM, Southern JF, Fuster V, Kantor HL. Magnetic resonance images lipid, fibrous, calcified, hemorrhagic, and thrombotic components of human atherosclerosis *in vivo*. *Circulation* 1996; **94**(5): 932–938.

14. Yuan C, Beach KW, Smith LH Jr, Hatsukami TS. Measurement of atherosclerotic carotid plaque size *in vivo* using high resolution magnetic resonance imaging. *Circulation* 1998; **98**(24): 2666–2671.

15. Hatsukami TS, Ross R, Polissar NL, Yuan C. Visualization of fibrous cap thickness and rupture in human atherosclerotic carotid plaque *in vivo* with high-resolution magnetic resonance imaging. *Circulation* 2000; **102**(9): 959–964.

16. Kim WY, Danias PG, Stuber M *et al.* Coronary magnetic resonance angiography for the detection of coronary stenoses. *N Engl J Med* 2001; **345**(26): 1863–1869.

17. Budoff MJ, Achenbach S, Duerinckx A. Clinical utility of computed tomography and magnetic resonance techniques for noninvasive coronary angiography. *J Am Coll Cardiol* 2003; **42**(11): 1867–1878.

18. van Geuns RJ, Wielopolski PA, de Bruin HG *et al.* MR coronary angiography with breath-hold targeted volumes: preliminary clinical results. *Radiology* 2000; **217**: 270–277.

19. Fayad ZA, Fuster V, Fallon JT *et al.* Noninvasive *in vivo* human coronary artery lumen and wall imaging using black-blood magnetic resonance imaging. *Circulation* 2000; **102**(5): 506–510.

20. Botnar RM, Stuber M, Kissinger KV, Kim WY, Spuentrup E, Manning WJ. Noninvasive coronary vessel wall and plaque imaging with magnetic resonance imaging. *Circulation* 2000; **102**(21): 2582–2587.

21. Rumberger JA, Simons DB, Fitzpatrick LA, Sheedy PF, Schwartz RS. Coronary artery calcium area by electron-beam computed tomography and coronary atherosclerotic plaque area. A histopathologic correlative study. *Circulation* 1995; **92**(8): 2157–2162.

22. O'Rourke RA, Brundage BH, Froelicher VF *et al.* American College of Cardiology/American Heart Association expert consensus document on electron-beam computed tomography for the diagnosis and prognosis of coronary artery disease. *J Am Coll Cardiol* 2000; **36**(1): 326–340.

23. Wong ND, Hsu JC, Detrano RC *et al.* Coronary artery calcium evaluation by electron beam computed tomography and its relation to new cardiovascular events. *Am J Cardiol* 2000; **86**: 498–508.

24. Arad Y, Spadaro LA, Goodman K, Newstein D, Guerci AD. Prediction of coronary events with electron beam computed tomography. *J Am Coll Cardiol* 2000; **36**(4): 1253–1260.

25. Detrano RC, Wong ND, Doherty TM *et al.* Coronary calcium does not accurately predict near-term future coronary events in high-risk adults. *Circulation* 1999; **99**(20): 2633–2638.

26. Raggi P, Cooil B, Callister TQ. Use of electron beam tomography data to develop models for prediction of hard coronary events. *Am Heart J* 2001; **141**(3): 375–382.

27. Kondos GT, Hoff JA, Sevrukov A *et al.* Electron-beam tomography coronary artery calcium and cardiac events: a 37-month follow-up of 5635 initially asymptomatic low- to intermediate-risk adults. *Circulation* 2003; **107**(20): 2571–2576. Epub May 12, 2003.

28. Shaw LJ, Raggi P, Schisterman E, Berman DS, Callister TQ. Prognostic value of cardiac risk factors and coronary artery calcium screening for all-cause mortality. *Radiology* 2003; **228**: 826–833.

29. Greenland PH, LaBree L, Azen SP, Doherty TM, Detrano RC. Coronary artery calcium score combined with framingham score for risk prediction in asymptomatic individuals. *JAMA* 2004; **291**: 210–215.

30. Greenland P, Abrams J, Aurigemma GP *et al.* Prevention conference V. Beyond secondary prevention: identifying the high-risk patient for primary prevention. Noninvasive tests of atherosclerotic burden: writing group III. *Circulation* 2000; **101**(1): E16–E22.

31. Becker CR, Knez A, Ohnesorge B, Schoepf UJ, Reiser MF. Imaging of noncalcified coronary plaques using helical CT with retrospective ECG gating. *AJR Am J Roentgenol* 2000; **175**(2): 423–424.

32. Becker CR, Nikolaou K, Muders M *et al.* Ex vivo coronary atherosclerotic plaque characterization with multi-detector-row CT. *Eur Radiol* 2003; **13**(9): 2094–2098. Epub Apr 12, 2003.

33. Estes JM, Quist WC, Lo Gerfo FW, Costello P. Noninvasive characterization of plaque morphology using helical computed tomography. *J Cardiovasc Surg (Torino)* 1998; **39**(5): 527–534.

34. Nikolaou K, Sagmeister S, Knez A *et al.* Multidetector-row computed tomography of the coronary arteries: predictive value and quantitative assessment of non-calcified vessel-wall changes. *Eur Radiol* 2003; **13**(11): 2505–2512.

35. Leber AW, Knez A, White CW *et al.* Composition of coronary atherosclerotic plaques in patients with acute myocardial infarction and stable angina pectoris determined by contrast-enhanced multislice computed tomography. *Am J Cardiol* 2003; **91**(6): 714–718.

36. Caussin C, Ohanessian A, Lancelin B *et al.* Coronary plaque burden detected by multislice computed tomography after acute myocardial infarction with near-normal coronary arteries by angiography. *Am J Cardiol* 2003; **92**(7): 849–852.

37. Schroeder S, Kopp AF, Baumbach A *et al*. Noninvasive detection and evaluation of atherosclerotic coronary plaques with multislice computed tomography. *J Am Coll Cardiol* 2001; **37**(5): 1430–1435.

38. Leber AW, Knez A, Becker A *et al*. Accuracy of multidetector spiral computed tomography in identifying and differentiating the composition of coronary atherosclerotic plaques; a comparative study with intracoronary ultrasound. *J Am Coll Cardiol* 2004; **43**(7): 1241–1247.

39. Achenbach S, Ropers D, Hoffmann U *et al*. Assessment of coronary remodeling in stenotic and nonstenotic coronary atherosclerotic lesions by multidetector spiral computed tomography. *J Am Coll Cardiol* 2004; **43**(5): 842–847.

40. Achenbach S, Moselewski F, Ropers D *et al*. Detection of calcified and non-calcified coronary atherosclerotic plaque by contrast-enhanced, submillimeter multidetector spiral computed tomography: a segment-based comparison with intravascular ultrasound. *Circulation* 2004; **109**(1): 14–17.

41. Mollet NR, Cademartiri F, Nieman K *et al*. Non-invasive assessment of coronary plaque burden using multislice computed tomography. *Am J Cardiol* 2005; **95**(10): 1165–1169.

42. Nieman K, Cademartiri F, Lemos PA *et al*. Reliable noninvasive coronary angiography with fast submillimeter multi-slice spiral computed tomography. *Circulation* 2002; **106**: 2051–2054.

43. Ropers D, Baum U, Pohle K *et al*. Detection of coronary artery stenoses with thin-slice multi-detector row spiral computed tomography and multi-planar reconstruction. *Circulation* 2003; **107**: 664–666.

44. Kuettner A, Trabold T, Schroeder S *et al*. Non-invasive detection of coronary lesions using 16-slice MDCT technology: initial clinical results. *J Am Coll Cardiol* 2004; **44**(6): 1230–1237.

45. Mollet, NR, Cademartiri F, Nieman K *et al*. Multi-slice spiral CT coronary angiography in patients with stable angina pectoris. *J Am Coll Cardiol* 2004; **43**(12): 2265–2270.

46. Martuscelli E, Romagnoli A, D'Eliseo, Razzini C *et al*. Accuracy of thin-slice computed tomography in the detection of coronary stenoses. *Eur Heart J* 2004; **25**: 1043–1048.

47. Mollet NR, Cademartiri F, Krestin GP *et al*. Improved diagnostic accuracy with 16-row multi-slice computed tomography coronary angiography. *J Am Coll Cardiol* 2005; **45**(1): 128–132.

48. Kuettner A, Beck T, Drosch T *et al*. Diagnostic accuracy of noninvasive coronary imaging using 16-slice spiral computed tomography with 188 ms temporal resolution. *JACC* 2005; **45**: 123–127.

49. Casscells W, Hathorn B, David M *et al*. Thermal detection of cellular infiltrates in living atherosclerotic plaques: possible implications for plaque rupture and thrombosis. *Lancet* 1996; **347**(9013): 1447–1451.

50. Verheye S, De Meyer GR, Van Langenhove G, Knaapen MW, Kockx MM. *In vivo* temperature heterogeneity of atherosclerotic plaques is determined by plaque composition. *Circulation* 2002; **105**(13): 1596–1601.

51. Stefanadis C, Diamantopoulos L, Vlachopoulos C *et al*. Thermal heterogeneity within human atherosclerotic coronary arteries detected *in vivo*: a new method of detection by application of a special thermography catheter. *Circulation* 1999; **99**(15): 1965–1971.

52. Stefanadis C, Toutouzas K, Tsiamis E *et al*. Increased local temperature in human coronary atherosclerotic plaques: an independent predictor of clinical outcome in

patients undergoing a percutaneous coronary intervention. *J Am Coll Cardiol* 2001; **37**(5): 1277–1283.

53. Diamantopoulos L, Liu X, De Scheerder I *et al.* The effect of reduced blood-flow on the coronary wall temperature. Are significant lesions suitable for intravascular thermography? *Eur Heart J* 2003; **24**(19): 1788–1795.

54. Cespedes EI, de Korte CL, van der Steen AF, von Birgelen C, Lancee CT. Intravascular elastography: principles and potentials. *Semin Interv Cardiol* 1997; **2**(1): 55–62.

55. de Korte CL, Pasterkamp G, van der Steen AF, Woutman HA, Bom N. Characterization of plaque components with intravascular ultrasound elastography in human femoral and coronary arteries *in vitro*. *Circulation* 2000; **102**(6): 617–623.

56. de Korte CL, Carlier SG, Mastik F *et al.* Morphological and mechanical information of coronary arteries obtained with intravascular elastography; feasibility study *in vivo*. *Eur Heart J* 2002; **23**(5): 405–413.

57. Schaar JA, de Korte CL, Mastik F *et al.* Intravascular palpography for high-risk vulnerable plaque assessment. *Herz* 2003; **28**(6): 488–495.

58. Schaar JA, de Korte CL, Mastik F *et al.* Characterizing vulnerable plaque features with intravascular elastography. *Circulation* 2003; **108**: 2636–2641.

59. Schaar JA, Regar E, Mastik F *et al.* Incidence of high-strain patterns in human coronary arteries: assessment with three-dimensional intravascular palpography and correlation with clinical presentation. *Circulation* 2004; **109**(22): 2716–2719. Epub May 24, 2004.

60. Nair A, Kuban BD, Tuzcu EM, Schoenhagen P, Nissen SE, Vince DG. Coronary plaque classification with intravascular ultrasound radiofrequency data analysis. *Circulation* 2002; **106**(17): 2200–2206.

61. Jang IK, Bouma BE, Kang DH *et al.* Visualization of coronary atherosclerotic plaques in patients using optical coherence tomography: comparison with intravascular ultrasound. *J Am Coll Cardiol* 2002; **39**: 604–609.

62. Brezinski ME, Tearney GJ, Weismann NJ *et al.* Assessing atherosclerotic plaque morphology: comparison of optical coherence tomography and high frequency intra-vascular ultrasound. *Heart* 1997; **77**: 397–403.

63. Yabushita H, Bouma BE, Houser SL *et al.* Characterization of human atherosclerosis by optical coherence tomography. *Circulation* 2002; **106**: 1640–1645.

64. Tearney GJ, Yabushita H, Houser SL *et al.* Quantification of macrophage content in atherosclerotic plaques by optical coherence tomography. *Circulation* 2003; **107**: 113–119.

65. Patwari P, Weissman NJ, Boppart SA *et al.* Assessment of coronary plaque with optical coherence tomography and high-frequency ultrasound. *Am J Cardiol* 2000; **85**: 641–644.

Section five:
Special groups of patients

CHAPTER 8

Acute coronary syndromes in special groups of patients

Piero O. Bonetti, Michael J. Zellweger, Christoph Kaiser, and Matthias E. Pfisterer

Atherosclerosis is a chronic, inflammatory disease, with acute coronary episodes. These episodes have different clinical expressions that can be modulated by several factors and particularly by their occurrence in special groups of patients. The goal of this chapter is to describe the particularities and the adapted treatment in these particular populations.

Women

Although, at any given age, the prevalence of coronary heart disease (CHD) is lower in women than in men, CHD represents the leading cause of mortality in both men and women in industrialized countries [1]. Importantly, during the last two decades, men, but not women, have experienced a decline in deaths due to cardiovascular disease [2]. Thus, acute coronary syndromes (ACSs) are not an uncommon event in the female population. However, despite the growing awareness that CHD is not only a "man's disease," management of women with ACS is still not optimal leading to missed diagnoses and inadequate treatment, resulting in excess mortality [3].

Similar to men, chest pain represents the most common symptom of ACS in women. However, compared with their male counterparts, women suffering from an ACS present more frequently with atypical symptoms including back and jaw pain, nausea and/or vomiting, dyspnea, indigestion, and palpitations [4]. Moreover, women are more likely to present with unstable angina than with acute myocardial infarction. Finally, it is widely recognized that noncardiac causes of chest pain are more prevalent in women than in men. Thus, recognition of ACS symptoms by both affected women and healthcare providers remains problematic, favoring underdiagnosis and delayed treatment of ACS in women.

It is well documented that, on average, women with ACS are older and have more comorbidities, such as hypertension, diabetes, and a history of congestive heart failure, despite a lower prevalence of previous myocardial infarction and left ventricular dysfunction than affected men, whereas the extent and severity of epicardial coronary stenoses tend to be lower in women than in men [5]. In contrast, given that women are underrepresented in the majority of published trials of ACS relative to their disease prevalence, there is only limited data regarding the optimal management of this large patient population [6]. Based on the current knowledge, women with ACS should be managed in a manner similar to men with regard to both drug therapy [aspirin and/or clopidogrel, β-blocker, unfractionated heparin or low molecular weight heparin (LMWH), platelet glycoprotein (GP) IIb/IIIa receptor antagonist] and invasive assessment/therapy [coronary angiography followed by percutaneous coronary intervention (PCI) or coronary artery bypass graft surgery (CABG) if necessary and feasible] [7,8]. Currently, however, women with ACS are less likely than men to receive recommended standard drug therapy as well as to undergo invasive diagnostic and therapeutic procedures, such as PCI and CABG [5,9]. Based on older studies, it is widely believed that women undergoing PCI or CABG fare worse than men. However, recently published trials suggest that advances in coronary revascularization techniques and adjunctive pharmacotherapy have led to a reduction of the morbidity and mortality associated with coronary revascularization procedures in women resulting in similar outcomes in both sexes. Thus, the female gender should no longer be a factor affecting decisions regarding revascularization [10].

In summary, women represent a considerable part of the ACS population. Affected women are older, have more comorbidities and more atypical presentations than their male counterparts. Based on currently available data, women and men with ACS should be managed similarly. Granted the use of current state-of-the-art diagnostic and therapeutic strategies, including both drug therapy and revascularization procedures, similar outcomes may be expected in women and men with ACS.

Patients with diabetes mellitus

Diabetic patients are substantially more likely to suffer stroke, myocardial infarction, or heart failure than nondiabetic patients, generally with a worse prognosis following any of these conditions. In patients who suffer an ACS, diabetes is an independent predictor of long-term mortality [11]. There is data suggesting that diabetic patients without previous myocardial infarction have a risk of myocardial infarction as high as nondiabetic patients with previous myocardial infarction [12]. Furthermore, diabetic patients often suffer silent myocardial infarction or complain about atypical symptoms [13].

Platelet aggregation is enhanced in diabetic patients, but antiplatelet drugs consistently reduce the incidence of thrombotic events in diabetic patients [14]. Aspirin is even recommended as primary prevention strategy in high-risk diabetics [15]. Also GP IIb/IIIa antagonists have been shown to be very effective in reducing target vessel revascularizations in diabetic patients [16].

Early treatment of myocardial infarction with β-blockers resulted in a 37% mortality reduction in diabetics compared with 13% in their nondiabetic counterparts. Long-term mortality reduction was 48% and 33%, respectively [17]. With respect to β-blocking agents, the fact should be stressed that deterioration in glycemic control or blunted counterregulatory response to hypoglycemia are rarely serious clinical problems, especially if cardio-selective β-blockers are used.

Angiotensin converting enzyme (ACE) inhibition has been shown to substantially reduce mortality in patients surviving myocardial infarction with reduced left ventricular ejection fraction. This is due to the fact that ACE inhibitors reduce infarct size and limit ventricular remodeling. The survival benefit of ACE inhibitors is also evident in diabetic patients [18] and may be particularly beneficial in the case of diabetic nephropathy [19].

Although similar success rates of PCI are observed in diabetic patients initially, diabetic patients have higher restenosis rates and a worse long-term outcome [20]. The use of drug eluting stents (sirolimus and paclitaxel) has dramatically reduced restenosis rates, and this is held true in diabetic subpopulations. However, more data are needed to elucidate this very important issue, especially in diabetic patients with ACS.

Tight glycemic control in patients with ACS plays a pivotal role. The randomized trial of insulin–glucose infusion followed by subcutaneous insulin treatment in diabetic patients with acute myocardial infarction (DIGAMI study) clearly demonstrated that insulin–glucose infusion followed by a multidose insulin regimen improved long-term prognosis in diabetic patients with acute myocardial infarction [21]. The DIGAMI study, however, could not answer the question whether this result was due to the initial insulin–glucose infusion or to the long-term subcutaneous treatment with insulin. This question is currently being investigated in the DIGAMI-2 study [22]. A study evaluating the administration of a glucose–insulin–potassium infusion at the time of primary PCI in diabetic patients with acute myocardial infarction demonstrated a significant mortality reduction in patients without evidence of heart failure. In contrast, patients with congestive heart failure at the time of PCI did not benefit from this intervention [23]. At this point in time, a specific study addressing glycemic control in non-ST-elevation myocardial infarction (NSTEMI) is lacking.

Taken together, these facts underscore the importance of a multidisciplinary management of diabetic patients with ACS to reach strict glycemic targets with an intensive insulin scheme and also demonstrate the remarkable advances in cardiovascular protection thanks to an optimized global pharmacological approach combined with modern revascularization strategies. Although the outcome of diabetic patients with ACS is generally worse than that of nondiabetic patients, diabetic patients seem to benefit equally from pharmacologic and interventional strategies and should receive them.

Elderly patients

Since the prevalence of coronary artery disease is increasing with age, ACSs are a common event in the elderly population. About four-fifth of the annual deaths from coronary artery disease occur in patients over 65 years of age with a significant increase in the female population, which is affected to a similar proportion compared with males [2]. Increased age has been identified as an independent important risk factor for death, recurrent myocardial infarction, heart failure, and stroke after ACS [24]. The increased mortality of ACS in the elderly can, however, only partly be explained by factors, such as important comorbidities, more extensive coronary artery disease, or impaired left ventricular systolic and diastolic function [24–26]. Other mechanisms that have been suggested include less catecholamine responsiveness, poor wound healing of infarcted myocardium, and reduced age-related tolerance of myocardial ischemia.

In contrast to younger patients with ACS, who most commonly present with acute chest pain at rest, elderly patients present often with atypical symptoms, such as dizziness, confusion, dyspnea, syncope, or acute confusion, which is especially common in octogenarians and may lead to undiagnosed cardiac ischemic events and to a substantial delay in the initiation of specific treatment [27].

In general, therapeutic options for ACS in the elderly do not differ from those in younger patients and include aspirin, clopidogrel, unfractionated heparin, LMWH, GP IIb/IIIa antagonists, and an early invasive approach to revascularization. It is important to know that most studies for the evaluation of therapeutic options in ACS were conducted in younger patients and that subanalyses of these trials used different cutoff ages, such as 65, 70, or 75 years for elderly patients. Clopidogrel was not studied in subsets of elderly patients, whereas the relative benefits of LMWH in patients greater than 65 years is particularly impressive [28,29]. The use of GP IIb/IIIa antagonists showed similar relative benefits in elderly patients compared with those in younger patients with, however, greater absolute benefits due to the higher event rate in older patients [30]. Despite a less favorable outcome of elderly patients after coronary revascularization in ACS, subgroup analyses of the TIMI (Thrombolysis in Myocardial Ischemia) IIIb and the FRISC (Fast Revascularization during Instability in Coronary artery disease) II trials in patients over 65 years demonstrated a greater benefit of an early invasive strategy in ACS compared with a conservative approach [31,32]. It is well known, however, that despite their substantially higher risk of adverse events, elderly patients are less likely to receive treatments of proven benefit or to be investigated in view of possible revascularization [33].

In summary, ACS is a very common and, due to atypical symptoms, often misdiagnosed condition in elderly patients. Despite a higher rate of comorbidities and more extensive coronary artery disease, advanced age is an independent risk factor in ACS. Treatment options do not differ substantially from those in younger patients. All of the drugs commonly used in younger patients are useful in elderly patients, provided that age-dependent dose adjustments are recognized and proper precautions related to comorbidities are taken [7]. In view of the underuse in diagnostic and therapeutic options in elderly patients, a more aggressive approach may be appropriate.

Patients with angiographically normal coronary arteries

Acute coronary syndromes may manifest in patients with angiographically normal or near normal coronary arteries. The pathophysiology of this condition remains unclear in many cases but may involve coronary vasospasm, endothelial dysfunction, hypercoagulable states, coronary thrombosis, coronary embolism, an imbalance between oxygen demand and supply, intense sympathetic stimulation, and coronary trauma.

Cocaine misuse
Use of cocaine is a well-described factor that may be associated with ACS in patients without obstructive CHD. The mechanisms involved in cocaine-induced ACS include coronary vasoconstriction, sympathetic activation, and platelet activation. Given the widespread use of cocaine, patients presenting with prolonged symptoms suggestive of myocardial ischemia should be questioned about the use of cocaine because its recognition mandates special management, including nitrates and calcium antagonists, whereas β-blockers should be avoided [34].

Cigarette smoking
There is strong evidence that cigarette smoking is an important predisposing risk factor for ACS in the presence of normal coronary arteries particularly in young patients. Presumed mechanisms are vasoconstriction associated with coronary endothelial dysfunction, platelet activation, and coronary thrombosis superimposed on endothelial erosions, or ruptured nonobstructive atherosclerotic plaques [35].

Variant angina
Variant angina (Prinzmetal's variant angina) represents a form of ACS that typically occurs in younger smokers without other classical coronary risk factors and is characterized by transient ST-segment elevation on the electrocardiogram (ECG) that is caused by focal coronary spasm. Coronary spasm may occur in angiographically normal coronary segments but is more often located at sites with nonobstructive atherosclerotic plaques. Chest pain typically occurs at rest without precipitating cause and shows a circadian pattern with clustering of attacks in the early morning. In most cases, the attacks

resolve spontaneously without progression to myocardial infarction, although cases of prolonged vasospasm with subsequent myocardial infarction and/or life-threatening arrhythmias have been reported. The exact pathogenesis of coronary spasm in variant angina is unclear, but may involve an imbalance between endothelium-derived vasoconstrictors and vasodilators due to endothelial dysfunction as well as a dysfunction of the autonomic nervous system. Therapy includes calcium antagonists and long-acting nitrates as well as elimination of cardiovascular risk factors (especially smoking) [36].

Syndrome X

Syndrome X is a condition defined by typical chest pain associated with electrocardiographic changes suggestive of myocardial ischemia during exercise despite angiographically normal epicardial coronary arteries. Rarely, episodes of prolonged chest pain may occur with moderate exercise or even at rest, suggesting ACS. The prevalence of syndrome X is significantly higher in women than in men. Although stress-induced myocardial perfusion defects can be detected in a proportion of affected patients, syndrome X is not associated with an increased mortality or an increased risk of cardiovascular events. However, episodes of chest pain may severely impair quality of life and lead to repeated unnecessary hospitalizations. Coronary microvascular dysfunction with a reduction in coronary blood flow reserve due to endothelial dysfunction has been implicated in the pathogenesis of syndrome X ("microvascular angina"). On the other hand, increased pain perception and psychiatric morbidity have been suggested to contribute to the symptoms of syndrome X [37]. Given its heterogeneity, treatment of syndrome X is challenging and needs to be tailored to the patient's needs. Therapy may include reassurance by demonstration of angiographically normal coronary arteries, drug therapy with antiischemic drugs (e.g. β-blockers, calcium antagonists, nitrates) and imipramine, as well as psychological intervention [38].

Transient left ventricular apical ballooning (Takotsubo cardiomyopathy)

Recently, an ACS characterized by the acute onset of reversible regional akinesia of the left ventricular apex and midventricle with hyperkinesis of the basal segments of the left ventricle in the absence of obstructive CHD has been described as "transient left ventricular apical ballooning syndrome" or "Takotsubo cardiomyopathy" [39]. The syndrome more often affects postmenopausal women and is typically preceded by an episode of emotional or physical stress. Patients present with chest pain and may show ECG findings similar to that of patients with ST-segment elevation myocardial infarction. Despite the extensive area of left ventricular dysfunction there is no or only minor elevation of cardiac enzymes. Because the cause of this syndrome is unknown there is currently no established therapy. Despite the dramatic initial presentation mimicking acute myocardial infarction, in-hospital mortality of patients with this syndrome is low and left ventricular wall motion abnormalities resolve completely in most patients within days to weeks after the initial presentation. Recurrence of the syndrome seems to be a rare event [40].

Conclusions

Acute coronary syndromes have different clinical expressions that are related not only to their occurrence in special group of patients but also to several underlying pathophysiological mechanisms. Obviously, these factors have to be considered with great attention for the management of these particular patients.

References

1. World Health Organization (WHO). The world health report 2004. Available at: http://www.who.int/whr/en/
2. American Heart Association. Heart disease and stroke statistics – 2005 update. Available at: http://www.americanheart.org
3. Pope JH, Aufderheide TP, Ruthazer R et al. Missed diagnoses of acute cardiac ischemia in the emergency department. *N Engl J Med* 2000; **342**: 1163–1170.
4. Patel H, Rosengren A, Ekman I. Symptoms in acute coronary syndromes: does sex make a difference? *Am Heart J* 2004; **148**: 27–33.
5. Hochman JS, McCabe CH, Stone PH et al. Outcome and profile of women and men presenting with acute coronary syndromes: a report from TIMI IIIB. *J Am Coll Cardiol* 1997; **30**: 141–148.
6. Lee PY, Alexander KP, Hammill BG et al. Representation of elderly persons and women in published randomized trials of acute coronary syndromes. *JAMA* 2001; **286**: 708–713.
7. Braunwald E, Antman EM, Beasley JW et al. ACC/AHA 2002 guideline update for the management of patients with unstable angina and non-ST-segment elevation myocardial infarction: a report of the American College of Cardiology/American Heart Association Task Force on Practice Guidelines (Committee on the Managment of Patients With Unstable Angina). Available at: http://www.acc.org/clinical/guidelines/unstable/unstable.pdf.
8. Bertrand ME, Simoons ML, Fox KAA et al. Management of acute coronary syndromes in patients presenting without persistent ST-segment elevation. *Eur Heart J* 2002; **23**: 1809–1840.
9. Stone PH, Thompson B, Anderson HV et al. Influence of race, sex, and age on management of unstable angina and non-Q-wave myocardial infarction: the TIMI III registry. *JAMA* 1996; **275**: 1104–1112.
10. Jacobs AK. Coronary revascularization in women in 2003. *Circulation* 2003; **107**: 375–377.
11. Lloyd-Jones DM, Camargo CA, Allen LA et al. Predictors of long-term mortality after hospitalization for primary unstable angina pectoris and non-ST-elevation myocardial infarction. *Am J Cardiol* 2003; **92**: 1155–1159.
12. Haffner SM, Lehto S, Ronnemaa T et al. Mortality from coronary heart disease in subjects with type 2 diabetes and in nondiabetic subjects with and without prior myocardial infarction. *N Engl J Med* 1998; **339**: 229–234.

13. Zellweger MJ, Hachamovitch R, Kang X *et al.* Prognostic relevance of symptoms versus objective evidence of coronary artery disease in diabetic patients. *Eur Heart J* 2004; **25**: 543–550.

14. Colwell JA, Nesto RW. The platelet in diabetes: focus on prevention of ischemic events. *Diabetes Care* 2003; **26**: 2181–2188.

15. Colwell JA. Aspirin therapy in diabetes. *Diabetes Care* 2003; **26**(Suppl. 1): S87–S88.

16. Arjomand H, Roukoz B, Surabhi SK *et al.* Platelets and antiplatelet therapy in patients with diabetes mellitus. *J Invasive Cardiol* 2003; **15**: 264–269.

17. Kendall MJ, Lynch KP, Hjalmarson A *et al.* Beta-blockers and sudden cardiac death. *Ann Intern Med* 1995; **123**: 358–367.

18. Zuanetti G, Latini R, Maggioni AP *et al.* Effect of the ACE inhibitor lisinopril on mortality in diabetic patients with acute myocardial infarction: data from the GISSI-3 study. *Circulation* 1997; **96**: 4239–4245.

19. Lewis EJ, Hunsicker LG, Bain RP *et al.* The effect of angiotensin-converting-enzyme inhibition on diabetic nephropathy. The Collaborative Study Group. *N Engl J Med* 1993; **329**: 1456–1462.

20. Kip KE, Faxon DP, Detre KM *et al.* Coronary angioplasty in diabetic patients. The National Heart, Lung, and Blood Institute Percutaneous Transluminal Coronary Angioplasty Registry. *Circulation* 1996; **94**: 1818–1825.

21. Malmberg K, Ryden L, Efendic S *et al.* Randomized trial of insulin–glucose infusion followed by subcutaneous insulin treatment in diabetic patients with acute myocardial infarction (DIGAMI study): effects on mortality at 1 year. *J Am Coll Cardiol* 1995; **26**: 57–65.

22. Malmberg K. Role of insulin–glucose infusion in outcomes after acute myocardial infarction: the diabetes and insulin-glucose infusion in acute myocardial infarction (DIGAMI) study. *Endocr Pract* 2004; **10**(Suppl. 2): 13–16.

23. van der Horst IC, Zijlstra F, van't Hof AW *et al.* Glucose–insulin–potassium infusion inpatients treated with primary angioplasty for acute myocardial infarction: the glucose-insulin-potassium study: a randomized trial. *J Am Coll Cardiol* 2003; **42**: 784–791.

24. Hasdai D, Holmes DR Jr, Criger DA *et al.* Age and outcome after acute coronary syndromes without persistent ST-segment elevation. *Am Heart J* 2000; **139**: 858–866.

25. Normad ST, Glickman ME, Sharma RG *et al.* Using admission characteristics to predict short-term mortality form myocardial infarction in elderly patients. Results from the Cooperative Cardiovascular Project. *JAMA* 1996; **275**: 1322–1328.

26. Pfisterer M. Long-term outcome in elderly patients with chronic angina managed invasively versus by optimized medical therapy: four-year follow-up of the randomized Trial of Invasive versus Medical therapy in Elderly patients (TIME). *Circulation* 2004; **110**: 1213–1218.

27. Bayer AJ, Chadha JS, Farag RR *et al.* Changing presentation of myocardial infarction with increasing old age. *J Am Geriatr Soc* 1986; **34**: 263–266.

28. Antman EM, McCabe CH, Gurfinkel EP *et al.* Enoxaparin prevents death and cardiac ischemic events in unstable angina/non-Q-wave myocardial infarction: results of the Thrombolysis In Myocardial Infarction (TIMI) 11B trial. *Circulation* 1999; **100**: 1593–1601.

29. Cohen M, Demers C, Gurfinkel EP *et al.* for the Efficacy and Safety of Subcutaneous Enoxaparin in Non-Q-Wave Coronary Events Study Group. A comparison of

low-molecular-weight heparin with unfractionated heparin for unstable coronary artery disease. *N Engl J Med* 1997; **337**: 447–452.

30. Mak KH, Effron MB, Moliterno DJ. Platelet glycoprotein IIb/IIIa receptor antagonists and their use in elderly patients. *Drugs Ageing*. 2000; **16**: 179–187.

31. Effects of tissue plasminogen activator and a comparison of early invasive and conservative strategies in unstable angina and non-Q-wave myocardial infarction: results of the TIMI IIIB trial. Thrombolysis In Myocardial Ischemia. *Circulation* 1994; **89**: 1545–1556.

32. FRagmin and Fast Revascularisation during InStability in Coronary artery disease Investigators. Invasive compared with non-invasive treatment in unstable coronary-artery disease: FRISC II prospective randomised multicentre study. *Lancet* 1999; **354**: 708–715.

33. Collinson J, Bakhai A, Flather MD *et al.* The management and investigation of elderly patients with acute coronary syndromes without ST elevation: an evidence-based approach? Results of the Prospective Registry of Acute Ischemic Syndromes in the United Kingdom (PRAIS-UK). *Age Ageing* 2005: **34**: 61–66.

34. Pitts WR, Lange RA, Cigarroa JE *et al.* Cocaine-induced myocardial ischemia and infarction: pathophysiology, recognition, and management. *Prog Cardiovasc Dis* 1997; **40**: 65–76.

35. Williams MJA, Restieaux NJ, Low CJS. Myocardial infarction in young people with normal coronary arteries. *Heart* 1998; **79**: 191–194.

36. Cannon PC, Braunwald E. Unstable angina and non-ST elevation myocardial infarction: Prinzmetal (variant) angina. In: Zipes DP, Libby P, Bonow RO, & Braunwald E, eds. *Braunwald's Heart Disease*, 7th edn. Elsevier Saunders, Philadelphia, PA, 2005: 1264–1267.

37. Kaski JC. Pathophysiology and management of patients with chest pain and normal coronary arteriograms (cardiac syndrome X). *Circulation* 2004; **109**: 568–572.

38. Kaski JC, Valenzuela Garcia LF. Therapeutic options for the management of patients with cardiac syndrome X. *Eur Heart J* 2001; **22**: 283–293.

39. Tsuchihashi K, Ueshima K, Uchida T *et al.* Transient left ventricular apical ballooning without coronary artery stenosis: a novel heart syndrome mimicking acute myocardial infarction. *J Am Coll Cardiol* 2001; **38**: 11–18.

40. Bybee KA, Kara T, Prasad A *et al.* Systematic review: transient left ventricular apical ballooning: a syndrome that mimics ST-segment elevation myocardial infarction. *Ann Intern Med* 2004; **141**: 858–865.

Section six:
Pharmacological treatment

CHAPTER 9

Antiischemic treatment (nitrates, β-blockers, calcium antagonists)

David McCarty, Colum G. Owens, and A.A. Jennifer Adgey

Introduction

Antiischemic therapy, including nitrates, β-blockers, and calcium channel antagonists, is commonly prescribed for patients with acute coronary syndromes (ACSs) [1,2]. In recent years, these syndromes have been redefined, with patients classified by the electrocardiogram at presentation into ST-segment elevation ACS (STE-ACS) and non-ST-segment elevation ACS (NSTE-ACS) groups [3]. The underlying pathophysiology of the syndromes has been increasingly elucidated, and treatment refined by critical analysis of evidence-based medicine [3]. Prescription of the various antiischemic therapies, particularly for patients with NSTE-ACS, has for many agents not been evaluated in contemporary clinical settings. Often the basis for their continuing use lies in extrapolation of data from previous trials in acute myocardial infarction (AMI), now reclassified as STE-ACS, together with consensus opinion [3]. This chapter will examine the pharmacology of these therapeutic agents, and consider the rationale and evidence for their use in the management of ACS patients.

Nitrates

Mode of action

The pharmacological actions of nitroglycerin and related compounds are principally mediated through nitric oxide donation. Stimulation of guanylate cyclase and increased cyclic guanosine monophosphate (GMP) levels in endothelial and vascular smooth muscle cells reduce vasomotor tone. Preload reduction, through decreased venous return and lowered left ventricular filling parameters, together with afterload reduction, from generalized vasodilatation and reduced systemic vascular resistance, serve to enhance cardiac function, and decrease myocardial oxygen demand [3–5]. Nitrates additionally relieve vascular spasm, and increase coronary collateral flow [3,5]. In AMI patients as well as in animal models, nitrates have been shown to limit infarct size, improve left ventricular function, and reduce remodeling [4,5]. In addition to their antiischemic effects, nitrates may also act to promote myocardial perfusion through antiplatelet properties [3].

Adverse effects
Adverse effects of nitrates include hypotension with consequent reflex tachycardia, increasing myocardial oxygen demand [5]. Dilation of nondiseased coronary segments may lead to coronary steal with redistribution of blood away from ischemic myocardium [5]. The development of tolerance to the vascular effects of nitrates is well recognized, due to the depletion of required sulphydryl groups [3,4].

Administration
Pharmacokinetic studies have not confirmed superiority of intravenous nitrate preparations over other routes of administration for ACS patients [3]. Angina at presentation is usually treated with sublingual or buccal preparations, with up to one-third of patients receiving intravenous therapy for ongoing ischemic pain in hospital [2].

Nitrates in NSTE-ACS
Evidence
No large-scale randomized data exist for nitrate use in NSTE-ACS patients [3]. Current guidelines extrapolate findings from earlier studies in AMI patients [3]. Only occasionally did these studies subdivide patients into ST-segment elevation MI or non ST-elevation MI. In ISIS-4, subgroup analysis of 10 388 patients with NSTE-ACS demonstrated no mortality reduction with nitrate therapy compared with placebo (5.3% versus 5.5%, $p = $ NS) [4].

Recommendations
The European Society of Cardiology (ESC) recommends nitrate use in patients with ACS to reduce ischemia (Class I recommendation, level of evidence: C) [3]. Consideration for initial intravenous therapy is recommended if no contraindications exist, with up titration of the dose until symptom relief or side effects occur. Transfer to a nonparenteral alternative is recommended when symptoms are controlled.

Calcium channel antagonists

Mode of action
The antiischemic properties of calcium antagonists are mediated by a reduction in afterload, myocardial contractility, and heart rate [3,6]. Inhibition of calcium entry to vascular smooth muscle cells in the peripheral circulation reduces vasomotor tone, producing vasodilatation and lowering systemic blood pressure. The agents decrease coronary spasm and increase collateral supply to ischemic myocardial territories. Direct action on myocardial cells

reduces intracellular calcium entry and contractility. This may result in adverse negative inotropy, but helps to protect the cell from calcium overload during ischemia/reperfusion [6]. Some calcium antagonists inhibit entry of calcium to cardiac conduction cells, prolonging repolarization and reducing heart rate [3]. Animal models of MI have suggested that administration of calcium antagonists reduces infarct size and preserves ventricular function [6].

Adverse effects

Adverse effects include reflex tachycardia with the dihydropyridine group, secondary to peripheral vasodilatation, which raises myocardial oxygen demand [6]. Headache, flushing, and hypotension may also occur. Atrioventricular (AV) block and cardiac failure may be exacerbated by these agents, which are contraindicated in such patients.

Calcium channel antagonists in NSTE-ACS
Evidence

The use of calcium antagonists in unstable angina has been examined in several small randomized controlled trials. A metaanalysis of these trials has shown no benefit in terms of mortality or progression to AMI [6]. However, they have shown equivalent efficacy to β-blockers in reducing symptoms and may prevent reinfarction in patients with NSTEMI [7,8].

Recommendations for use

The ESC recommends calcium antagonist use in patients with NSTE-ACS to reduce ischemia and for the prevention of death or infarction (Class II recommendation; level of evidence: B) [3]. Dihydropyridine administration without concurrent β blockade is not advised [3]. In particular, prescription is recommended for patients intolerant of β-blockade or those with variant angina. The agents may be harmful in the presence of left ventricular impairment or AV conduction disease.

β-blockers

β-adrenergic antagonist therapy (β-blockers) play a major role in the treatment of patients with cardiovascular disease as they have antiischemic, antiarrhythmic, and antihypertensive properties [3,9–12], as well as their established role in patients with left ventricular dysfunction post-AMI [13].

Mode of action

β-blockers bind selectively to the β-adrenoceptors producing a competitive and reversible antagonism of the effects of β-adrenergic stimuli on various organs [9]. They can be classified according to their cardioselectivity (i.e. the degree of effect on β_1-adrenoceptors in the heart compared with that on the β_2-adrenoceptors in the other tissues), degree of α_1-adrenoceptor blockade, and intrinsic sympathomimetic activity (exerting a weak β-agonist

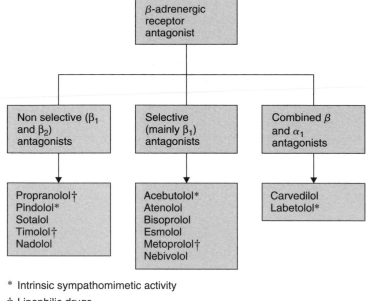

* Intrinsic sympathomimetic activity

† Lipophilic drugs

Figure 9.1 Classification of β-blockers.

response) (see Figure 9.1). Additionally, they can be classified as either lipophilic or hydrophilic.

Lipophilic drugs

Lipophilic drugs (metoprolol, propranolol) are rapidly absorbed from the gastrointestinal tract, but have an extensive first pass effect and so have a low oral bioavailability. They have short half-lives (1–5 h) and readily cross the blood–brain barrier, accounting for their greater incidence of central side effects. These drugs may accumulate in patients with reduced hepatic blood flow (elderly, congestive heart failure, liver disease) [9].

Hydrophilic drugs

These drugs (atenolol, esmolol) are absorbed incompletely from the gastrointestinal tract and are renally excreted. They have longer half-lives (6–24 h) and do not readily cross the blood–brain barrier. Elimination is decreased in patients with reduced glomerular filtration rates [9].

Balanced clearance drugs

Bisoprolol has a low first-pass metabolism, is excreted equally by hepatic and renal routes and crosses the blood–brain barrier. Carvedilol has an extensive first-pass effect (thus low oral bioavailability), binds to plasma proteins, and is eliminated by hepatic metabolism. Esmolol is an i.v. preparation with an ultrashort half-life (9 min) and is hydrolyzed by red cell esterases [9].

Mode of action
The mechanisms of action of β-blockers are diverse and incompletely understood, but may be considered as follows:

Antihypertensive action. β-blockers decrease cardiac output, and cause inhibition of release of renin and production of angiotensin II [9].

Antiischemic action. β-blockers reduce heart rate, cardiac contractility, and systolic blood pressure thus reducing myocardial oxygen demand. Prolongation of diastole by reduction in heart rate may increase myocardial perfusion by increasing coronary diastolic perfusion time [3,9–11].

Improvement of left ventricular structure and function. β-blockers may improve cardiac function because of reduced heart rate, improved coronary diastolic filling, upregulation of β-adrenergic receptors, and reduction of myocardial oxidative stress. In the presence of chronic ischemia, they improve ejection fraction particularly during exercise and improve left ventricular function [9,10].

Antiarrhythmic effect. β-blockers exert their antiarrhythmic effect by reducing heart rate, decreasing spontaneous firing of ectopic pacemakers, increasing refractory period of the AV node, and reducing sympathetic overstimulation of the ventricular myocardium [9,12].

Adverse effects
Cardiovascular
Bradycardia and AV block are principally seen in patients with sinus node dysfunction or AV nodal disease and should be avoided in these patients. Other peripheral effects (cold extremities, worsening of claudication) occur due to peripheral blockade of β_2-receptors and unopposed stimulation of vascular α-adrenoceptors [9].

Pulmonary
β-blockers can cause a life-threatening increase in airway resistance in patients with asthma and bronchospastic chronic obstructive pulmonary disease (COPD) and should be used with extreme caution in these groups of patients [9].

Central effects
These are more common with lipophilic drugs and include fatigue, headache, vivid dreams, and depression [9].

β-blockers in NSTE-ACS
Evidence
Few randomized studies exist for the use of β-blockers in NSTE-ACS patients. A metaanalysis suggested a 13% relative risk reduction in risk of progression to

AMI in patients with unstable angina treated with β-blockers [9]. Retrospective data from the Cooperative Cardiovascular Project demonstrated a 40% mortality reduction in patients with non-Q-wave AMI [14].

Recommendations

The ESC recommends that patients with NSTE-ACS should be treated with β-blockers as soon as possible to control ischemia and prevent AMI/reinfarction (Class I recommendation, level of evidence: B) [3,9]. After the acute phase, all patients should receive β-blockers during long-term secondary prevention (Class I recommendation, level of evidence: A) [9].

References

1. Fox KAA, Cokkinos DV, Deckers J *et al*. The ENACT study: a pan-European survey of acute coronary syndromes. European Network for Acute Coronary Treatment. *Eur Heart J* 2000; **21**: 1440–1449.
2. Collinson J, Flather MD, Fox KAA *et al*. Clinical outcomes, risk stratification and practice patterns of unstable angina and myocardial infarction without ST elevation: Prospective Registry of Acute Ischaemic Syndromes in the U.K. (PRAIS-UK). *Eur Heart J* 2000; **21**: 1450–1457.
3. Bertrand ME, Simoons ML, Fox KAA *et al*. Management of acute coronary syndromes in patients presenting without persistent ST-segment elevation. *Eur Heart J* 2002; **23**: 1809–1840.
4. ISIS-4 Collaborative Group. ISIS-4: a randomised factorial trial assessing early oral captopril, oral mononitrate, and intravenous magnesium sulphate in 58 050 patients with suspected acute myocardial infarction. *Lancet* 1995; **345**: 669–685.
5. Yusuf S, Collins R, MacMahon S *et al*. Effect of intravenous nitrates on mortality in acute myocardial infarction: an overview of the randomised trials. *Lancet* 1988; i: 1088–1092.
6. Held PH, Yusuf S, Furberg CD. Calcium channel blockers in acute myocardial infarction and unstable angina: an overview. *Br Med J* 1989; **299**: 1187–1192.
7. Theroux P, Taeymans Y, Morissette D *et al*. A randomized study comparing propranolol and diltiazem in the treatment of unstable angina. *J Am Coll Cardiol* 1985; **5**: 717–722.
8. Gibson RS, Boden WE, Theroux P *et al*. Diltiazem and reinfarction in patients with non-Q-wave myocardial infarction. Results of a double-blind, randomized, multicenter trial. *N Engl J Med* 1986; **315**: 423–429.
9. The Task Force on Beta-blockers of the European Society of Cardiology. Expert Consensus document on β-adrenergic receptor blockers. *Eur Heart J* 2004; **25**: 1341–1362.
10. Lip GYH, Lydakis C, Beevers DG. Management of patients with myocardial infarction and hypertension. *Eur Heart J* 2000; **21**: 1125–1134.
11. Gluckman TJ, Sachdev M, Schulman SP *et al*. A simplified approach to the management of non-ST-segment elevation acute coronary syndromes. *JAMA* 2005; **293**: 349–357.

12. Hjalmarson A. Effects of beta blockade on sudden cardiac death during acute myocardial infarction and the post-infarction period. *Am J Cardiol* 1997; **80**: 35J–39J.
13. The CAPRICORN Investigators. Effect of carvedilol on outcome after myocardial infarction in patients with left-ventricular dysfunction: the CAPRICORN randomised trial. *Lancet* 2001; **357**: 1385–1390.
14. Gottlieb SS, McCarter RJ, Vogel RA. Effect of betablockade on mortality among high-risk and low-risk patients after myocardial infarction. *N Engl J Med* 1998; **339**: 489–497.

CHAPTER 10

Antiplatelet therapies: aspirin, thienopyridines, and glycoprotein IIb/IIIa receptor inhibitors

Jaydeep Sarma and Keith A.A. Fox

Cellular events in acute atherothrombosis

Acute atherothrombosis, thrombus formation on ruptured vulnerable atherosclerotic plaques, is at the pathological root of acute coronary syndromes (ACSs) [1]. Although culprit lesions may not be hemodynamically flow limiting, degradation of plaque shoulder regions exposes prothrombotic matrix materials triggering local clotting cascades [2]. In the coronary tree, the resultant thrombus load may cause transient or permanent vessel occlusion, clinically manifesting as myocardial ischemia or infarction.

Plaque pathophysiology

Atherosclerosis is a chronic inflammatory disease, and atherosclerotic plaque rupture bears hallmarks of a dynamic inflammatory cellular process [3]. Leukocyte-mediated inflammation induces endothelial damage and disrupts plaque structure, leading to plaque rupture [4]. Vascular wall damage may be exacerbated by acute insults including altered shear stress [5] and enhanced systemic inflammatory responses [6].

In advanced or complex atheromatous lesions (Stary type IV and V) [7], the plaque lipid core contains apoptotic macrophage, smooth muscle cell and mesenchymal cell debris, and free cholesterol crystals [8]. Plaque rupture exposes the tissue-factor-rich lipid core to circulating blood initiating the coagulation cascade and thrombin generation [9]. Tissue factor levels from activated plaque macrophages are increased further by extrinsic stimuli including cigarette smoking. Plaque vulnerability is related to lipid core size, fibrous cap thickness, activity and density of macrophages [10,11] and local matrix metalloproteinases [12]. Resultant local thrombus deposition reduces flow with resultant tissue ischemia, potential vessel closure, and myocyte death. Alternatively, local thrombus may resolve and the artery remodeled, restoring luminal patency [13].

Thrombus pathophysiology

Plaque rupture exposes subendothelial collagen promoting platelet activation, adhesion, granule release, and aggregation [14]. The platelet surface glycoprotein (GP) IIb/IIIa changes to an active conformation, binding to activated platelets via fibrinogen bridges, and also binds platelets to subendothelial von Willebrand factor [15]. Tissue factor interacts with factor VII to activate factor X, causing conversion of prothrombin to thrombin in the prothrombinase complex [16]. Thrombin, a serine protease, cleaves fibrinopeptides from fibrinogen allowing fibrin monomer polymerization, and converts factor XIII to XIIIa, which crosslinks the fibrin clot. Fibrin molecules trap platelets, erythrocytes, and leukocytes, forming thrombus, slowing blood flow, and exacerbating further platelet and erythrocyte deposition. Thrombin binds the extracellular domain of platelet-surface protease-activated receptors (PARs) initiating a signaling cascade that promotes platelet activation. Platelets change shape, expose integrins, and release α-granule contents including ADP, thromboxane A2, and platelet factor 4, leading to further platelet activation and aggregation, and leukocyte recruitment. Increased vascular permeability enhances inflammatory leukocyte entry to vascular injury sites. Exposure of negatively charged phosphatidylserine at the platelet cell membrane provides a focus for thrombus formation [17]. ADP acts as a cofactor for many platelet agonists, including thromboxane A_2 (TxA_2), collagen, and thrombin. Platelet activation is triggered by ADP binding to G-protein coupled receptors, first the $P2Y_1$ receptor and then the $P2Y_{12}$ receptor [18], with the latter receptor being the target for current thienopyridine drugs.

Pharmacology of individual agents

Aspirin

Aspirin is a key agent in acute and chronic atherosclerosis management. Selective blockade of TxA_2 enables the use of low-dose aspirin in long-term therapy, but the need to rapidly reach effective levels of platelet inhibition in acute phases of treatment still requires the use of higher doses.

Biochemical mechanism of action of aspirin

Aspirin irreversibly inhibits cyclooxygenase-1 (COX-1) activity [19] by acetylation of a serine domain. This blocks platelet production of thromboxane TxA_2, a potent inducer of platelet aggregation and vasoconstriction [20]. Production of PGI_2 (an inhibitor of platelet aggregation and a vasodilator) is blocked only at higher aspirin doses [21]. Aspirin in common with nonsteroidal antiinflammatory agents is capable of inhibiting COX-2, suggesting a direct antiinflammatory effect. Subgroup analysis of the Physicians' Health Study [22] found that the reduction in the risk of a first myocardial infarction (MI) with the use of 325 mg of aspirin on alternate days appeared related to CRP levels, suggesting antiinflammatory as well as antiplatelet effects [23].

However, the doses required for this are significantly higher than those for antithrombotic and antiplatelet activity.

Aspirin: pharmacokinetics and dynamics

Aspirin is rapidly absorbed in the stomach and upper intestine achieving peak plasma levels of 30–40 min after ingestion, and platelet inhibition within 1 h. Enteric-coated aspirin delays absorption and should be avoided in acute treatment: if only enteric-coated tablets are available, tablets should be chewed. Plasma aspirin has a half-life of 15–20 min, but platelet inhibition lasts for the lifespan of the platelet (~10 days), because irreversible COX-1 inactivation [24] affects both platelets and megakaryocytes [25].

Aspirin dosing

Aspirin is an effective antithrombotic in doses possibly as low as 30 mg/day. Aspirin at 75 mg/day is effective in reducing the risk of acute myocardial infraction (AMI) or death in patients with unstable angina [26] and chronic stable angina [27]. Higher dose aspirin can enhance fibrinolysis [28] and suppression of thrombin formation at doses of 3–500 mg/day [29]. Even higher doses of 1500 mg/day cause antivitamin K anticoagulant effects [30]. However, there is no evidence that low doses (i.e. 50–100 mg/day) are less clinically effective than high doses (i.e. 650–1500 mg/day) for atherothrombotic protection, and data from the Antiplatelet Trialists' Collaboration overview support this conclusion [31]. There is also evidence that low-dose aspirin produces fewer gastrointestinal (GI) side effects than 300 mg/day [32]. In summary, biochemical studies and the dose dependence of side effects support the use of lower-dose aspirin [33].

Aspirin nonresponders, "resistance"

Aspirin resistance describes the inability of aspirin (1) to protect individuals from thrombotic complications; (2) to cause prolongation of the bleeding time; or (3) to produce an effect on *in vitro* tests of platelet function. Nonresponse to aspirin, or to other antiplatelet agents, may be due to a variety of factors aside from true resistance (ranging from the impact of an overwhelming thrombotic stimulus to poor patient compliance). Variable platelet responses to aspirin also have been described in up to 25% of patients with ischemic heart disease [34], peripheral arterial disease [35], and cerebrovascular disease, with *COX-1* gene mutations being raised as a possible explanation [36]. Aspirin nonresponders have been identified in 40% of patients undergoing elective coronary artery bypass grafting (CABG) who showed no prolongation of bleeding time [37]. In contrast, repeated measurements of platelet aggregation in the Research Group on Instability in Coronary Artery Disease in southeast Sweden (RISC) study [38] had consistently reduced platelet aggregation. *In vitro* data suggests plaque macrophages or endothelial cells may generate TXA$_2$ via a COX-2 pathway, thus limiting aspirin efficacy in atherosclerosis, but the clinical relevance of this is as yet unclear [39]. Variable results from studies using different techniques to assess aspirin efficacy highlight methodological difficulties surrounding the measurement of aspirin resistance, and should be interpreted with caution. Until aspirin resistance is better defined, no single test of platelet function is currently recommended to assess the antiplatelet effect of aspirin in the individual patients.

Thienopyridines
Biochemical mechanism of action of thienopyridines
Thienopyridines irreversibly inhibit ADP binding to the platelet surface purinergic receptor, P2Y12 [40]. Previous agents, such as ticlopidine, induced adverse effects including thrombocytopenia and bone marrow failure necessitating frequent routine hematological monitoring [41]. Clopidogrel, with a better safety profile, is the current thienopyridine of choice [42]. Structural analysis suggests that irreversible modification of the ADP-receptor site is caused by disulfide bridge formation between reactive thiol groups and a cysteine residue of the platelet ADP receptor [43], explaining the irreversible activity that clopidogrel has upon platelet function, a clinical consideration in the context of hemorrhagic risk.

Clopidogrel: pharmacokinetics and dynamics
Clopidogrel, like ticlopidine, is inactive *in vitro*. Absorbed in the upper GI tract, clopidogrel is converted to an active metabolite by the hepatic cytochrome P450 system [43]. Clopidogrel requires a loading dose to attain effective plasma levels of the active metabolite in an acute setting. Clopidogrel causes a maximum of 60% inhibition of ADP-induced aggregation after 3–5 days if administered without a loading dose. Bleeding time is significantly prolonged with both agents reaching a maximum of 1.5- to 2-fold over baseline at 3–7 days [44,45]. Recovery of platelet function requires 3–5 days, due to the need to synthesize new platelets [46,47].

Clopidogrel dosing
Clopidogrel inhibits platelet aggregation in a dose-dependent fashion. A single dose of 400 mg induces 40% inhibition of platelet aggregation detectable after 2 h [48]. Regular daily dosing of 50–100 mg clopidogrel inhibits platelet aggregation from the second day of treatment (25–30% inhibition) reaching 50–60% inhibition after 4–7 days. As would be expected from these pharmacokinetic and pharmacodynamic features, a loading dose of clopidogrel results in a much more rapid onset of platelet inhibition than that achieved by regular low doses [49], and recommended loading doses in ACS management are 300 mg followed by 75 mg once daily [50]. However, larger loading doses (450–600 mg) used in the context of percutaneous coronary intervention (PCI) have been proved effective and safe in recent studies [51]. Like aspirin, clopidogrel induces a permanent defect in a platelet protein only recoverable by new platelet synthesis, allowing a repeated once-daily regimen with low doses despite a short chemical half-life.

Newer ADP receptor antagonists

Newer agents have been assessed for ADP receptor blockade. Data presented at the ACC Annual Scientific Session 2005 showed that the oral agent prasugrel (CS-747, LY640315, Lilly) induces safe and effective *in vivo* platelet inhibition beyond that offered by clopidogrel. Further definitive large-scale clinical data are awaited from the ongoing TRITON TIMI-38 study that aims to recruit 13 000 patients with ACS undergoing interventional treatment, directly comparing prasugrel to clopidogrel. Of further interest has been the intravenous agent cangrelor (AR-C69931MX, AstraZeneca), a potent selective and reversible P2Y12 receptor antagonist that has been demonstrated to be effective in animal models of PCI [52], and in phase II clinical studies in patients with ACSs [53].

GP IIb/IIIa blockade
Biochemical mechanism of action of GP IIb/IIIa antagonists

Blockade of platelet surface GP IIb/IIIa molecules limits platelet aggregation and also may limit the interactions between platelets, endothelium, and leukocytes. Two principal groups of drugs are in use currently: monoclonal antibodies and small peptide inhibitors. The humanized murine monoclonal antibody 7E3, abciximab (Lilly), recognizes the active conformational state of GP IIb/IIIa, limiting platelet–platelet binding [54]. Abciximab may decrease thrombin formation because of reduced thrombus formation, and can inhibit tissue-factor-induced thrombin generation [55]. Abciximab binds to the $\alpha v \beta_3$ integrin [56], and modulates the expression of Mac-1 by limiting platelet–leukocyte binding [57] and appears to bind directly to leukocyte surface Mac-1 (CD11b/CD18) [58] thereby contributing to an antiinflammatory and potentially antirestenotic effect, although clinical studies have not supported the latter hypothesis [59].

Small synthetic molecules, such as tirofiban and eptifibatide, are designed to competitively bind at Arg-Gly-Asp (RGD) amino acid sites [60], causing transient GP IIb/IIIa blockade. Tirofiban (MK-383, Aggrastat; Merck, USA) is a nonpeptide tyrosine derivative that selectively inhibits the GP IIb/IIIa receptor, with minimal effects on the $\alpha v \beta_3$ vitronectin receptor [61,62]. Eptifibatide (Integrilin) is a synthetic disulfide-linked cyclic heptapeptide modeled on the Lys-Gly-Asp sequence seen in the snake venom disintegrin from *Sistrurus m barbouri* (barbourin). It also has a high specificity for the GP IIb/IIIa receptor but binds the $\alpha v \beta_3$ vitronectin receptor much less avidly [63]. The use of both monoclonal antibody and small peptide molecule GP IIb/IIIa blockade reduces platelet–leukocyte binding, platelet activation, and soluble CD40L in patients with ACS undergoing PCI [64].

GP IIb/IIIa pharmacokinetics and dynamics: abciximab

Abciximab binds with high affinity to the GP IIb/IIIa ligand binding site. Following a loading IV bolus, plasma concentrations decrease rapidly with an initial half-life of 30 min, due to rapid binding to platelet GP IIb/IIIa.

Of the injected bolus 65% attaches to circulating and splenic platelets [65]. Peak effects on receptor blockade, platelet aggregation, and bleeding time are observed 2 h after bolus administration of 0.25 mg/kg. Bleeding times return to near-normal values by 12 h [65] and full platelet function including aggregation recovers over the course of 48 h, although platelet-bound abciximab remains in circulation for 15 days [66]. Maintenance of platelet blockade may be achieved by administering a 0.125 g/kg/min (maximum 10 g/min) infusion following bolus administration [65]. Once the infusion has finished, unbound plasma levels fall rapidly over 6 h. This regimen was chosen for the Evaluation of 7E3 for the Prevention of Ischemic Complications (EPIC) trial [67], which showed that the addition of abciximab to conventional antithrombotic therapy reduced the incidence of ischemic events in patients undergoing PTCA. The increased major hemorrhage with abciximab treatment noted in EPIC has been subsequently reduced by limiting heparin doses and ensuring rapid sheath removal [59]. Thrombocytopenia represents the other important side effect of abciximab treatment. Of the patients treated with abciximab, 1–2% develop platelet counts less than 50 000/μL, with 0.5–1% of these reflecting rapid decreases within 2 h of administration. Platelet counts should be obtained 2–4 h after initiating therapy, permitting the rapid identification of this latter group. Thrombocytopenia can be treated effectively by immediate cessation of abciximab therapy, with recovery occurring over several days [68]. In the EPIC trial, 6% of abciximab-treated patients developed antibodies to the agent raising potential risks of reinjecting abciximab [69] including anaphylaxis, neutralization of abciximab, and thrombocytopenia.

GP IIb/IIIa pharmacokinetics and dynamics; adverse reactions: tirofiban

Both IV bolus and IV infusions of tirofiban produce rapid inhibition of platelet aggregation in a dose responsive manner. Early data showed that tirofiban infused at 0.15 μg/kg/min over 4 h inhibited 97% of ADP-induced platelet aggregation, prolonging the bleeding time by 2.5-fold [70], with a plasma half-life of 1.6 h [71]. Bleeding times normalize 4 h after stopping tirofiban, with 80% recovery of platelet aggregatory function. Further increases in bleeding time of 4.1 ± 1.5-fold occur if aspirin is coadministered despite constant tirofiban plasma levels, suggesting synergistic antiplatelet effects [70]. In patients receiving aspirin and heparin during PCI a 10 μg/kg bolus dose of tirofiban inhibits 93% of platelet aggregation within 5 min. A tirofiban infusion of 0.10 μg/kg/min increases bleeding times to over 30 min within 2 h [73], with 87% inhibition of platelet aggregation following a 16–24 h infusion.

Severe but reversible thrombocytopenia has been reported in a small percentage of patients treated with tirofiban, for which an immunologic mechanism has been proposed [73], mediated by preformed antibodies to a conformation of the GP IIb/IIIa receptor induced by the binding of tirofiban to the receptor [74]. No data are available on the safety of reinfusing tirofiban.

GP IIb/IIIa pharmacokinetics and dynamics; adverse reactions

Early clinical studies, on patients pretreated with aspirin and heparin undergoing elective PCI, showed 85% inhibition of platelet aggregation 1 h after a 90 μg/kg IV bolus of eptifibatide. Similar levels of platelet inhibition were seen 4 h after a 1 μg/kg/min IV infusion [75], but significant variation in responses occurred between subjects. Median bleeding times were prolonged to over 26 min with eptifibatide infusion, but returned towards normal, 1 h after stopping the drug. A later study [76] in 54 patients undergoing coronary interventions who were pretreated with aspirin and heparin showed that a 180 μg/kg IV bolus inhibited ADP-induced platelet aggregation by greater than 95% within 15 min, and this effect was sustained by a 1 μg/kg/min infusion given for 18–24 h. However, over 50% of baseline aggregatory function was recovered 4 h after stopping treatment. Patients receiving heparin plus eptifibatide had longer activated clotting times than patients on heparin alone [76], suggesting that eptifibatide, like abciximab [55], can inhibit thrombin generation *in vitro*. In keeping with this, a modest increase in hemorrhagic complications was reported in patients treated with eptifibatide in the Platelet IIb/IIIa in Unstable Angina: Receptor Suppression Using Integrilin Therapy (PURSUIT) trial [77].

Eptifibatide treatment has not been associated with an increased frequency of cases of overall thrombocytopenia, but it may be associated with a small increase in cases of profound thrombocytopenia [77]. All patients receiving parenteral GP IIb/IIIa blockers should be monitored within 24 h of the initiation of therapy for development of thrombocytopenia.

GP IIb/IIIa dosing

Abciximab

A bolus dose of 0.25 mg/kg abciximab blocks over 80% of platelet receptors and reduces ADP-induced platelet aggregation to less than 20% of baseline [65], which is maintained by a 0.125 μg/kg/min (maximum 10 μg/min) continuous intravenous infusion. For unstable ACS patients, treatment should be started up to 24 h prior to the possible intervention. For the prevention of ischemic complications in patients undergoing PCI, and who are not currently receiving abciximab, the bolus should be administered 10–60 min prior to PCI followed by a 12-h infusion.

Heparin cotherapy with abciximab produces an added risk of bleeding, and must be carefully administered to maintain an activated clotting time (ACT) of 200 s. Modified heparin doses should be used in conjunction with abciximab if administered pre-PCI. Initial heparin bolus doses should not exceed 7000 U, with 70 U/kg of heparin to correct an ACT less than 150 s, and 50 U/kg heparin to correct an ACT of 150–199 s. The ACT should be checked no earlier than 2 min after the initial bolus and every 30 min during the procedure. If the ACT remains less than 200 s, additional heparin boluses of 20 U/kg may be administered until an ACT greater than or equal to 200 s is achieved.

Eptifibatide
For medical treatment of ACS, an intravenous bolus of 180 mcg/kg should be administered, followed by a continuous infusion of 2.0 mcg/kg/min for up to 72 h, until revascularization is considered, or clinical stabilization has occurred.

Stable patients undergoing PCI, who are not already receiving the drug, should receive an intravenous bolus of 180 mcg/kg immediately prior to the procedure, followed by a second bolus of 180 mcg/kg 10 min after the first bolus injection. A continuous infusion should be started simultaneously with the first bolus, at a dose of 2.0 mcg/kg/min. Eptifibatide infusion for 16 h appears adequate to reduce ischemic complications after nonurgent PCI [79]. If PCI is performed urgently, the eptifibatide infusion should be continued for 20–24 h post-PCI for an overall maximum duration of therapy of 96 h. Heparin should be discontinued postprocedure to optimize the safety of sheath removal.

Heparin therapy must be rigorously monitored if coadministered with epti-fibatide. For medical therapy of ACS patients weighing greater than or equal to 70 kg, a bolus dose of 5000 U it is recommended, followed by a constant intravenous infusion of 1000 U/h. For patients weighing less than 70 kg, a bolus dose of 60 U/kg followed by an infusion of 12 U/kg/h is recommended. The activated partial thromboplastin time (aPTT) must be maintained between 50 and 70 s to avoid potential excessive bleeding.

For PCI in the setting of ACS, the ACT must be maintained at a value between 300 and 350 s. For patients undergoing nonurgent PCI and who have not been treated with heparin within 6 h before intervention, an initial heparin bolus of 60 U/kg is recommended, to achieve a target ACT of 200–300 s.

Tirofiban
Tirofiban is currently administered with a loading dose of 0.4 mcg/kg/min for 30 min, and continued at 0.1 mcg/kg/min. The dose should be halved in patients with severe renal insufficiency, and is contraindicated in patients with severe hypertension (systolic BP >200 mm Hg); active internal bleeding; a history of intracranial haemorrhage, or intracranial neoplasm, arterio-venous malformation, or aneurysm; acute pericarditis; bleeding diathesis; trauma or stroke within the previous 30 d; platelet count <100 000/mm^3; and a history of thrombocytopenia following previous tirofiban exposure. As with eptifibatide, if heparin is co-administered, careful monitoring of coagulation must be maintained. It is suggested that an aPTT of between 50–70 s unless PCI needs to be performed; maintain ACT between 300–350 s during PCI; if platelet count decreases to <100 000/mm^3, perform additional

platelet counts to exclude pseudothrombocytopenia; if thrombocytopenia is confirmed, discontinue GP IIb/IIIa inhibitors and heparin and appropriately monitor and treat the condition.

Treatment: evidence base for current practice

Acute therapy for coronary ischemia involves immediate analgesia and oxygenation. Antiplatelet therapy should be initiated as soon as possible, as it is crucial in optimizing patient outcomes. Aspirin, thienopyridines, and GP IIb/IIIa receptor antagonists still form the currently accepted repertoire of antiplatelet treatments, and remain under investigation in clinical studies.

Aspirin
Aspirin immediate treatment: medical
Aspirin (300 mg) should be administered by paramedic or emergency room medical staff, as soon as suspicion of an ACS is raised. Evidence from the Antithrombotic Trialist's Collaboration metaanalysis presents compelling evidence of a reduction in vascular death, MI, and stroke for patients taking aspirin following ACS [31]. The benefits of prompt aspirin therapy have been noted in previous studies of AMI as well as ACS: the Second International Study of Infarct Survival (ISIS-2) [79] used 162.5 mg aspirin to significantly reduce vascular mortality, nonfatal reinfarction, and nonfatal stroke in AMI patients without increasing hemorrhagic stroke or GI bleeding. Aspirin should be administered to virtually all patients with suspected AMI [80,81] and ACS given the overlap in clinical presentation and clinical benefits. Immediate use of aspirin for ACS has been demonstrated to be beneficial in multiple studies looking at cotherapy with anticoagulants [82,83] as well as adjunctive antiplatelet agents [84–86].

Aspirin immediate treatment: interventional
Aspirin pretreatment reduces the frequency of ischemic complications when started promptly. In an early study of elective balloon angioplasty, a large reduction in periprocedural Q-wave MI was achieved if antiplatelet therapy was started 24 h before the procedure [87]. Although aspirin treatment alone is surprisingly effective at limiting stent thrombosis [88], adjunctive antiplatelet therapy is needed to optimize outcomes [89].

Aspirin chronic treatment: medical
Long-term aspirin therapy offers a 20–25% risk reduction of MI, stroke, or vascular death in patients with chronic stable angina, [90] and patients with prior MI [31], and in unstable angina [82,84,85] risk reductions of greater than or equal to 50% have been observed [91]. A widespread consensus exists in defining a narrow range of recommended daily doses (i.e. 75–160 mg) for MI,

stroke, and vascular death prevention [92,93]. This is supported by separate trial data in over 20 000 patients randomized to treatment with low-dose aspirin or placebo as well as by an overview of all antiplatelet trials showing no dose dependence for the protective effects of aspirin [31].

Aspirin chronic treatment: interventional

Continued treatment with aspirin is recommended following intervention with or without stent placement in patients who have suffered ACS. In a randomized trial of long-term aspirin therapy following angioplasty, 325 mg daily aspirin given for 6 months significantly reduced the incidence of MI [94]. Given the compeling data from medically treated patients, only those who are aspirin intolerant should not be offered the drug, and the potential substitution of long-term clopidogrel considered.

Clopidogrel
Acute clopidogrel treatment: medical

Loading with a thienopyridine following aspirin increases antiplatelet activity. Clopidogrel (300 mg oral) should be offered once a clinical diagnosis of ACS is confirmed by electrocardiogram (ECG) and/or biochemical marker (troponin) criteria, with daily clopidogrel 75 mg thereafter. The Clopidogrel in Unstable angina to prevent Recurrent ischemic Events (CURE) trial showed that clopidogrel significantly reduced the composite endpoint of cardiovascular death, MI, or stroke, which occurred in all patient subgroups presenting with acute unstable coronary syndromes [95]. Fewer recurrent ischemic episodes were noted within the first few hours after randomization, although there was no significant difference in the incidence of non-ST-elevation MI (NSTEMI). There was a significant but small increase in bleeding risk with clopidogrel. Although data initially suggested increased bleeding in patients who underwent early CABG within 5 days, subsequent analysis shows that even this group have greater benefit than hazard as many of the thrombotic events occur prior to surgery [96]. There appears to be no significant increase in life-threatening major hemorrhage in patients receiving clopidogrel who go on to surgical CABG [97]. It is therefore reasonable to suggest that all ACS patients should be commenced on clopidogrel treatment at the time of diagnosis. For the small minority of patients with a high likelihood of very early CABG, platelet inhibition with aspirin and small molecule IIb/IIIa inhibitor would be appropriate.

The CLARITY ($n = 3491$) and COMMIT ($n = 45\,852$) trials have tested the use of clopidogrel with lytic therapy in ST-elevation ACS. CLARITY [97] demonstrated a highly significant reduction in the frequency of occluded arteries (clopidogrel 15.0%; placebo 21.7%; 95% CI, 0.53–0.76; $p < .0001$). COMMIT (ACC Hotline 2005) conducted in China and without a loading dose of clopidogrel, nevertheless, found a highly significant reduction in the risk of death (8.1% death versus 7.5%, a 7% relative risk reduction, $p = .03$) and for death, re-MI, or stroke a 9% relative risk reduction ($p = 0.002$). Clopidogrel will therefore be part of acute treatment for ST-elevation MI.

Acute clopidogrel treatment: interventional

Evidence from several studies in acute and elective coronary intervention suggests that early treatment with clopidogrel improves outcomes during and after PCI. The PCI CURE study showed that pretreatment with clopidogrel and aspirin therapy compared with placebo and aspirin prior to PCI; caused a 44% reduction in the primary endpoint of cardiovascular death, MI, or urgent revascularization at 30 days [89]. After PCI, over 80% of patients in both treatment arms received open-label thienopyridine for a median of 30 days, mainly because of stent placement, and as such, the 30-day risk reduction reflects the effects of clopidogrel pre-treatment. Studies of elective percutaneous intervention further strengthen the case for adequate pretreatment with clopidogrel. In the Clopidogrel for the Reduction of Events During Observation (CREDO) study, patients who received a loading dose of 300 mg clopidogrel at least 6 h before PCI experienced a significant relative risk reduction of 38.6% for death, MI, and target vessel revascularization compared with no reduction with treatment less than 6 h before PCI. Rapid antiplatelet effects can be safely achieved using a 600 mg dose of clopidogrel [98]. Recent data from the Antiplatelet therapy for Reduction of MYocardial Damage during Angioplasty (ARMYDA-2) study confirm the safety and efficacy of high-dose clopidogrel loading in elective PCI with benefits seen within 2 h of administration [99]. This strategy may be an option to enable adequate antiplatelet activity during urgent PCI. Moreover, loading with high-dose (600 mg) clopidogrel enhances antiplatelet activity even in patients already on long-term clopidogrel therapy, suggesting that the antiplatelet effects of 75 mg clopidogrel may be improved further during intervention [100].

Chronic clopidogrel treatment: medical

The CURE study showed major clinical benefits at 30 days with further benefits over the subsequent 8-month treatment period, arguing for prolonged clopidogrel therapy in ACS patients treated medically. More recent cost analyses confirm the economic as well as clinical gain from this strategy [101], data that should allay concerns regarding the added expenditure that this involves. ACS represent a prothrombotic state not just confined to the coronary arterial tree, with evidence of generalized platelet activation [102]. Multiple vulnerable plaques in nonculprit vessels have been angioscopically identified during cardiac catheterization in ACS subjects undergoing invasive investigation and treatment [103]. Protracted treatment with clopidogrel offers antiplatelet activity to ensure that early benefits are not lost, and may limit thrombotic events while other secondary prevention therapies including statins and angiotensin converting enzyme inhibitors act to pacify plaque over the months following an index coronary event.

Chronic clopidogrel treatment: interventional

For patients undergoing interventional management, there are data to suggest that aggressive antiplatelet strategies are just as important. In the PCI-CURE study, 2658 patients underwent PCI after double-blinded randomization to clopidogrel or placebo [89]. All patients received aspirin, and following a post-PCI 4-week treatment period on open-label thienopyridine (clopidogrel or ticlopidine), the study drug (placebo or clopidogrel) was again administered for an average of 8 months. Further analysis of cardiovascular events before and after PCI showed that clopidogrel caused a highly significant 31% reduction in cardiovascular death or MI. Prolonged clopidogrel treatment for 12 months has been examined in the CREDO study [104], with evidence of a significant 26.9% relative reduction in the combined risk of death, MI, or stroke. Current changes in stent technology toward the use of drug eluting stents demands longer periods of combination antiplatelet therapy of up to 12 months, to counteract the prothrombotic nature of drug eluting polymers. The increasing use of drug eluting stents is likely to prolong clopidogrel treatment duration post-PCI. Economic analyses support protracted treatment periods post-PCI despite the added costs, with the benefit being most pronounced in high-risk patients [105].

Thus in ACS patients on aspirin and undergoing PCI, a strategy of clopidogrel pretreatment followed by at least 1 month and preferably longer-term therapy of 9–12 months is beneficial in reducing major cardiovascular events [89].

GP IIb/IIIa inhibition in ACS

The use of GP IIb/IIIa antagonists is a rapidly changing area within ACS management, especially in the context of PCI. Risks of significant bleeding must be balanced against benefits of immediate antiplatelet activity, which is of critical importance when dealing with acute lesions bearing high thrombus loads.

Acute GP IIb/IIIa treatment: medical

Use of GP IIb/IIIa inhibitors in the acute medical management of ACS patients is variable often being dictated by local practice and economic considerations [106,107].

Metaanalysis of GP IIb/IIIa antagonist use across six large, randomized, placebo-controlled trials showed a small nonsignificant reduction in the odds of death or MI in the active treatment limbs for patients undergoing noninvasive management [108]. Reductions in the endpoints of death or nonfatal MI considered individually did not achieve statistical significance [77,109,110].

Early treatment with aspirin, more aggressive loading doses of clopidogrel, and the increasingly widespread use of low molecular weight heparin may encourage more selective use of GP IIb/IIIa inhibitors in risk stable ACS patients. Patients who continue to display signs of ischemia despite aspirin, thienopyridine, and heparin treatment should receive GP IIb/IIIa blockade and early intervention [111,112].

Acute GP IIb/IIIa treatment: interventional

Glycoprotein IIb/IIIa inhibitors are frequently used routinely in percutaneous intervention, supported by current AHA/ACC guidelines [113]. Late follow-up of abciximab trial metaanalysis shows reductions in both periprocedural MIs and 1-year mortality [114] across age, gender, clinical, and lesion subgroups, excluding vein grafts [115], with pronounced benefits in diabetic patients [116]. However, the advantage of IIb/IIIa inhibitors has been questioned by recent large randomized trials albeit focusing predominantly on a stable elective target population. The Intracoronary Stenting and Antithrombotic Regimen-Rapid Early Action for Coronary Treatment (ISAR-REACT) study [117] randomized over 2000 patients with stable angina, who received a 600 mg dose of clopidogrel at least 2 h before PCI or were treated with abciximab during their procedure. The use of abciximab produced no difference in the combined endpoint of death, MI and urgent TVR (target vessel revascularization) at 30 days, but did increase the incidence of thrombocytopenia and significant hemorrhage. The lack of advantage of IIb/IIIa inhibitors was also present in diabetic patients, both in these trials and in the recently reported trial, Is Abciximab a Superior Way to Eliminate Elevated Thrombotic Risk in Diabetics (ISAR-SWEET) [118]. These trials, however, excluded enrolment of patients with highly unstable syndromes. The ongoing ISAR-REACT II trial will specifically address the need of IIb/IIIa inhibitors in patients with unstable angina and NSTEMI pretreated with high-dose clopidogrel.

In the Enhanced Suppression of the Platelet IIb/IIIa Receptor with Integrilin Therapy (ESPRIT) trial, the primary composite endpoint of death, MI, target-vessel revascularization, and "bailout" GP IIb/IIIa antagonist therapy during coronary stenting was significantly reduced with eptifibatide treatment at the expense of a small increase in major bleeds, but no increase in the need for transfusions.

In the Do Tirofiban and ReoPro Give similar Efficacy? (TARGET) Trial, tirofiban was directly compared with abciximab in 5308 patients undergoing coronary stenting [119]. The primary composite endpoint of death, nonfatal MI, and urgent TVR at 30 days occurred less frequently in those given abciximab. The dose of tirofiban may have been suboptimal resulting in inadequate platelet inhibition, although by 6 months, there was no significant difference in the primary endpoint between the two agents.

In high-risk unstable ACS patients displaying recurrent ischemia, with ECG changes and elevated troponin levels, IIb/IIIa inhibitors remain indicated [120–122]. If IIb/IIIa blockade is required immediately before PCI and especially if target lesions are complex or disease is diffuse, abciximab may be the agent of choice.

Role of bivalirudin: implications for GP IIb/IIIa use

Direct thrombin inhibitors in place of unfractionated heparin may reduce bleeding risks. The Randomized Evaluation in PCI Linking Angiomax to

Reduced Clinical Events (REPLACE)-2 trial, an interventional study including urgent and elective revascularization procedures showed bivalirudin to be non-inferior to GP IIb/IIIa blockade, as well as reducing risks of major hemorrhage [123]. This extended to complex subsets such as patient with renal failure [124]. The Acute Catheterization and Urgent Intervention Triage strategy (ACUITY) trial [125] will randomize 13 800 patients with ACS undergoing an invasive strategy, to assess the role that bivalirudin may have to play in combination with, or as a replacement for, current anticoagulant and antiplatelet agents. The use of bivalirudin may reduce the future use of GP IIb/IIIa blockade in invasive management strategies.

Use of antiplatelet agents in ACS: summary

Medical management

1 Aspirin and clopidogrel treatment should be commenced promptly in patients presenting with clinical features of ACS.

2 In higher-risk patients, including those with ongoing ischemia, a GP IIb/IIIa inhibitor and invasive management are indicated. Thienopyridine treatment may lessen the need for GP IIb/IIIa blockade in lower risk patients.

3 Long-term aspirin therapy should be offered to all ACS patients, with clopidogrel being substituted if there is evidence of intolerance to aspirin, for example, upper GI irritation.

4 Clopidogrel should be continued for up to 12 months to maximize clinical benefit in medically managed patients.

Invasive and interventional management

1 Aspirin and clopidogrel treatment should be commenced as early as possible.

2 Patients undergoing angiography who may proceed electively to CABG are safe to commence clopidogrel, but individual operators may wish to defer clopidogrel until angiography is complete. If patients have been fully loaded with clopidogrel, individual physicians may wish to consider stopping clopidogrel therapy for 5–7 days prior to CABG if surgical revascularization can be deferred.

3 In proceeding to PCI without prior clopidogrel, an aggressive loading dose, for example, 600 mg p.o. should be considered.

4 Early use of GP IIb/IIIa antagonists are indicated in patients with ongoing ischemia where catheterization and PCI are planned. For patients deemed high risk, GP IIb/IIIa antagonists should be administered prior to PCI.

5 Clopidogrel treatment post-PCI should be continued for at least 1 month in non-ACS patients after bare metal stenting, 6–12 months after drug eluting stenting.

Management pathway for antiplatelet therapies

A simple flow chart to illustrate the order of antiplatelet therapies in the management of ACS is given below.

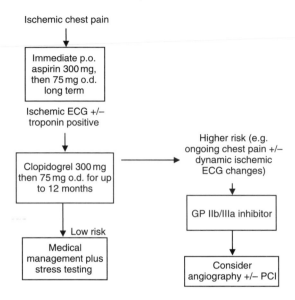

References

1. Fuster V, Badimon JJ, Chesebro JH. Atherothrombosis: mechanisms and clinical therapeutic approaches 321. *Vasc Med* 1998; **3**(3): 231–239.
2. Kullo IJ, Edwards WD, Schwartz RS. Vulnerable plaque: pathobiology and clinical implications 324. *Ann Intern Med* 1998; **129**(12): 1050–1060.
3. Fuster V, Stein B, Ambrose JA, Badimon L, Badimon JJ, Chesebro JH. Athero-sclerotic plaque rupture and thrombosis. Evolving concepts 494. *Circulation* 1990; **82**(Suppl. 3): II47–II59.
4. Libby P, Geng YJ, Aikawa M *et al.* Macrophages and atherosclerotic plaque stability 385. *Curr Opin Lipidol* 1996; **7**(5): 330–335.
5. Davies PF. Flow-mediated endothelial mechanotransduction. *Physiol Rev* 1995; **75**(3): 519–560.
6. Tousoulis D, Davies G, Stefanadis C, Toutouzas P, Ambrose JA. Inflammatory and thrombotic mechanisms in coronary atherosclerosis 86. *Heart* 2003; **89**(9): 993–997.
7. Stary HC, Chandler AB, Dinsmore RE *et al.* A definition of advanced types of ather-osclerotic lesions and a histological classification of atherosclerosis: a report from the committee on vascular lesions of the council on arteriosclerosis, American Heart Association. *Arterioscler Thromb Vasc Biol* 1995; **15**(9): 1512–1531.
8. Fernandez-Ortiz A, Badimon JJ, Falk E *et al.* Characterization of the rel-ative thrombogenicity of atherosclerotic plaque components: implications for consequences of plaque rupture. *J Am Coll Cardiol* 1994; **23**(7): 1562–1569.

9. Toschi V, Gallo R, Lettino M *et al*. Tissue factor modulates the thrombogenicity of human atherosclerotic plaques. *Circulation* 1997; **95**(3): 594–599.

10. Moreno PR, Falk E, Palacios IF, Newell JB, Fuster V, Fallon JT. Macrophage infiltration in acute coronary syndromes. Implications for plaque rupture. *Circulation* 1994; **90**(2): 775–778.

11. van der Wal AC, Becker AE, van der Loos CM, Das PK. Site of intimal rupture or erosion of thrombosed coronary atherosclerotic plaques is characterized by an inflammatory process irrespective of the dominant plaque morphology. *Circulation* 1994; **89**(1): 36–44.

12. Shah PK. Mechanisms of plaque vulnerability and rupture 113. *J Am Coll Cardiol* 2003; **41**(4 Suppl. S): 15S–22S.

13. Rauch U, Osende JI, Fuster V, Badimon JJ, Fayad Z, Chesebro JH. Thrombus formation on atherosclerotic plaques: pathogenesis and clinical consequences. *Ann Intern Med* 2001; **134**(3): 224–238.

14. Corti R, Farkouh ME, Badimon JJ. The vulnerable plaque and acute coronary syndromes 124. *Am J Med* 2002; **113**(8): 668–680.

15. Fressinaud E, Baruch D, Girma JP, Sakariassen KS, Baumgartner HR, Meyer D. von Willebrand factor-mediated platelet adhesion to collagen involves platelet membrane glycoprotein IIb–IIIa as well as glycoprotein Ib. *J Lab Clin Med* 1988; **112**(1): 58–67.

16. Lawson JH, Kalafatis M, Stram S, Mann KG. A model for the tissue factor pathway to thrombin I. An empirical study. *J Biol Chem* 1994; **269**(37): 23357–23366.

17. Heemskerk JW, Bevers EM, Lindhout T. Platelet activation and blood coagulation. *Thromb Haemost* 2002; **88**(2): 186–193.

18. Hardy AR, Conley PB, Luo J, Benovic JL, Poole AW, Mundell SJ. P2Y1 and P2Y12 receptors for ADP desensitize by distinct kinase-dependent mechanisms. *Blood* 2005; 105(9): 3552–3560.

19. Burch JW, Stanford N, Majerus PW. Inhibition of platelet prostaglandin synthetase by oral aspirin. *J Clin Invest* 1978; **61**(2): 314–319.

20. Majerus PW. Arachidonate metabolism in vascular disorders. *J Clin Invest* 1983; **72**(5): 1521–1525.

21. Taylor DW, Barnett HJ, Haynes RB *et al*. Low-dose and high-dose acetylsalicylic acid for patients undergoing carotid endarterectomy: a randomised controlled trial. *Lancet* 1999; **353**(9171): 2179–2184.

22. Final report on the aspirin component of the ongoing physicians' health study. Steering Committee of the Physicians' Health Study Research Group. *N Engl J Med* 1989; **321**(3): 129–135.

23. Ridker PM, Cushman M, Stampfer MJ, Tracy RP, Hennekens CH. Inflammation, aspirin, and the risk of cardiovascular disease in apparently healthy men. *N Engl J Med* 1997; **336**(14): 973–979.

24. Frishman WH. Cyclooxygenase inhibition in patients with coronary artery disease. *J Am Coll Cardiol* 2004; **43**(4): 532–533.

25. van Pampus EC, Huijgens PC, Zevenbergen A, Twaalfhoven H, van Kamp GJ, Langenhuijsen MM. Influence of aspirin on human megakaryocyte prostaglandin synthesis. *Eur J Haematol* 1993; **50**(5): 264–268.

26. The RISC Group. Risk of myocardial infarction and death during treatment with low dose aspirin and intravenous heparin in men with unstable coronary artery disease. *Lancet* 1990; **336**(8719): 827–830.

27. Juul-Moller S, Edvardsson N, Jahnmatz B, Rosen A, Sorensen S, Omblus R. Double-blind trial of aspirin in primary prevention of myocardial infarction in patients with stable chronic angina pectoris. The Swedish Angina Pectoris Aspirin Trial (SAPAT) Group. *Lancet* 1992; **340**(8833): 1421–1425.
28. Bjornsson TD, Schneider DE, Berger HJ. Aspirin acetylates fibrinogen and enhances fibrinolysis. Fibrinolytic effect is independent of changes in plasminogen activator levels. *J Pharmacol Exp Ther* 1989; **250**(1): 154–161.
29. Szczeklik A, Musial J, Undas A *et al.* Inhibition of thrombin generation by aspirin is blunted in hypercholesterolemia. *Arterioscler Thromb Vasc Biol* 1996; **16**(8): 948–954.
30. Kessels H, Beguin S, Andree H, Hemker HC. Measurement of thrombin generation in whole blood – the effect of heparin and aspirin. *Thromb Haemost* 1994; **72**(1): 78–83.
31. Collaboration AT. Collaborative meta-analysis of randomised trials of antiplatelet therapy for prevention of death, myocardial infarction, and stroke in high risk patients. *BMJ* 2002; **324**(7329): 71–86.
32. The Dutch TIA Trial Study Group. A comparison of two doses of aspirin (30 mg vs. 283 mg a day) in patients after a transient ischemic attack or minor ischemic stroke. *N Engl J Med* 1991; **325**(18): 1261–1266.
33. Ridker PM, Hennekens CH, Tofler GH, Lipinska I, Buring JE. Anti-platelet effects of 100 mg alternate day oral aspirin: a randomized, double-blind, placebo-controlled trial of regular and enteric coated formulations in men and women. *J Cardiovasc Risk* 1996; **3**(2): 209–212.
34. Wang JC, Aucoin-Barry D, Manuelian D *et al.* Incidence of aspirin nonresponsiveness using the Ultegra Rapid Platelet Function Assay-ASA. *Am J Cardiol* 2003; **92**(12): 1492–1494.
35. Mueller MR, Salat A, Stangl P *et al.* Variable platelet response to low-dose ASA and the risk of limb deterioration in patients submitted to peripheral arterial angioplasty. *Thromb Haemost* 1997; **78**(3): 1003–1007.
36. Hillarp A, Palmqvist B, Lethagen S, Villoutreix BO, Mattiasson I. Mutations within the cyclooxygenase-1 gene in aspirin non-responders with recurrence of stroke. *Thrombosis Res* 2003; **112**(5–6): 275–283.
37. Buchanan MR, Brister SJ. Individual variation in the effects of ASA on platelet function: implications for the use of ASA clinically. *Can J Cardiol* 1995; **11**(3): 221–227.
38. The RISC Group. Risk of myocardial infarction and death during treatment with low dose aspirin and intravenous heparin in men with unstable coronary artery disease. *Lancet* 1990; **336**(8719): 827–830.
39. Maclouf J, Folco G, Patrono C. Eicosanoids and iso-eicosanoids: constitutive, inducible and transcellular biosynthesis in vascular disease. *Thromb Haemost* 1998; **79**(4): 691–705.
40. Foster CJ, Prosser DM, Agans JM *et al.* Molecular identification and characterization of the platelet ADP receptor targeted by thienopyridine antithrombotic drugs. *J Clin Invest* 2001; **107**(12): 1591–1598.
41. Love BB, Biller J, Gent M. Adverse haematological effects of ticlopidine. Prevention, recognition and management. *Drug Saf* 1998; **19**(2): 89–98.
42. Quinn MJ, Fitzgerald DJ. Ticlopidine and clopidogrel. *Circulation* 1999; **100**(15): 1667–1672.

43. Savi P, Pereillo JM, Uzabiaga MF *et al.* Identification and biological activity of the active metabolite of clopidogrel. *Thromb Haemost* 2000; **84**(5): 891–896.
44. Gachet C, Cazenave JP, Ohlmann P *et al.* The thienopyridine ticlopidine selectively prevents the inhibitory effects of ADP but not of adrenaline on cAMP levels raised by stimulation of the adenylate cyclase of human platelets by PGE1. *Biochem Pharmacol* 1990; **40**(12): 2683–2687.
45. Mills DC, Puri R, Hu CJ *et al.* Clopidogrel inhibits the binding of ADP analogues to the receptor mediating inhibition of platelet adenylate cyclase. *Arterioscler Thromb* 1992; **12**(4): 430–436.
46. Di Minno G, Cerbone AM, Mattioli PL, Turco S, Iovine C, Mancini M. Functionally thrombasthenic state in normal platelets following the administration of ticlopidine. *J Clin Invest* 1985; **75**(2): 328–338.
47. Boneu B, Destelle G. Platelet anti-aggregating activity and tolerance of clopidogrel in atherosclerotic patients. *Thromb Haemost* 1996; **76**(6): 939–943.
48. Herbert JM, Frehel D, Vallee E *et al.* Clopidogrel, a novel antiplatelet and antithrombotic agent. *Cardiovasc Drug Rev* 1993; **11**(2): 180–198.
49. Savcic M, Hauert J, Bachmann F, Wyld PJ, Geudelin B, Cariou R. Clopidogrel loading dose regimens: kinetic profile of pharmacodynamic response in healthy subjects. *Semin Thromb Hemost* 1999; **25**(Suppl. 2): 15–19.
50. Bertrand ME, Rupprecht HJ, Urban P, Gershlick AH, Investigators FT. Double-blind study of the safety of clopidogrel with and without a loading dose in combination with aspirin compared with ticlopidine in combination with aspirin after coronary stenting: the clopidogrel aspirin stent international cooperative study (CLASSICS). *Circulation* 2000; **102**(6): 624–629.
51. Seyfarth HJ, Koksch M, Roethig G *et al.* Effect of 300- and 450-mg clopidogrel loading doses on membrane and soluble P-selectin in patients undergoing coronary stent implantation. *Am Heart J* 2002; **143**(1): 118–123.
52. Wang K, Zhou X, Zhou Z *et al.* Blockade of the platelet P2Y12 receptor by AR-C69931MX sustains coronary artery recanalization and improves the myocardial tissue perfusion in a canine thrombosis model. *Arterioscler Thromb Vasc Biol* 2003; **23**(2): 357–362.
53. Storey RF, Wilcox RG, Heptinstall S. Comparison of the pharmacodynamic effects of the platelet ADP receptor antagonists clopidogrel and AR-C69931MX in patients with ischaemic heart disease. *Platelets* 2002; **13**(7): 407–413.
54. Kohmura C, Gold HK, Yasuda T *et al.* A chimeric murine/human antibody Fab fragment directed against the platelet GP IIb/IIIa receptor enhances and sustains arterial thrombolysis with recombinant tissue-type plasminogen activator in baboons. *Arterioscler Thromb* 1993; **13**(12): 1837–1842.
55. Reverter JC, Beguin S, Kessels H, Kumar R, Hemker HC, Coller BS. Inhibition of platelet-mediated, tissue factor-induced thrombin generation by the mouse/human chimeric 7E3 antibody potential implications for the effect of c7E3 Fab treatment on acute thrombosis and "clinical restenosis." *J Clin Invest* 1996; **98**(3): 863–874.
56. Tam SH, Sassoli PM, Jordan RE, Nakada MT. Abciximab (ReoPro, chimeric 7E3 Fab) demonstrates equivalent affinity and functional blockade of glycoprotein IIb/IIIa and alpha(v)beta3 integrins. *Circulation* 1998; **98**(11): 1085–1091.
57. Neumann FJ, Zohlnhofer D, Fakhoury L, Ott I, Gawaz M, Schomig A. Effect of glycoprotein IIb/IIIa receptor blockade on platelet–leukocyte interaction and

surface expression of the leukocyte integrin Mac-1 in acute myocardial infarction. *J Am Coll Cardiol* 1999; **34**(5): 1420–1426.

58. Schwarz M, Nordt T, Bode C, Peter K. The GP IIb/IIIa inhibitor abciximab (c7E3) inhibits the binding of various ligands to the leukocyte integrin Mac-1 (CD11b/CD18, [alpha]M[beta]2). *Thrombosis Res* 2002; **107**(3–4): 121–128.

59. Lincoff AM *et al.*, for the EPILOG Investigators. Platelet glycoprotein IIb/IIIa receptor blockade and low-dose heparin during percutaneous coronary revascularization. *N Engl J Med* 1997; **336**(24): 1689–1697.

60. Andrieux A, Rabiet MJ, Chapel A, Concord E, Marguerie G. A highly conserved sequence of the Arg-Gly-Asp-binding domain of the integrin beta 3 subunit is sensitive to stimulation. *J Biol Chem* 1991; **266**(22): 14202–14207.

61. Hartman GD, Egbertson MS, Halczenko W *et al.* Non-peptide fibrinogen receptor antagonists. 1. Discovery and design of exosite inhibitors. *J Med Chem* 1992; **35**(24): 4640–4642.

62. Egbertson MS, Chang CT, Duggan ME *et al.* Non-peptide fibrinogen receptor antagonists. 2. Optimization of a tyrosine template as a mimic for Arg-Gly-Asp. *J Med Chem* 1994; **37**(16): 2537–2551.

63. Scarborough RM, Naughton MA, Teng W *et al.* Design of potent and specific integrin antagonists. Peptide antagonists with high specificity for glycoprotein IIb–IIIa. *J Biol Chem* 1993; **268**(2): 1066–1073.

64. Furman MI, Krueger LA, Linden MD *et al.* GP IIb–IIIa antagonists reduce thromboinflammatory processes in patients with acute coronary syndromes undergoing percutaneous coronary intervention. *J Thromb Haemost* 2005; **3**(2): 312–320.

65. Tcheng JE, Ellis SG, George BS *et al.* Pharmacodynamics of chimeric glycoprotein IIb/IIIa integrin antiplatelet antibody Fab 7E3 in high-risk coronary angioplasty. *Circulation* 1994; **90**(4): 1757–1764.

66. Mascelli MA, Lance ET, Damaraju L, Wagner CL, Weisman HF, Jordan RE. Pharmacodynamic profile of short-term abciximab treatment demonstrates prolonged platelet inhibition with gradual recovery from GP IIb/IIIa receptor blockade. *Circulation* 1998; **97**(17): 1680–1688.

67. Califf RM for the EPIC Investigators. Use of a monoclonal antibody directed against the platelet glycoprotein IIb/IIIa receptor in high-risk coronary angioplasty. *N Engl J Med* 1994; **330**(14): 956–961.

68. Berkowitz SD, Harrington RA, Rund MM, Tcheng JE. Acute profound thrombocytopenia after c7E3 Fab (Abciximab) therapy. *Circulation* 1997; **95**(4): 809–813.

69. Tcheng JE, Kereiakes DJ, Braden GA *et al.* Readministration of abciximab: interim report of the ReoPro readministration registry. *Am Heart J* 1999; **138**(1 Pt 2): S33–S38.

70. Barrett JS, Murphy G, Peerlinck K *et al.* Pharmacokinetics and pharmacodynamics of MK-383, a selective non-peptide platelet glycoprotein-IIb/IIIa receptor antagonist, in healthy men. *Clin Pharmacol Ther* 1994; **56**(4): 377–388.

71. Peerlinck K, De Lepeleire I, Goldberg M *et al.* MK-383 (L-700,462), a selective nonpeptide platelet glycoprotein IIb/IIIa antagonist, is active in man. *Circulation* 1993; **88**(4): 1512–1517.

72. Kereiakes J, Kleiman NS, Ambrose J *et al.* Randomized, double-blind, placebo-controlled dose-ranging study of tirofiban (MK-383) platelet IIb/IIIa blockade in

high risk patients undergoing coronary angioplasty. *J Am Coll Cardiol* 1996; **27**(3): 536–542.

73. Bednar B, Cook JJ, Holahan MA *et al.* Fibrinogen receptor antagonist-induced thrombocytopenia in chimpanzee and rhesus monkey associated with preexisting drug-dependent antibodies to platelet glycoprotein IIb/IIIa. *Blood* 1999; **94**(2): 587–599.

74. Madan M, Berkowitz SD. Understanding thrombocytopenia and antigenicity with glycoprotein IIb–IIIa inhibitors. *Am Heart J* 1999; **138**(4 Pt 2): 317–326.

75. Tcheng JE, Harrington RA, Kottke-Marchant K *et al.* Multicenter, randomized, double-blind, placebo-controlled trial of the platelet integrin glycoprotein IIb/IIIa blocker integrelin in elective coronary intervention. *Circulation* 1995; **91**(8): 2151–2157.

76. Harrington RA, Kleiman NS, Kottke-Marchant K *et al.* Immediate and reversible platelet inhibition after intravenous administration of a peptide glycoprotein IIb/IIIa inhibitor during percutaneous coronary intervention. *Am J Cardiol* 1995; **76**(17): 1222–1227.

77. Harrington HA for the PURSUIT Trial Investigators. Inhibition of platelet glycoprotein IIb/IIIa with eptifibatide in patients with acute coronary syndromes. *N Engl J Med* 1998; **339**(7): 436–443.

78. Rebeiz AG, Dery JP, Tsiatis AA *et al.* Optimal duration of eptifibatide infusion in percutaneous coronary intervention (An ESPRIT substudy). *Am J Cardiol* 2004; **94**(7): 926–929.

79. ISIS-2 (Second International Study of Infarct Survival) Collaborative Group 1. Randomised trial of intravenous streptokinase, oral aspirin, both, or neither among 17,187 cases of suspected acute myocardial infarction: ISIS-2. *Lancet* 1988; **2**(8607): 349–360.

80. Hennekens CH, Dyken ML, Fuster V. Aspirin as a therapeutic agent in cardiovascular disease: a statement for healthcare professionals from the American heart association. *Circulation* 1997; **96**(8): 2751–2753.

81. Hennekens CH. Update on aspirin in the treatment and prevention of cardiovascular disease. *Am J Manag Care* 2002; **8**(Suppl. 22): S691–S700.

82. Theroux P, Ouimet H, McCans J *et al.* Aspirin, heparin, or both to treat acute unstable angina. *N Engl J Med* 1988; **319**(17): 1105–1111.

83. Oler A, Whooley MA, Oler J, Grady D. Adding heparin to aspirin reduces the incidence of myocardial infarction and death in patients with unstable angina. A meta-analysis. *JAMA* 1996; **276**(10): 811–815.

84. Lewis HD, Davis JW, Archibald DG *et al.* Protective effects of aspirin against acute myocardial infarction and death in men with unstable angina. Results of a veterans administration cooperative study. *N Engl J Med* 1983; **309**(7): 396–403.

85. Cairns JA, Gent M, Singer J *et al.* Aspirin, sulfinpyrazone, or both in unstable angina. Results of a Canadian multicenter trial. *N Engl J Med* 1985; **313**(22): 1369–1375.

86. The clopidogrel in unstable angina to prevent recurrent events (CURE) trial investigators. Effects of clopidogrel in addition to aspirin in patients with acute coronary syndromes without ST-segment elevation. *N Engl J Med* 2001; **345**(7): 494–502.

87. Schwartz L, Bourassa MG, Lesperance J *et al.* Aspirin and dipyridamole in the prevention of restenosis after percutaneous transluminal coronary angioplasty. *N Engl J Med* 1988; **318**(26): 1714–1719.

88. Hall P, Nakamura S, Maiello L *et al.* A randomized comparison of combined ticlopidine and aspirin therapy versus aspirin therapy alone after successful intravascular ultrasound-guided stent implantation. *Circulation* 1996; **93**(2): 215–222.
89. Mehta SR, Yusuf S, Peters RJ *et al.* Effects of pretreatment with clopidogrel and aspirin followed by long-term therapy in patients undergoing percutaneous coronary intervention: the PCI-CURE study. *Lancet* 2001; **358**(9281): 527–533.
90. Juul-Moller S, Edvardsson N, Jahnmatz B, Rosen A, Sorensen S, Omblus R. Double-blind trial of aspirin in primary prevention of myocardial infarction in patients with stable chronic angina pectoris. The Swedish Angina Pectoris Aspirin Trial (SAPAT) Group. *Lancet* 1992; **340**(8833): 1421–1425.
91. The RISC Group. Risk of myocardial infarction and death during treatment with low dose aspirin and intravenous heparin in men with unstable coronary artery disease. *Lancet* 1990; **336**(8719): 827–830.
92. Patrono C. Aspirin as an antiplatelet *Drug. N Engl J Med* 1994; **330**(18): 1287–1294.
93. Patrono C, Coller B, Dalen JE *et al.* Platelet-active drugs: the relationships among dose, effectiveness, and side effects. *Chest* 2001; **119**(90010): 39S–63.
94. Savage MP, Goldberg S, Bove AA *et al.* Effect of thromboxane A2 blockade on clinical outcome and restenosis after successful coronary angioplasty: Multi-Hospital Eastern Atlantic Restenosis Trial (M-HEART II). *Circulation* 1995; **92**(11): 3194–3200.
95. Peters RJG, Mehta SR, Fox KAA *et al.* Effects of aspirin dose when used alone or in combination with clopidogrel in patients with acute coronary syndromes: observations from the Clopidogrel in Unstable angina to prevent Recurrent Events (CURE) study. *Circulation* 2003; **108**(14): 1682–1687.
96. Fox KAA, Mehta SR, Peters R *et al.* Benefits and risks of the combination of Clopidogrel and aspirin in patients undergoing surgical revascularization for non-ST-elevation acute coronary syndrome: the Clopidogrel in Unstable angina to prevent Recurrent ischemic Events (CURE) trial. *Circulation* 2004; **110**(10): 1202–1208.
97. Sabatine MS, Cannon CP, Gibson CM *et al.* Addition of Clopidogrel to aspirin and fibrinolytic therapy for myocardial infarction with ST-segment elevation. *N Engl J Med* 2005. **352**(12): 1179–1189.
98. Muller I, Seyfarth M, Rudiger S *et al.* Effect of a high loading dose of clopidogrel on platelet function in patients undergoing coronary stent placement. *Heart* 2001; **85**(1): 92–93.
99. Patti G, Colonna G, Pasceri V, Pepe LL, Montinaro A, Di Sciascio G. Randomized trial of high loading dose of Clopidogrel for reduction of periprocedural myocardial infarction in patients undergoing coronary intervention: results From the ARMYDA-2 (Antiplatelet therapy for Reduction of MYocardial Damage during Angioplasty) study. *Circulation* 2005; **111**(16): 2099–2106.
100. Kastrati A, von Beckerath N, Joost A, Pogatsa-Murray G, Gorchakova O, Schomig A. Loading with 600 mg Clopidogrel in patients with coronary artery disease with and without chronic clopidogrel therapy. *Circulation* 2004; **110**(14): 1916–1919.
101. Lindgren P, Jonsson B, Yusuf S. Cost-effectiveness of clopidogrel in acute coronary syndromes in Sweden: a long-term model based on the CURE trial. *J Intern Med* 2004; **255**(5): 562–570.

102. Bahit MC, Granger CB, Wallentin L. Persistence of the prothrombotic state after acute coronary syndromes: implications for treatment. *Am Heart J* 2002; **143**(2): 205–216.
103. Asakura M, Ueda Y, Yamaguchi O *et al.* Extensive development of vulnerable plaques as a pan-coronary process in patients with myocardial infarction: an angioscopic study. *J Am Coll Cardiol* 2001; **37**(5): 1284–1288.
104. Steinhubl SR, Berger PB, Mann III JT *et al.* Early and sustained dual oral antiplatelet therapy following percutaneous coronary intervention: a randomized controlled trial. *JAMA* 2002; **288**(19): 2411–2420.
105. Cowper PA, Udayakumar K, Sketch J, Peterson ED. Economic effects of prolonged clopidogrel therapy after percutaneous coronary intervention. *J Am Coll Cardiol* 2005; **45**(3): 369–376.
106. Cohen MG, Pacchiana CM, Corbalan R *et al.* Variation in patient management and outcomes for acute coronary syndromes in Latin America and North America: results from the Platelet IIb/IIIa in Unstable Angina: Receptor Suppression Using Integrilin Therapy (PURSUIT) trial. *Am Heart J* 2001; **141**(3): 391–401.
107. Fox KAA, Goodman SG, Anderson FA, Jr *et al.* From guidelines to clinical practice: the impact of hospital and geographical characteristics on temporal trends in the management of acute coronary syndromes: the Global Registry of Acute Coronary Events (GRACE). *Eur Heart J* 2003; **24**(15): 1414–1424.
108. Boersma E, Harrington RA, Moliterno DJ *et al.* Platelet glycoprotein IIb/IIIa inhibitors in acute coronary syndromes: a meta-analysis of all major randomised clinical trials. *Lancet* 2002; **359**(9302): 189–198.
109. Ottervanger JP, Armstrong P, Barnathan ES *et al.* Long-term results after the glycoprotein IIb/IIIa inhibitor abciximab in unstable angina: one-year survival in the GUSTO IV-ACS (Global Use of Strategies To Open Occluded Coronary Arteries IV – Acute Coronary Syndrome) trial. *Circulation* 2003; **107**(3): 437–442.
110. The platelet receptor inhibition in ischemic syndrome management in patients limited by unstable signs and symptoms (PRISM-PLUS) study investigators. Inhibition of the platelet glycoprotein IIb/IIIa receptor with tirofiban in unstable angina and non-Q-wave myocardial infarction. *N Engl J Med* 1998; **338**(21): 1488–1497.
111. Neumann FJ, Kastrati A, Pogatsa-Murray G *et al.* Evaluation of prolonged antithrombotic pretreatment ("cooling off" strategy) before intervention in patients with unstable coronary syndromes: a randomized controlled trial. *JAMA* 2003; **290**(12): 1593–1599.
112. Cantor WJ, Goodman SG, Cannon CP *et al.* Early cardiac catheterization is associated with lower mortality only among high-risk patients with ST- and non-ST-elevation acute coronary syndromes: observations from the OPUS-TIMI 16 trial. *Am Heart J* 2005; **149**(2): 275–283.
113. Smith SC, Jr, Dove JT, Jacobs AK *et al.* ACC/AHA guidelines for percutaneous coronary intervention (revision of the 1993 PTCA guidelines) – executive summary: a report of the American College of Cardiology/American Heart Association taskforce on practice guidelines (committee to revise the 1993 guidelines for percutaneous transluminal coronary angioplasty) endorsed by the Society for Cardiac Angiography and Interventions. *Circulation* 2001; **103**(24): 3019–3041.
114. The EPISTENT Investigators. Randomised placebo-controlled and balloon-angioplasty-controlled trial to assess safety of coronary stenting with use of platelet glycoprotein-IIb/IIIa blockade. Evaluation of platelet IIb/IIIa inhibitor for stenting. 1. *Lancet* 1998; **352**(9122): 87–92.

115. Roffi M, Mukherjee D, Chew DP *et al.* Lack of benefit from intravenous platelet glycoprotein IIb/IIIa receptor inhibition as adjunctive treatment for percutaneous interventions of aortocoronary bypass grafts: a pooled analysis of five randomized clinical trials. *Circulation* 2002; **106**(24): 3063–3067.

116. Marso SP, Lincoff AM, Ellis SG *et al.* Optimizing the percutaneous interventional outcomes for patients with diabetes mellitus : results of the EPISTENT (Evaluation of Platelet IIb/IIIa Inhibitor for Stenting Trial) diabetic substudy. *Circulation* 1999; **100**(25): 2477–2484.

117. Kastrati A, Mehilli J, Schuhlen H *et al.* A clinical trial of abciximab in elective percutaneous coronary intervention after pretreatment with Clopidogrel. *New Engl J Med* 2004; **350**(3): 232–238.

118. Mehilli J, Kastrati A, Schuhlen H *et al.* Randomized clinical trial of abciximab in diabetic patients undergoing elective percutaneous coronary interventions after treatment with a high loading dose of Clopidogrel. *Circulation* 2004; **110**(24): 3627–3635.

119. Topol EJ, Moliterno DJ, Herrmann HC *et al.* Comparison of two platelet glycoprotein IIb/IIIa inhibitors, tirofiban and abciximab, for the prevention of ischemic events with percutaneous coronary revascularization. *N Engl J Med* 2001; **344**(25): 1888–1894.

120. Montalescot G, Barragan P, Wittenberg O *et al.* Platelet glycoprotein IIb/IIIa inhibition with coronary stenting for acute myocardial infarction 1. *N Engl J Med* 2001; **344**(25): 1895–1903.

121. Antoniucci D, Migliorini A, Parodi G *et al.* Abciximab-supported infarct artery stent implantation for acute myocardial infarction and long-term survival: a prospective, multicenter, randomized trial comparing infarct artery stenting plus abciximab with stenting alone. *Circulation* 2004; **109**(14): 1704–1706.

122. Kastrati A, Mehilli J, Schlotterbeck K *et al.* Early administration of reteplase plus abciximab vs abciximab alone in patients with acute myocardial infarction referred for percutaneous coronary intervention: a randomized controlled trial 1. *JAMA* 2004; **291**(8): 947–954.

123. Lincoff AM, Bittl JA, Harrington RA *et al.* Bivalirudin and provisional glycoprotein IIb/IIIa blockade compared with heparin and planned glycoprotein IIb/IIIa blockade during percutaneous coronary intervention: REPLACE-2 randomized trial. *JAMA* 2003; **289**(7): 853–863.

124. Chew DP, Lincoff AM, Gurm H *et al.* Bivalirudin versus heparin and glycoprotein IIb/IIIa inhibition among patients with renal impairment undergoing percutaneous coronary intervention (a subanalysis of the REPLACE-2 trial). *Am J Cardiol* 2005; **95**(5): 581–585.

125. Stone GW, Bertrand M, Colombo A *et al.* Acute Catheterization and Urgent Intervention Triage strategY (ACUITY) trial: study design and rationale. *Am Heart J* 2004; **148**(5): 7764–775.

CHAPTER 11

Antithrombin drugs: LMWH, unfractionated heparin, direct thrombin inhibitors

Raphaelle Dumaine and Gilles Montalescot

Introduction

Acute coronary syndromes (ACSs) are, in most cases, the clinical manifestation of intracoronary thrombosis following the disruption of an atherosclerotic plaque. The contact between circulating blood procoagulant molecules and structures of the vessel wall, such as fibronectin, collagen, and von Willebrand factor, results in tissue factor expression and coagulation factors activation. Thrombin is a key enzyme of the coagulation cascade, as it controls the ultimate step: the conversion of fluid-phase fibrinogen into fibrin, which polymerizes into crosslinked fibrin polymers that form the basis of the clot. Furthermore, thrombin sustains the clotting process by two mechanisms: amplification of its own production by activating the intrinsic pathway, particularly factors XI, IX, VIII, and X; and platelet activation. Thrombin binds to fibrin, fibrin degradation products, as well as subendothelial matrix, and remains active once bound. However, bound thrombin cannot be inactivated by antithrombin–heparin complex [1]. Thus thrombin-rich clot represents a powerful reservoir of prothrombotic thrombin.

Unfractionated heparin (UFH) has long been the only thrombin inhibitor used in unstable angina patients, despite the lack of definitive proven benefit over placebo in ACS patients treated with aspirin [2,3]. In addition, as will be developed further, several pharmacological characteristics limit the antithrombin activity of UFH. This, associated with the necessity of close monitoring of anticoagulant activity, as well as a high incidence of heparin-induced thrombocytopenia [4] encouraged the development of alternative antithrombin strategies.

The present chapter discusses the evidence surrounding the use of low molecular weight heparins (LMWHs) and direct thrombin inhibitors (DTIs) as alternative thrombin inhibitors to UFH in the setting of ACS.

Mechanisms of action of the different thrombin inhibitors

Thrombin has an active site and two exosites, one of which – exosite 1 – binds to its fibrin substrate, orientating it toward the active site.

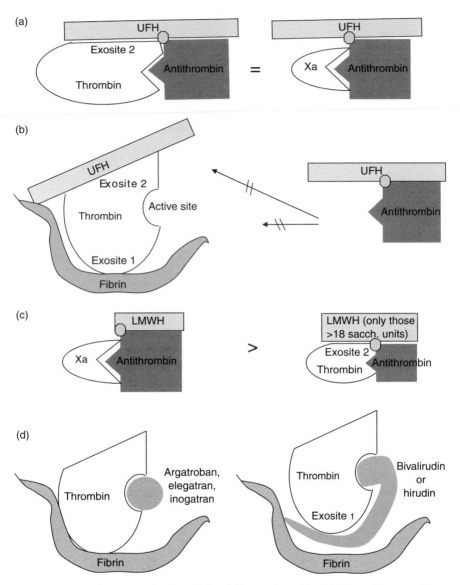

Figure 11.1 Mechanisms of action of the different thrombin inhibitors (See text for details regarding the part figures). Adapted in part from Ref. [1].

Figure 11.1 displays the mechanisms of action of the different thrombin inhibitors.

Unfractionated heparin

Unfractionated Heparin binds to exosite 2 on thrombin and also to antithrombin, forming a ternary complex. This ternary complex is necessary for the inhibition of thrombin by antithrombin (Figure 11.1(a), left). Contrary to thrombin inhibition, inactivation of factor Xa does not require the formation of a ternary complex. UFH inhibits thrombin and factor Xa in the same proportion (the ratio antiXa/IIa activity equals 1) (Figure 11.1(a), right). The interaction of the heparins (UFH as well as LMWH) with antithrombin is mediated by a unique pentasaccharide sequence, present in approximately one-third of the UFH chains [5].

In addition, UFH also binds simultaneously to fibrin and thrombin. The heparin–thrombin–fibrin complex lessens the ability of the heparin–antithrombin complex to inhibit thrombin and increases the affinity of thrombin for its fibrin substrate. This results in a protection of fibrin-bound thrombin from inactivation by the heparin–antithrombin complex [1] (Figure 11.1(b)).

Low molecular weight heparins

Low molecular weight heparins result from the depolymerization of UFH chains and contain approximatively 20% of the chains of the critical pentasaccharide unit needed for their interaction with antithrombin [5]. Contrary to UFH, LMWH action is primarily directed against factor Xa because most of the chains are not sufficiently long to form the ternary complex necessary for the inactivation of thrombin (<50% of the chains contain at least the 18 saccharide units needed for the formation of the ternary heparin–thrombin–antithrombin complex) (Figure 11.1(c)). Depending on LMWH, the antithrombin/anti-Xa activity ratio varies from 1.9 (tinzaparin) to 3.8 (enoxaparin) [5].

Direct thrombin inhibitors

Direct thrombin inhibitors either bind selectively to the active site of thrombin (active site directed inhibitors) or bind both to the active site and exosite 1 (bivalent inhibitors). The former inhibitors, such as argatroban, efegatran, and inogatran, inhibit fibrin-bound thrombin without displacing it (Figure 11.1(d), left). The latter inhibitors, such as hirudin and bivalirudin, remove thrombin from its fibrin substrate [1] (Figure 11.1(d), right).

Potential advantages of the new thrombin inhibitors over UFH

A comparison of the pharmacological properties of the main classes of thrombin inhibitors is shown in Table 11.1.

The antithrombin action of UFH is limited by variable efficacy and stability, mainly due to a poor bioavailability, nonspecific protein binding, neutralization by platelet factor-4, and a lack of efficacy on fibrin-bound thrombin [6]. Moreover, UFH exhibits prothrombotic properties related to a poor control of von Willebrand factor release, as well as platelet activation, platelet aggregation through binding and upregulation of the platelet GP IIb-IIIa receptor, and thrombin generation rebound after discontinuation [7–11].

Table 11.1 Comparison of pharmacological properties of the different thrombin inhibitors.

	UFH	LMWH	DTI
Presence of cofactor required	+++	+++	−
Renal clearance	±	++	+
Predictability in pharmacological profile	−	++	++
Inhibition of thrombin generation	+	++	−
Control of von Willebrand factor release	+	+++	++
TFPI release	+	++	−
Inhibition of bound thrombin	−	−	+++
Rebound of thrombin generation after discontinuation	+++	+	++
Platelet activation	+++	+	−
Nonspecific protein binding	+++	+	−
Neutralization by platelet factor-4	+++	+	−
Immuno-thrombocytopenia	+++	+	−

Fractionated LMWH have a more predictable pharmacological profile than UFH, removing the need for therapeutic drug monitoring. This is mainly due to reduced nonspecific protein binding and reduced neutralization by platelet factor-4. Other properties such as reduced induction of von Willebrand factor release and reduced platelet activation are of crucial importance in the setting of ACS. The release of von Willebrand factor has been shown to be a strong predictor of outcome in ACS without ST-segment elevation [8,9], as well as in acute myocardial infarction with ST-segment elevation [12,13]. LMWH has shown repeatedly to reduce this marker of outcome significantly [8,9,13]. Furthermore, LMWH produces enhanced release of tissue factor pathway inhibitor (TFPI), a glycoprotein that forms a quaternary complex with the factor VIIa–tissue factor complex and factor Xa, thus inhibiting the factor VIIa–tissue factor complex [6]. This extended action on the coagulation cascade, upstream from thrombin, is a theoretical advantage over UFH, especially in the setting of ACS, where limiting the amplification of clot formation by inhibiting thrombin generation is a key element of the treatment strategy. Heparin-induced thrombocytopenia is also much less common with LMWH than UFH [4].

Direct thrombin inhibitors do not bind to plasma proteins, providing a more predictable pharmacological response than UFH. They are not affected by platelet factor-4, have a low immunogenic propensity, and thus are very unlikely to induce thrombocytopenia. Furthermore, bivalirudin blocks thrombin signaling to the platelet receptors, protease activated receptors (PARs), thus limiting platelet activation.

Contrary to heparins, DTIs are active against fibrin-bound thrombin. However, because they exert a direct action on thrombin, in a 1 : 1 stoichiometric fashion, the amount of thrombin inhibited is parallel to the concentration of DTI. This is the main limitation of their action, as increasing their concentration to achieve a greater inhibition of thrombin is associated with prohibitive bleeding rates [6].

LMWH in ACS

Comparison of LMWH and UFH

Several randomized clinical trials have compared the efficacy and safety of LMWH and UFH among medically managed patients presenting with ACS [14–17]. Among those, enoxaparin was the only LMWH to demonstrate a significant and sustained benefit over UFH. In the metaanalysis of the TIMI (Thrombolysis in Myocardial Infarction) 11B and ESSENCE trials, enoxaparin was associated with a significant reduction of death and MI at 8, 14, and 43 days (OR 0.77, 95% CI = 0.62–0.95; OR 0.79, 95% CI = 0.65–0.96; and OR 0.82, 95% CI = 0.69–0.97, respectively) [18].

More recently, safety and efficacy of these two antithrombin regimens have been compared among patients receiving up-to-date anthrombotic regimens, with tirofiban [A to Z [19], ACUTE (Antithrombotic Combination using Tirofiban and Enoxaparin) II [20]], or eptifibatide [INTERACT [21]], and among patients undergoing an early invasive strategy [SYNERGY (Superior Yield of the New Strategy of Enoxaparin Revascularization and Glycoprotein IIb/IIIa Inhibitors) [22]].

In the ACUTE II trial [20], 525 patients with non-ST-segment elevation ACS and treated with tirofiban and aspirin were randomized to receive either UFH (5000 U bolus followed by an infusion of 1000 U/h adjusted to a therapeutic aPTT, $n = 210$) or enoxaparin [1.0 mg/kg subcutaneous (SC) injection every 12 h, $n = 315$] in a double-blind fashion, during 24–96 h. The primary safety endpoint of total bleeding incidence (TIMI major + TIMI minor + loss without any identified site) occurred among 4.8% versus 3.5% of patients receiving UFH versus enoxaparin (OR 1.4, 95% CI = 0.6–3.4). There was no difference in the incidence of death/MI between the UFH and enoxaparin groups (1.9% versus 2.5%; and 7.1% versus 6.7% respectively; $p = $ NS for both). However, refractory ischemia and rehospitalization due to unstable angina occurred more often in the UFH group (4.3% versus 0.6%; and 7.1% versus 1.6%, respectively, $p < .05$ for both).

The A to Z trial (phase A) was an open-label randomized noninferiority trial comparing enoxaparin ($n = 2026$) with weight and aPTT-adjusted intravenous UFH ($n = 1961$) in non-ST-segment elevation ACS receiving aspirin and tirofiban [19]. The prespecified criterion for noninferiority was met for the primary efficacy endpoint of death/MI/refractory ischemia at 7 days (9.4% in the UFH group versus 8.4% in the enoxaparin group, HR 0.88, 95% CI = 0.71–1.08). When stratifying patients per prerandomization treatment, the authors observed a trend toward a lower incidence of the primary endpoint in the enoxaparin arm when no prior anticoagulant had been administered (HR 0.77, 95% CI = 0.53–1.11, $p = .38$ for interaction). Enoxaparin was as safe as UFH regarding the incidence of TIMI minor or major bleeding (3.0% versus 2.2%, $p = $ NS).

The INTERACT trial was a randomized open-label trial comparing enoxaparin ($n = 380$) with intravenous aPTT-adjusted UFH ($n = 366$) in high-risk non-ST-segment elevation ACS receiving aspirin and eptifibatide [21]. The primary safety endpoint of major non-CABG (coronary artery bypass grafting) related bleeding at 96 h occurred significantly less often among enoxaparin treated patients (1.8% versus 4.6%, $p = .03$). Minor bleeding was more frequent in the enoxaparin group (30.3% versus 20.8%, $p = .003$). The primary efficacy outcome of ischemia detected by continuous electrocardiogram monitoring was significantly less frequent in the enoxaparin group during the initial (14.3% versus 25.4%, $p = .0002$) and subsequent (12.7% versus 25.9%, $p < .0001$) 48 h monitoring periods. Finally, death/MI at 30 days occurred significantly less among enoxaparin treated patients (5% versus 9%, $p = .031$).

The SYNERGY trial [22] was a randomized, open-label, international trial comparing enoxaparin and UFH among 10 027 high-risk patients with non-ST-segment elevation ACS to be treated with an intended early invasive strategy. The incidence of the composite primary efficacy endpoint (death/MI at 30 days) was similar in enoxaparin and UFH-treated patients (14.0% versus 14.5% respectively, OR 0.96; 95% CI = 0.86–1.06). There was no difference in the rate of ischemic events during percutaneous coronary intervention (PCI) between the two groups. The primary safety outcome was major bleeding or stroke. There was no difference between the two groups with respect to stroke incidence; the incidence of major bleeding was modestly increased in the enoxaparin group when using the TIMI bleeding classification (9.1% versus 7.6%, $p = .008$) but not when using the GUSTO (Global Use of Strategies To Open Occluded Coronary Arteries) classification (2.7% versus 2.2%, $p = .08$). The need for transfusions was similar among the two groups (17.0% versus 16.0%, $p = .16$).

A pooled analysis was performed among 21 946 patients included in six randomized trials comparing UFH and enoxaparin in the setting of non-ST-segment elevation ACS [23]. Death at 30 days was similar for both antithrombin strategies (3.0% for both), but enoxaparin treatment was associated with lower incidence of death/MI at 30 days than UFH populations (10.1% versus 11.0%; OR 0.91; 95% CI = 0.83–0.99; number needed to treat = 107). The benefit of enoxaparin was even higher among patients receiving no prerandomization antithrombin therapy (8.0% versus 9.4%; OR 0.81; 95% CI = 0.70–0.94; number needed to treat = 72). No significant difference was found in blood transfusion (OR, 1.01; 95% CI = 0.89–1.14) or major bleeding (OR 1.04; 95% CI = 0.83–1.30) at 7 days after randomization.

In all these trials, enoxaparin was administered at the dose of 1 mg/kg SC every 12 h, in order to achieve therapeutic anti-Xa levels. This is of importance as it has been demonstrated that low anti-Xa activity (<0.5 IU/mL) was an independent predictor of poor outcome among ACS patients; conversely, anti-Xa activity, within the target range of 0.5–1.2 IU/mL, is not related to bleeding events [24]. Among patients with impaired creatinine clearance (chronic kidney disease, elderly patients), the therapeutic range is safely achieved by reducing enoxaparin dose [25].

LMWH for PCI in the setting of ACS

There is very few literature on LMWH management in the transition from medical to interventional therapy.

Collet *et al.* examined the safety and efficacy of performing PCI in the setting of ACS on enoxaparin therapy without interruption of, or addition of, anticoagulation for PCI [26]. The only rule was to perform PCI within 8 h of the last SC enoxaparin injection, when the anti-Xa levels are close to the peak of activity. Four hundred fifty-one consecutive patients with non-ST-segment elevation ACS received at least 48 h treatment with SC enoxaparin (1 mg/kg/12 h). Of the patients, 293 (65%) underwent coronary angiography within 8 h of the morning enoxaparin SC injection, with PCI in 132 (28%) patients with no further enoxaparin. The mean anti-Xa activity at the time of catheterization was >0.5 IU/mL in 97.6% patients. There were no instances of in-hospital acute vessel closure or urgent revascularization following PCI. Death/MI at 30 days occurred in 3.0% in the PCI group, but 6.2% in the whole population, and 10.8% in patients not undergoing catheterization. The 30-day major-bleeding rate was 0.8% in the PCI group, which was comparable to that in the medically managed patients (1.3%).

Recent data drawn from more than 350 patients indicate that similar anti-Xa levels to those found after 48 h of SC treatment are achieved after just two SC doses of enoxaparin [27].

In the NICE-3 study [28], 661 ACS patients were treated with enoxaparin SC 1 mg/kg plus abciximab, eptifibatide, or tirofiban at standard doses. For the transition from the ward to the catheter laboratory, the following strategies were followed: no interruption and no addition of enoxaparin for PCI within 8 h of the last SC injection and an additive IV bolus of 0.3 mg/kg was provided when PCI was performed between 8 and 12 h of the last enoxaparin SC injection. The major bleeding rate was 4.5% and the in-hospital death/MI/urgent TVR rate was 5.7%.

In the SYNERGY trial described above, on comparing enoxaparin and UFH in more than 10 000 ACS patients who were managed with current early invasive strategy, 92% patients underwent coronary angiography, PCI was performed in 47%, and 57% received GP IIb-IIIa inhibitors. When stratifying by prerandomization therapy, the benefit of enoxaparin was the highest among patients either receiving enoxaparin or no antithrombin therapy before randomization. The authors stated that "as a first-line agent in the absence of changing antithrombin therapy during treatment, enoxaparin appears to be superior to UFH without an increased bleeding risk" [22].

Data from the abovementioned trials are becoming integrated into current recommendations. A recent expert consensus concluded that substantial evidence exists that patients receiving SC LMWH in the management of ACS can safely undergo cardiac catheterization and PCI, and that concerns about transition of medical to interventional management "should not impede upstream use of LMWH" [29]. The anticoagulation management is recommended as follows: in patients undergoing PCI within 8 h of the previous SC dose no additional antithrombin regimen is required; when PCI is performed within 8–12 h following a SC LMWH injection, supplemental treatment with either a lower dose of IV LMWH bolus (enoxaparin 0.3 mg IV bolus) or UFH could be given. It was furthermore concluded that LMWH and GP IIb/IIIa antagonists can be safely used in combination without any apparent increase in the risk of major bleeding [29].

Direct thrombin inhibitors

Phase III ACS trials with DTIs are limited to hirudin and bivalirudin.

Recombinant hirudin

The GUSTO-IIb [30] trial randomized 8011 patients with NSTE-ACS between UFH (5000 U bolus, followed by a 1000 U/h infusion) and hirudin (0.1 mg/kg bolus, followed by a 0.1 mg/kg/h infusion) during 3–5 days. Incidence of the composite of death/MI at 30 days was similar for the two groups (9.1% versus 8.3%, $p = $ NS), but hirudin was associated with an increased risk of severe bleeding (1.3% versus 0.9%, $p = .06$) and intracranial bleeding (0.2% versus 0.02%, $p = .06$).

After the OASIS (Organization to Assess Strategies for Ischemic Syndromes) pilot dose-finding study [31], the OASIS-2 was a double-blind randomized trial comparing UFH (5000 U bolus then 15 U/kg/h; $n = 5058$) and hirudin (0.4 mg/kg bolus then 0.15 mg/kg/h, $n = 5083$) for 72 h among ACS patients [32]. The composite of cardiovascular death or new MI at 7 days (primary endpoint) tended to be less frequent among hirudin-treated patients than among UFH-treated patients [3.6% versus 4.2%, relative risk (RR) 0.84 (95% CI $= 0.69–1.02$); $p = .077$]. Hirudin was associated with lower rate of cardiovascular death/new MI/refractory angina at 7 days as compared with UFH [5.6% versus 6.7%, RR 0.82 (0.70–0.96); $p = .0125$]. These efficacy results were, however, balanced by an excess of major bleeding requiring transfusion with hirudin (1.2% versus 0.7%; $p = .01$).

The safety concerns were then raised against the use of hirudin, and probably caused the interruption of further development of this agent. Conversely, bivalirudin seems to be associated with less bleeding than UFH.

Bivalirudin (or hirulog)

Bivalirudin is to date the only DTI indicated for use as an anticoagulant in patients with unstable angina undergoing PCI.

The first trial assessing hirulog as antithrombin therapy in the setting of ACS was the dose-finding, randomized, double-blind TIMI 7 trial [33]. This trial included 410 patients, with unstable angina, who were to receive a 72 h infusion of hirulog at four different doses: 0.02, 0.25, 0.5, and 1 mg/kg/h. No statistical difference was observed among the four groups with respect to the primary efficacy endpoint of death/MI/rapid clinical deterioration/recurrent ischemia by 72 h (8.1%, 6.2%, 11.4%, and 6.2%, p = NS). However, the secondary endpoint of death/MI at discharge was more frequent in the lowest dose group than in all three higher dose hirulog groups (10.0% versus 3.2%, in the 0.25, 0.5, and 1 mg/kg/h groups, p = .008). Incidence of major bleeding was attributed to low hirulog (2/410, 0.5%).

A comparison between hirulog and UFH was performed in the Bivalirudin (Hirulog) Angioplasty Study [34]. In this randomized, double-blind trial, 4098 patients undergoing PCI for unstable or postinfarction angina were allocated to the following procedural anticoagulant strategies: UFH at the dose of 175 U/kg IV bolus followed by 18–24 h infusion of 15 U/kg/h plus a bolus of 60 U/kg if ACT was <350 s or bivalirudin as an IV bolus of 1 mg/kg followed by a 4 h infusion of 2.5 mg/kg/h and a 14–20 h infusion of 0.2 mg/kg/h. The primary endpoint of death/MI/abrupt vessel closure or clinical deterioration of cardiac origin was similar in both therapies by on-treatment analysis (bivalirudin 11.4%, UFH 12.2%, p = NS), however, major bleeding was significantly reduced with bivalirudin (3.8% versus 9.8%, p < .001). In a prospectively defined subgroup of 704 postinfarction angina patients, the primary endpoint was significantly reduced (9.1% versus 14.2% p = .04) and bleeding rates were still lower among bivalirudin-treated as compared to UFH-treated patients (3% versus 11.1%, p < .001).

Reanalysis of the Bivalirudin Angioplasty Study [35], including the entire intention-to-treat cohort of 4312 patients – and not just the 4098 patients treated as per protocol – indicated a significant benefit of bivalirudin in the new endpoint of death/MI/repeat revascularization at 7 days (6.2% versus 7.9%, p = .04) and 90 days (15.7% versus 18.5%, p = .01). At 180 days, the absolute risk reduction was maintained but this was not significant (23.0% versus 24.7%, p = .15). Major bleeding was again less frequent with bivalirudin than UFH (3.5% versus 9.3% p < .001) [35].

On the basis of these trials bivalirudin does appear to be more effective and safer than UFH in ACS patients undergoing PCI. However, the high dose of heparin described above resulted in a median ACT of 383 s in the UFH group (as compared to 346 s in the bivalirudin group, p < .001), which is higher than the recommended ACT, and this might have handicapped the UFH arm. Contemporary guidelines for UFH use in patients undergoing PCI and not receiving intravenous GP IIb-IIIa inhibitors recommend a bolus of 60 or 70 U/kg to a maximum of 100 U/kg with a target ACT of 300–350 s with the Hemochron device (International Technidyne, Edison, NJ) [36] used in the present study.

The results of the PROTECT-TIMI 30 trial have been presented at the 2004 American Heart Association scientific session. This randomized, open-label, multicenter study compared eptifibatide in combination with heparin (UFH or enoxaparin) with bivalirudin plus provisional eptifibatide in 857 high-risk ACS patients undergoing PCI. The primary endpoint of coronary flow reserve (angiographic endpoint) was similar in both groups. The myocardial perfusion post-PCI as assessed by TIMI myocardial perfusion grade was significantly improved in eptifibatide-treated patients (grade 3 in 57.9% eptifibatide-treated patients versus 50.9% bivalirudin-treated patients, $p = .048$). In addition, duration of ischemia among patients with an event was significantly reduced in the eptifibatide groups (36 versus 169 minutes in the bivalirudin group, $p = .013$). No major bleeding occurred in the bivalirudin group, as compared to 0.7% in the eptifibatide group ($p = $ NS); minor bleedings were less frequent among bivalirudin-treated patients (0.4% versus 2.5%, $p = .027$).

On the basis of these pilot studies, it appears that the safety and efficacy potential benefits of bivalirudin during PCI may be extended to contemporary practice with planned or provisional GP IIb-IIIa blockade. Results of the ongoing ACUITY trial should provide more definitive conclusions in the specific setting of ACS. The ACUITY trial is a phase III randomized open-label parallel group study designed to assess noninferiority of bivalirudin with or without GP IIb-IIIa inhibitors versus enoxaparin with GP IIb-IIIa inhibitors among more than 13 000 patients undergoing early invasive management for NSTE-ACS.

Other DTIs have only been studied in phase II ACS trials. Efegatran and inogatran have been compared with UFH in unstable angina patients without significant benefit [37,38]. Argatroban has only been compared with UFH as adjunctive antithrombin therapy to thrombolysis in patients with acute MI [39].

Conclusion

There is now a substantial evidence base that so far supports the use of LMWH, and more specifically enoxaparin, over UFH in ACS patients undergoing currently recommended early invasive strategy, as antithrombin strategy before and during angiography. From a practical point of view, LMWH use is safe, simple, does not need adjustment for IIb-IIIa antagonist use and requires no monitoring. The use and optimal dose of LMWH during PCI still needs to be defined more precisely. A number of studies are underway to address these issues.

If emerging evidence suggests that bivalirudin is a safe anticoagulant during urgent PCI, more definitive conclusions are awaited with respect to its efficacy in the specific setting of ACS. The results of the ongoing ACUITY trial comparing the two antithrombin strategies among ACS patients should be of great importance in that regard.

References

1. Weitz JI, Buller HR. Direct thrombin inhibitors in acute coronary syndromes: present and future. *Circulation* 2002; **105**: 1004–1011.
2. Theroux P, Ouimet H, McCans J *et al.* Aspirin, heparin, or both to treat acute unstable angina. *N Engl J Med* 1988; **319**: 1105–1111.
3. Oler A, Whooley MA, Oler J, Grady D. Adding heparin to aspirin reduces the incidence of myocardial infarction and death in patients with unstable angina. A meta-analysis. *JAMA* 1996; **276**: 811–815.
4. Warkentin TE, Levine MN, Hirsh J *et al.* Heparin-induced thrombocytopenia in patients treated with low-molecular-weight heparin or unfractionated heparin. *N Engl J Med* 1995; **332**: 1330–1335.
5. Weitz JI. Low-molecular-weight heparins. *N Engl J Med* 1997; **337**: 688–698.
6. Antman EM. The search for replacements for unfractionated heparin. *Circulation* 2001; **103**: 2310–2314.
7. Montalescot G, Bal-dit-Sollier C, Chibedi D *et al.* Comparison of effects on markers of blood cell activation of enoxaparin, dalteparin, and unfractionated heparin in patients with unstable angina pectoris or non-ST-segment elevation acute myocardial infarction (the ARMADA study). *Am J Cardiol* 2003; **91**: 925–930.
8. Montalescot G, Collet JP, Lison L *et al.* Effects of various anticoagulant treatments on von Willebrand factor release in unstable angina. *J Am Coll Cardiol* 2000; **36**: 110–114.
9. Montalescot G, Philippe F, Ankri A *et al.* Early increase of von Willebrand factor predicts adverse outcome in unstable coronary artery disease: beneficial effects of enoxaparin. French Investigators of the ESSENCE Trial. *Circulation* 1998; **98**: 294–299.
10. Sobel M, Fish WR, Toma N *et al.* Heparin modulates integrin function in human platelets. *J Vasc Surg* 2001; **33**: 587–594.
11. Xiao Z, Theroux P. Platelet activation with unfractionated heparin at therapeutic concentrations and comparisons with a low-molecular-weight heparin and with a direct thrombin inhibitor. *Circulation* 1998; **97**: 251–256.
12. Collet JP, Montalescot G, Vicaut E *et al.* Acute release of plasminogen activator inhibitor-1 in ST-segment elevation myocardial infarction predicts mortality. *Circulation* 2003; **108**: 391–394.
13. Ray KK, Morrow DA, Gibson CM, Murphy S, Antman EM, Braunwald E. Predictors of the rise in vWF after ST elevation myocardial infarction: implications for treatment strategies and clinical outcome: an ENTIRE-TIMI 23 substudy. *Eur Heart J* 2005; **26**: 440–446.
14. Antman EM, McCabe CH, Gurfinkel EP *et al.* Enoxaparin prevents death and cardiac ischemic events in unstable angina/non-Q-wave myocardial infarction. Results of the thrombolysis in myocardial infarction (TIMI) 11B trial. *Circulation* 1999; **100**: 1593–1601.
15. Cohen M, Demers C, Gurfinkel EP *et al.* A comparison of low-molecular-weight heparin with unfractionated heparin for unstable coronary artery disease. Efficacy and safety of subcutaneous enoxaparin in non-Q-wave coronary events study group. *N Engl J Med* 1997; **337**: 447–452.
16. Klein W, Buchwald A, Hillis SE *et al.* Comparison of low-molecular-weight heparin with unfractionated heparin acutely and with placebo for 6 weeks in the

management of unstable coronary artery disease. Fragmin in unstable coronary artery disease study (FRIC). *Circulation* 1997; **96**: 61–68.

17. For the FRAXIS investigators Comparison of two treatment durations (6 days and 14 days) of a low molecular weight heparin with a 6-day treatment of unfractionated heparin in the initial management of unstable angina or non-Q wave myocardial infarction: FRAX.I.S. (FRAxiparine in Ischaemic Syndrome). *Eur Heart J* 1999; **20**: 1553–1562.

18. Antman EM, Cohen M, Radley D *et al.* Assessment of the treatment effect of enoxaparin for unstable angina/non-Q-wave myocardial infarction. TIMI 11B-ESSENCE meta-analysis. *Circulation* 1999; **100**: 1602–1608.

19. Blazing MA, de Lemos JA, White HD *et al.* Safety and efficacy of enoxaparin vs unfractionated heparin in patients with non-ST-segment elevation acute coronary syndromes who receive tirofiban and aspirin: a randomized controlled trial. *JAMA* 2004; **292**: 55–64.

20. Cohen M, Theroux P, Borzak S *et al.* Randomized double-blind safety study of enoxaparin versus unfractionated heparin in patients with non-ST-segment elevation acute coronary syndromes treated with tirofiban and aspirin: the ACUTE II study. The antithrombotic combination using tirofiban and enoxaparin. *Am Heart J* 2002; **144**: 470–477.

21. Goodman SG, Fitchett D, Armstrong PW, Tan M, Langer A. Randomized evaluation of the safety and efficacy of enoxaparin versus unfractionated heparin in high-risk patients with non-ST-segment elevation acute coronary syndromes receiving the glycoprotein IIb/IIIa inhibitor eptifibatide. *Circulation* 2003; **107**: 238–244.

22. Ferguson JJ, Califf RM, Antman EM *et al.* Enoxaparin vs unfractionated heparin in high-risk patients with non-ST-segment elevation acute coronary syndromes managed with an intended early invasive strategy: primary results of the SYNERGY randomized trial. *JAMA* 2004; **292**: 45–54.

23. Petersen JL, Mahaffey KW, Hasselblad V *et al.* Efficacy and bleeding complications among patients randomized to enoxaparin or unfractionated heparin for antithrombin therapy in non-ST-segment elevation acute coronary syndromes: a systematic overview. *JAMA* 2004; **292**: 89–96.

24. Montalescot G, Collet JP, Tanguy ML *et al.* Anti-Xa activity relates to survival and efficacy in unselected acute coronary syndrome patients treated with enoxaparin. *Circulation* 2004; **110**: 392–398.

25. Collet JP, Montalescot G, Fine E *et al.* Enoxaparin in unstable angina patients who would have been excluded from randomized pivotal trials. *J Am Coll Cardiol* 2003; **41**: 8–14.

26. Collet JP, Montalescot G, Lison L *et al.* Percutaneous coronary intervention after subcutaneous enoxaparin pretreatment in patients with unstable angina pectoris. *Circulation* 2001; **103**: 658–663.

27. Collet JP, Montalescot G, Golmard JL *et al.* Subcutaneous enoxaparin with early invasive strategy in patients with acute coronary syndromes. *Am Heart J* 2004; **147**: 655–661.

28. Ferguson JJ, Antman EM, Bates ER *et al.* Combining enoxaparin and glycoprotein IIb/IIIa antagonists for the treatment of acute coronary syndromes: final results of the National Investigators Collaborating on Enoxaparin-3 (NICE-3) study. *Am Heart J* 2003; **146**: 628–634.

29. Kereiakes DJ, Montalescot G, Antman EM *et al.* Low-molecular-weight heparin therapy for non-ST-elevation acute coronary syndromes and during

percutaneous coronary intervention: an expert consensus. *Am Heart J* 2002; **144**: 615–624.

30. The GUSTO IIb investigators. A comparison of recombinant hirudin with heparin for the treatment of acute coronary syndromes. The Global Use of Strategies to Open Occluded Coronary Arteries. *N Engl J Med* 1996; **335**: 775–782.

31. The Organization to Assess Strategies for Ischemic Syndromes (OASIS) Investigators. Comparison of the effects of two doses of recombinant hirudin compared with heparin in patients with acute myocardial ischemia without ST elevation: a pilot study. *Circulation* 1997; **96**: 769–777.

32. The Organisation to Assess Strategies for Ischemic Syndromes (OASIS-2) Investigators. Effects of recombinant hirudin (lepirudin) compared with heparin on death, myocardial infarction, refractory angina, and revascularisation procedures in patients with acute myocardial ischaemia without ST elevation: a randomised trial. *Lancet* 1999; **353**: 429–438.

33. Fuchs J, Cannon CP. Hirulog in the treatment of unstable angina. Results of the Thrombin Inhibition in Myocardial Ischemia (TIMI) 7 trial. *Circulation* 1995; **92**: 727–733.

34. Bittl JA, Strony J, Brinker JA *et al.* Treatment with bivalirudin (Hirulog) as compared with heparin during coronary angioplasty for unstable or postinfarction angina. Hirulog Angioplasty Study Investigators. *N Engl J Med* 1995; **333**: 764–769.

35. Bittl JA, Chaitman BR, Feit F, Kimball W, Topol EJ. Bivalirudin versus heparin during coronary angioplasty for unstable or postinfarction angina: final report reanalysis of the Bivalirudin Angioplasty Study. *Am Heart J* 2001; **142**: 952–959.

36. Popma JJ, Ohman EM, Weitz J, Lincoff AM, Harrington RA, Berger P. Antithrombotic therapy in patients undergoing percutaneous coronary intervention. *Chest* 2001; **119**: 321S–336S.

37. Klootwijk P, Lenderink T, Meij S *et al.* Anticoagulant properties, clinical efficacy and safety of efegatran, a direct thrombin inhibitor, in patients with unstable angina. *Eur Heart J* 1999; **20**: 1101–1111.

38. Andersen K, Dellborg M. Heparin is more effective than inogatran, a low-molecular weight thrombin inhibitor in suppressing ischemia and recurrent angina in unstable coronary disease. Thrombin Inhibition in Myocardial Ischemia (TRIM) Study Group. *Am J Cardiol* 1998; **81**: 939–944.

39. Vermeer F, Vahanian A, Fels PW *et al.* Argatroban and alteplase in patients with acute myocardial infarction: the ARGAMI Study. *J Thromb Thrombolysis* 2000; **10**: 233–240.

CHAPTER 12

Statin therapy in ACS

François Schiele

Introduction

Statins, 3-hydroxy-3-methylglutaryl coenzyme A reductase, are the drugs available for the effective prevention and treatment of atherosclerotic disease. Many randomized trials have demonstrated a 20–30% reduction in cardiovascular events linked to low-density lipoprotein cholesterol (LDL-C) reduction; the time to event curves diverging after 1 year of treatment. Thus, statins have become the first-choice drug for the treatment of hypercholesterolemia and for secondary prevention in patients with atherosclerosis.

Until recently, their interest in the setting of acute coronary syndromes (ACSs) was controversial. The update of the executive summary in the third report of the National Cholesterol Education Program (NCEP) on Detection and Treatment of High Blood Cholesterol in Adults (ATP III) included the conclusions of five major clinical trials with statin therapy and reported the implications for the treatment of high-risk patients, namely patients with ACS [1] (Table 12.1).

The conclusions can be summarized in four points (Table 12.1):

1 "Intensive therapy should be considered for all patients admitted to the hospital for acute coronary syndromes."

2 The recommended target for LDL-C is <100 mg/dL, "but <70 mg/dL is a therapeutic option on the basis of available clinical trial evidence."

3 "Choice of drug and dosage should be guided in part by measurement of LDL-C within 24 h of admission" and "modification of therapy can be made at follow up if necessary to achieve the desired LDL-C level."

4 "If the baseline is higher (than 0.70 mg/dL) a high dose of statin or the combination of standard dose of statins with ezetimibe, bile acid sequestrant or nicotinic acid may be required."

Thus, aggressive lipid-lowering treatment, namely high doses of statins, are now part of the efficient interventions in ACS, in addition to double or triple antiplatelet and antithrombotic therapy or early invasive strategy.

These changes in recommendations are the repercussion of the demonstration of the biological effects on the one hand, and the results of clinical trials showing the benefit from early treatment with statins on the other hand. The new recommendation is to treat early, taking into account the potential interest of biological targets for these treatments.

Table 12.1 NCEP, Adult Treatment Panel III guidelines on cholesterol management.

Risk category	LDL-C Goal	Initiate TLC	Consider drug therapy**
High risk: CHD* or CHD risk equivalents† (10-year risk > 20%)	<100 mg/dL (optional goal: <70 mg/dL)‖	≥100 mg/dL#	≥100 mg/dL†† (<100 mg/dL: consider drug options)**
Moderately high risk: 2 + risk factors‡ (10-year risk 10% to 20%)§§	<130 mg/dL¶	≥130 mg/dL#	≥130 mg/dL (100–129 mg/dL; consider drug options)‡‡
Moderate risk: 2 + risk factors‡ (10-year risk <10%)§§	<130 mg/dL	≥130 mg/dL	≥160 mg/dL
Lower risk: 0–1 risk factor§	<160 mg/dL	≥160 mg/dL	≥190 mg/dL (160–189 mg/dL: LDL-lowering drug optional)

*CHD includes history of myocardial infarction, unstable angina, coronary artery procedures (angioplasty or bypass surgery), or evidence of clinically significant myocardial ischemia.
Source. Reproduced from Ref.1, with permission.

Rationale for the beneficial effect of statins in ACS

Acute coronary syndromes are related to plaque complication, platelet activation, and thrombus formation. Thus, the key role of a double or triple antiplatelet therapy combined with antithrombotic agents has been extensively demonstrated.

Inflammation plays a major role in the occurrence of plaque complication and acute coronary events. The term "vulnerable plaque" corresponds to histopathologic characteristics where inflammation is one of the most important elements, including presence of macrophages, monocytes, and lymphocytes. The activation of macrophages in the fibrous cap of the atherosclerotic plaque contributes through matrix metalloprotease, other cytokines, and proinflammatory mediators to the degradation of the fibrous cap, its rupture, and the initiation of the thrombotic process [2].

Besides the reduction in LDL-C, statins have several biological effects, so-called pleiotropic effects that explain their potential interest in patients with ACS: restoration of the endothelial function, antiinflammatory and antiproliferative effects, platelet inhibition and, as a result, plaque stabilization [3].

Restoration of endothelial dysfunction

Impairment of endothelial function is commonly observed in patients with multiple risk factors [4] or atherosclerosis [5] and is related to a decrease in nitric oxide (NO) production [6]. NO has various biological effects such as vasodilatation and inhibition of platelet aggregation, thrombin formation, leukocyte adhesion, and smooth muscle cells proliferation [7].

Independently of the decrease in LDL-C, statins fight against endothelial dysfunction by restoring NO release [6–9]. This improvement in endothelial function has been demonstrated after 6 months treatment [10–12], but is also effective earlier, within 24 h after treatment initiation [13,14].

Antiinflammatory effects of statins

In vitro studies have shown numerous biological effects of statins leading to plaque stabilization. The decrease in lipid content and the increase in collagen contained in the plaque [15,16] contribute to plaque stabilization. However, statins also have a direct antiinflammatory effect [17] (related to a reduction in inflammatory mediators): (1) neointimal inflammation [18]; (2) production of interleukin (IL)8, IL6, and monocyte chemotactic protein [19]; (3) CD40 ligand production [20]; NF-κB activation; (5) chemokine expression in vascular smooth muscle cells [21] and metalloproteases [16]; and last but not least, (6) reduction in high-sensitive C-reactive protein (CRP) levels [22–24]. Whether CRP is a marker of inflammation or a mediator of atherosclerosis remains unclear, but statins significantly decrease its concentration, independently of the cholesterol lowering effect [25].

Antithrombotic effect, plaque regression, and other effects

Hyperlipidemia increases platelet aggregation and thromboxane B2 formation [26–29] and platelet thrombus deposition is twice as high in patients with hypercholesterolemia [30]. Thus, statins reduce platelet activation through their lipid-lowering effect, but also exert a direct effect on the production of thromboxane B2 [29] and platelet thrombus deposition [30].

A reduction in the progression of the atherosclerotic plaque has been demonstrated with statins, either when assessed by the carotid intima-media thickness [31–33], or in coronary arteries, measured by intravascular ultrasound [34].

Additional beneficial effects, such as the reduction of life-threatening ventricular arrhythmias, have also been observed with statins in patients with atherosclerotic heart disease, and could explain the reduction in mortality after ACS [35,36].

Benefit of early statin therapy in ACS

A significant reduction in mortality has been extensively demonstrated with statins in patients with stable coronary disease [4S (Scandinavian Simvastatin Survival Study), CARE (Cholesterol and Recurrent Events), LIPID (Long-term Prevention with Pravastatin in Ischemic Disease) [37–39]] or patients with multiple risk factors [AFCAPS-TEXCAPS (Airforce/Texas Coronary Atherosclerosis Prevention Study), WOSCOPS (West of Scotland Coronary

Prevention Study), HPS [37,40,41]]. In these trials, patients with recent ACS were excluded and, where previous ACS existed, the interval between ACS and inclusion was at least 6 months in 4S [39], and 3 months in CARE [37] and in LIPID [38].

In these trials, the beneficial effect of statin therapy appeared only after 1 or 2 years and therefore, guidelines for the management of ACS did not recommend lipid-lowering agents early after onset of symptoms. In the light of observational, and later randomized studies, we moved toward recommended introduction of statins early and at high doses after ACS.

Post hoc and observational studies

The effect of early statin therapy after ACS was initially demonstrated in retrospective observational studies, where patients treated with statins had more favorable outcome after ACS than those who were not.

A post hoc observational study, pooling the data from two large trials, showed that lipid-lowering therapy, prescribed early after ACS, yielded a dramatic 50% reduction in mortality, 6 months after ACS [42].

Subsequently, large prospective studies confirmed the beneficial effect of early statin therapy in patients with ACS. In the prospective, observational study from the Swedish Register of Cardiac Intensive Care, the use of statins before discharge after myocardial infarction lowered 1 year mortality by 25% [43].

Moreover, in a subgroup analysis from the Platelet Receptor Inhibition in Ischemic Syndrome Management (PRISM) study; the rate of death and myocardial infarction after ACS was halved at 30 days in patients previously treated with statins, and interestingly, patients in whom statins were withdrawn on admission had the highest mortality [44].

Specific randomized studies

These have directly addressed the question of early use of statins with apparently divergent results. The Pravastatin Acute Coronary Treatment (PACT) study failed to demonstrate a clinical benefit, but this study was stopped early, after only 3408 patients were included instead of the 10 000 planned. Thus, only a nonsignificant reduction in the combined endpoint was observed. Although inconclusive, these results did not disprove the theory of benefit with early (within 24 h) introduction of statins after ACS, but showed the safety of this approach [45].

The Fluvastatin On Risk Diminishing after Acute myocardial Infarction (FLORIDA) study was also underpowered to demonstrate a clinical benefit of fluvastatin, given one day after myocardial infarction [46].

Lastly, the Myocardial Ischemia Reduction with Aggressive Cholesterol Lowering (MIRACL) study demonstrated a 16% reduction in the primary endpoint at 4 months between patients receiving either high doses atorvastatin (80 mg/day) early (24–96 h) after onset of ACS or placebo [47]. This study was nevertheless somewhat disappointing since the reduction of the composite endpoint was mainly the result of a reduction in the incidence of revascularization, and statin therapy did not show any reduction in mortality or myocardial infarction.

Again, the Aggrastat to Zocor (A to Z) study [48] results seemed disappointing: early and aggressive statin therapy was associated with a nonsignificant trend for reduction in the primary endpoint. However, when you look at mortality (all cause death or cardiovascular mortality), the trend for reduction with early and aggressive treatment was nearly significant (p-value .08 and .05, respectively). One concern with these results was the lack of difference during the first months, which contrasted with the results of the MIRACL or of the Pravastatin or Atorvastatin Evaluation and Infection Therapy-Thrombolysis in Myocardial Infarction 22 (PROVE IT-TIMI 22) studies [49].

The PROVE IT-TIMI 22 study included patients with recent (<10 days) ACS and three quarters of them were actively treated with multiple secondary prevention medications, such as antiplatelets, angiotensin converting enzyme inhibitors, β-blockers, and statins. Thus this study evaluated the benefit of early aggressive versus early moderate lipid-lowering therapy, on top of efficient treatments. Another important finding was the early reduction in clinical events; the event curves started to diverge at 30 days and the difference reached statistical significance at 180 days (Figure 12.1).

Early and aggressive statin therapy and the dual biological target

Contrary to previous trials, PROVE IT-TIMI 22 did not really validate the concept of early statin therapy, but rather that of "early aggressive statin" therapy in ACS. Two studies, PROVE IT-TIMI 22 and REVERSAL (Reversal of Atherosclerosis with Aggressive Lipid Lowering) [34] compared aggressive (atorvastatin 80 mg/day) with moderate (pravastatin 40 mg/day) LDL-C lowering. Only PROVE IT-TIMI 22 included patients with recent ACS, but both studies showed a benefit with the aggressive regimen.

In PROVE IT-TIMI 22, aggressive statin therapy led to a reduction in the combined endpoint, and in REVERSAL, similar therapy resulted in a reduction of coronary atherosclerotic plaque volume. One link between these two studies may be the relation between the efficacy on the endpoint and the reduction in both LDL-C and CRP concentrations [50,51].

Statin therapy provides greater clinical benefit in patients with elevated CRP [24] and the lowering effect of CRP is largely independent of LDL-C level [25]. Thus a double biological target for statin therapy (LDL-C and CRP levels) could be an important goal for prognosis. The data from the PROVE IT-TIMI 22 study fully confirmed this hypothesis, showing the difference in clinical outcome according to an LDL-C level above or below 0.70 mg/L

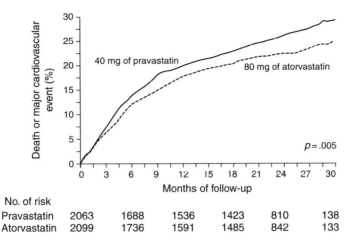

Figure 12.1 Early separation of event curves between patients with or without early aggressive statins therapy after ACS in the PROVE IT-TIMI 22 study. Reproduced from Ref. 49, with permission.

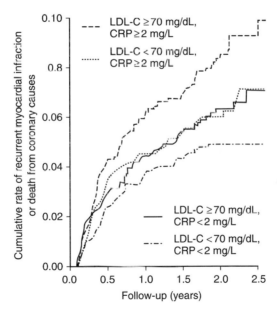

Figure 12.2 Cumulative rate of cardiovascular death or nonfatal myocardial infarction according to the quartiles of CRP and LDL-cholesterol. Reproduced from ref. 51, with permission.

and a CRP above or below 2 mg/L, both assessed 30 days after the initiation of statins (Figure 12.2) [51].

Interestingly, although atorvastatin provided better outcomes than pravastatin in the PROVE IT-TIMI 22 study, after stratification on the levels of LDL-C

Table 12.2 Rates of progression according to the change in LDL-C and CRP levels.*

Subgroup	No. of Patients	Percent atheroma volume†			Total atheroma volume (mm³)†		
		Median	95% CI	Mean ± SD	Median	95% CI	Mean ± SD
Reduction in LDL-C and CRP both greater than median	141	0.24 (−2.8 to 3.5)‡	−0.77 to 0.54	0.33 ± 5.3	−1.98 (−23.0 to 10.8)‡	−6.26 to 3.67	−2.41 ± 31.6
Reduction in LDL-C greater than median, reduction in CRP less than median	106	0.81 (−2.0 to 4.8)	−0.32 to 1.81	1.62 ± 4.7	2.06 (−12.8 to 21.5)	−3.26 to 6.41	4.04 ± 28.7
Reduction in LDL-C less than median, reduction in CRP greater than median	108	1.21 (−2.0 to 4.0)	−0.31 to 2.08	0.91 ± 4.9	−1.04 (−18.6 to 22.5)	−6.78 to 8.74	1.42 ± 29.2
Reduction in LDL-C and CRP both less than median	141	1.82 (−1.5 to 5.1)	1.0 to 2.84	2.25 ± 5.0	8.21 (−11.8 to 27.5)	0.40 to 13.05	7.49 ± 27.5

*CRP levels were not available for six patients at baseline or follow-up. The subgroups were formed on the basis of the median percent change in LDL cholesterol of −37.1% and the median percent change in CRP of −21.4%.

† Values in parentheses are interquartile ranges. Confidence intervals (CIs) are for the medians.

‡$p = .001$ for the comparison with the subgroup in which the reduction in the levels of both LDL-C and CRP was less than the median reduction (by Wilcoxon's rank-sum test).

Source: Reproduced from Ref. 50, with permission.

and CRP, there was no residual effect of the type of statin, suggesting that only the two biological targets are important, whatever the statin used.

These findings were confirmed in patients in a stable condition in the REVERSAL study: both LDL-C and CRP were independent predictors of the magnitude of plaque progression (Table 12.2) [50].

Conclusion

The benefit of giving statins early after ACS is based on a robust biological rationale and demonstrated by clinical evidence, despite possible side effects. All taken together, the results of clinical trials also show that the beneficial effect of statins is more likely achieved with aggressive treatment, namely high doses of statins. Little is known about the efficacy of other lipid-lowering treatments in ACS, but the benefit cannot be predicted only by the LDL-C reduction. Early clinical benefits from statins derive from antiinflammatory effects, whereas the mid- and long-term benefits are the reflection of lipid-lowering properties.

Thus, not only has early stain therapy become one of the recommended medications in ACS, but the question now is, what low should both the CRP and the LDL-C levels be, in order to avoid the recurrence of acute vascular events and the progression of the atherosclerosis.

Last, patients' long-term adherence to statin therapy and other evidence-based therapies will also play an important role and need careful attention [52].

References

1. Grundy SM, Cleeman JI, Merz CN et al. Implications of recent clinical trials for the National Cholesterol Education Program Adult Treatment Panel III guidelines. *J Am Coll Cardiol* 2004; **44**: 720–732.
2. Ross R. Atherosclerosis – an inflammatory disease. *N Engl J Med* 1999; **340**(2): 115–126.
3. Davies MJ. Going from immutable to mutable atherosclerotic plaques. *Am J Cardiol* 2001; **88**(4A): 2F–9F.
4. Vita JA, Yeung AC, Winniford M et al. Effect of cholesterol-lowering therapy on coronary endothelial vasomotor function in patients with coronary artery disease. *Circulation* 2000; **102**(8): 846–851.
5. Egashira K, Inou T, Hirooka Y et al. Impaired coronary blood flow response to acetylcholine in patients with coronary risk factors and proximal atherosclerotic lesions. *J Clin Invest* 1993; **91**(1): 29–37.
6. Endres M, Laufs U, Huang Z et al. Stroke protection by 3-hydroxy-3-methylglutaryl (HMG)-CoA reductase inhibitors mediated by endothelial nitric oxide synthase. *Proc Natl Acad Sci USA* 1998; **95**(15): 8880–8885.
7. Di Napoli P, Taccardi AA, Oliver M, De Caterina R. Statins and stroke: evidence for cholesterol-independent effects. *Eur Heart J* 2002; **23**(24): 1908–1921.
8. Davis ME, Harrison DG. Cracking down on caveolin: role of 3-hydroxy-3-methylglutaryl coenzyme A reductase inhibitors in modulating edothelial cell nitric oxide production. *Circulation* 2001; **103**(1): 2–4.

9. Laufs U. Beyond lipid-lowering: effects of statins on endothelial nitric oxide. *Eur J Clin Pharmacol* 2003; **58**(11): 719–731.

10. Treasure CB, Klein JL, Weintraub WS *et al*. Beneficial effects of cholesterol-lowering therapy on the coronary endothelium in patients with coronary artery disease. *N Engl J Med* 1995; **332**(8): 481–487.

11. Anderson TJ, Meredith IT, Charbonneau F *et al*. Endothelium-dependent coronary vasomotion relates to the susceptibility of LDL to oxidation in humans. *Circulation* 1996; **93**(9): 1647–1650.

12. Egashira K, Hirooka Y, Kai H *et al*. Reduction in serum cholesterol with pravastatin improves endothelium-dependent coronary vasomotion in patients with hypercholesterolemia. *Circulation* 1994; **89**(6): 2519–2524.

13. Wassmann S, Faul A, Hennen B, Scheller B, Bohm M, Nickenig G. Rapid effect of 3-hydroxy-3-methylglutaryl coenzyme a reductase inhibition on coronary endothelial function. *Circ Res* 2003; **93**(9): e98–e103.

14. Laufs U, La Fata V, Plutzky J, Liao JK. Upregulation of endothelial nitric oxide synthase by HMG CoA reductase inhibitors. *Circulation* 1998; **97**(12): 1129–1135.

15. Weissberg PL, Clesham GJ, Bennett MR. Is vascular smooth muscle cell proliferation beneficial? *Lancet* 1996; **347**(8997): 305–307.

16. Crisby M, Nordin-Fredriksson G, Shah PK, Yano J, Zhu J, Nilsson J. Pravastatin treatment increases collagen content and decreases lipid content, inflammation, metalloproteinases, and cell death in human carotid plaques: implications for plaque stabilization. *Circulation* 2001; **103**(7): 926–933.

17. Ridker PM. Should statin therapy be considered for patients with elevated C-reactive protein? The need for a definitive clinical trial. *Eur Heart J* 2001; **22**(23): 2135–2137.

18. Bustos C, Hernandez-Presa MA, Ortego M *et al*. HMG-CoA reductase inhibition by atorvastatin reduces neointimal inflammation in a rabbit model of atherosclerosis. *J Am Coll Cardiol* 1998; **32**(7): 2057–2064.

19. Yoshida M, Sawada T, Ishii H *et al*. Hmg-CoA reductase inhibitor modulates monocyte-endothelial cell interaction under physiological flow conditions *in vitro*: involvement of Rho GTPase-dependent mechanism. *Arterioscler Thromb Vasc Biol* 2001; **21**(7): 1165–1171.

20. Wagner AH, Gebauer M, Guldenzoph B, Hecker M. 3-hydroxy-3-methylglutaryl coenzyme A reductase-independent inhibition of CD40 expression by atorvastatin in human endothelial cells. *Arterioscler Thromb Vasc Biol* 2002; **22**(11): 1784–1789.

21. Ortego M, Bustos C, Hernandez-Presa MA *et al*. Atorvastatin reduces NF-kappaB activation and chemokine expression in vascular smooth muscle cells and mononuclear cells. *Atherosclerosis* 1999; **147**(2): 253–261.

22. Jialal I, Stein D, Balis D, Grundy SM, Adams-Huet B, Devaraj S. Effect of hydroxymethyl glutaryl coenzyme a reductase inhibitor therapy on high sensitive C-reactive protein levels. *Circulation* 2001; **103**(15): 1933–1935.

23. Kinlay S, Schwartz GG, Olsson AG *et al*. High-dose atorvastatin enhances the decline in inflammatory markers in patients with acute coronary syndromes in the MIRACL study. *Circulation* 2003; **108**(13): 1560–1566.

24. Ridker PM, Rifai N, Clearfield M *et al*. Measurement of C-reactive protein for the targeting of statin therapy in the primary prevention of acute coronary events. *N Engl J Med* 2001; **344**(26): 1959–1965.

25. Albert MA, Danielson E, Rifai N, Ridker PM. Effect of statin therapy on C-reactive protein levels: the pravastatin inflammation/CRP evaluation (PRINCE): a randomized trial and cohort study. *JAMA* 2001; **286**(1): 64–70.

26. Stuart MJ, Gerrard JM, White JG. Effect of cholesterol on production of thromboxane b2 by platelets *in vitro*. *N Engl J Med* 1980; **302**(1): 6–10.

27. Carvalho AC, Colman RW, Lees RS. Platelet function in hyperlipoproteinemia. *N Engl J Med* 1974; **290**(8): 434–438.

28. Davi G, Averna M, Catalano I *et al*. Increased thromboxane biosynthesis in type IIa hypercholesterolemia. *Circulation* 1992; **85**(5): 1792–1798.

29. Notarbartolo A, Davi G, Averna M *et al*. Inhibition of thromboxane biosynthesis and platelet function by simvastatin in type IIa hypercholesterolemia. *Arterioscler Thromb Vasc Biol* 1995; **15**(2): 247–251.

30. Lacoste L, Lam JY, Hung J, Letchacovski G, Solymoss CB, Waters D. Hyperlipidemia and coronary disease. Correction of the increased thrombogenic potential with cholesterol reduction. *Circulation* 1995; **92**(11): 3172–3177.

31. Taylor AJ, Kent SM, Flaherty PJ, Coyle LC, Markwood TT, Vernalis MN. ARBITER: Arterial Biology for the Investigation of the Treatment Effects of Reducing Cholesterol. A randomized trial comparing the effects of atorvastatin and pravastatin on carotid intima medial thickness. *Circulation* 2002; **106**(16): 2055–2060.

32. Crouse JR, III, Grobbee DE, O'Leary DH *et al*. Measuring Effects on intima media Thickness: an Evaluation Of Rosuvastatin in subclinical atherosclerosis – the rationale and methodology of the METEOR study. *Cardiovasc Drugs Ther* 2004; **18**(3): 231–238.

33. Smilde TJ, van Wissen S, Wollersheim H, Trip MD, Kastelein JJ, Stalenhoef AF. Effect of aggressive versus conventional lipid lowering on atherosclerosis progression in familial hypercholesterolaemia (ASAP): a prospective, randomised, double-blind trial. *Lancet* 2001; **357**(9256): 577–581.

34. Nissen SE, Tuzcu EM, Schoenhagen P *et al*. Effect of intensive compared with moderate lipid-lowering therapy on progression of coronary atherosclerosis: a randomized controlled trial. *JAMA* 2004; **291**(9): 1071–1080.

35. Mitchell LB, Powell JL, Gillis AM, Kehl V, Hallstrom AP. Are lipid-lowering drugs also antiarrhythmic drugs? An analysis of the Antiarrhythmics versus Implantable Defibrillators (AVID) trial. *J Am Coll Cardiol* 2003; **42**(1): 81–87.

36. De Sutter J, Tavernier R, De Buyzere M, Jordaens L, De Backer G. Lipid lowering drugs and recurrences of life-threatening ventricular arrhythmias in high-risk patients. *J Am Coll Cardiol* 2000; **36**(3): 766–772.

37. Sacks FM, Pfeffer MA, Moye LA *et al*. The effect of pravastatin on coronary events after myocardial infarction in patients with average cholesterol levels. Cholesterol and Recurrent Events Trial investigators. *N Engl J Med* 1996; **335**(14): 1001–1009.

38. Tonkin AM, Colquhoun D, Emberson J *et al*. Effects of pravastatin in 3260 patients with unstable angina: results from the LIPID study. *Lancet* 2000; **356**(9245): 1871–1875.

39. Scandinavian Simvastatin Survival Study Group. Randomised trial of cholesterol lowering in 4444 patients with coronary heart disease: the Scandinavian Simvastatin Survival Study (4S). *Lancet* 1994; **344**(8934): 1383–1389.

40. Shepherd J, Cobbe SM, Ford I *et al*. Prevention of coronary heart disease with pravastatin in men with hypercholesterolemia. West of Scotland Coronary Prevention Study Group. *N Engl J Med* 1995; **333**(20): 1301–1307.

41. ALLHAT Officers and Coordinators for the ALLHAT Collaborative Research Group. Major outcomes in moderately hypercholesterolemic, hypertensive patients randomized to pravastatin vs usual care: the Antihypertensive and Lipid-Lowering Treatment to Prevent Heart Attack Trial (ALLHAT-LLT). *JAMA* 2002; **288**(23): 2998–3007.

42. Aronow HD, Topol EJ, Roe MT *et al.* Effect of lipid-lowering therapy on early mortality after acute coronary syndromes: an observational study. *Lancet* 2001; **357**(9262): 1063–1068.

43. Stenestrand U, Wallentin L. Early statin treatment following acute myocardial infarction and 1-year survival. *JAMA* 2001; **285**(4): 430–436.

44. Heeschen C, Hamm CW, Laufs U, Snapinn S, Bohm M, White HD. Withdrawal of statins increases event rates in patients with acute coronary syndromes. *Circulation* 2002; **105**(12): 1446–1452.

45. Thompson PL, Meredith I, Amerena J, Campbell TJ, Sloman JG, Harris PJ. Effect of pravastatin compared with placebo initiated within 24 hours of onset of acute myocardial infarction or unstable angina: the Pravastatin in Acute Coronary Treatment (PACT) trial. *Am Heart J* 2004; **148**(1): e2.

46. Liem AH, van Boven AJ, Veeger NJ *et al.* Effect of fluvastatin on ischaemia following acute myocardial infarction: a randomized trial. *Eur Heart J* 2002; **23**(24): 1931–1937.

47. Schwartz GG, Olsson AG, Ezekowitz MD *et al.* Effects of atorvastatin on early recurrent ischemic events in acute coronary syndromes: the MIRACL study: a randomized controlled trial. *JAMA* 2001; **285**(13): 1711–1718.

48. de Lemos JA, Blazing MA, Wiviott SD *et al.* Early intensive vs a delayed conservative simvastatin strategy in patients with acute coronary syndromes: phase Z of the A to Z trial. *JAMA* 2004; **292**(11): 1307–1316. Epub 2004 Aug 30.

49. Cannon CP, Braunwald E, McCabe CH *et al.* Intensive versus moderate lipid lowering with statins after acute coronary syndromes. *N Engl J Med* 2004; **350**(15): 1495–1504. Epub 2004 Mar 08.

50. Nissen SE, Tuzcu EM, Schoenhagen P *et al.* Statin therapy, LDL cholesterol, C-reactive protein, and coronary artery disease. *N Engl J Med* 2005; **352**(1): 29–38.

51. Ridker PM, Cannon CP, Morrow D *et al.* C-reactive protein levels and outcomes after statin therapy. *N Engl J Med* 2005; **352**(1): 20–8.

52. Eagle KA, Kline-Rogers E, Goodman SG *et al.* Adherence to evidence-based therapies after discharge for acute coronary syndromes: an ongoing prospective, observational study. *Am J Med* 2004; **117**(2): 73–81.

Section seven:
Myocardial revascularization

CHAPTER 13

Percutaneous coronary interventions and stenting/CABG in non-ST-segment elevation acute coronary syndromes

Nicolas Meneveau and Jean-Pierre Bassand

Introduction

The optimal early management of patients presenting with non-ST-segment elevation acute coronary syndromes (NSTE-ACSs) has been studied extensively over the past 10 years. Treatment of patients presenting with an NSTE-ACS aims at immediate relief of ischemia, and the prevention of serious adverse events, such as death, myocardial (re)infarction, and life-threatening arrhythmias.

Eight randomized trials have assessed the merits of an invasive strategy involving routine cardiac catheterization, with revascularization if feasible, versus a conservative strategy where angiography and revascularization are reserved for patients who have evidence of recurrent ischemia either at rest or on provocative testing [1–8]. The first three of these trials failed to demonstrate a significant benefit in patients who underwent early invasive strategy [1–3]. However, the subsequent five trials, in which glycoprotein IIb/IIIa inhibitors (GP IIb/IIIa inhibitors) and intracoronary stents were used extensively, have shown a significant benefit of an early invasive approach in high-risk patients [4–8].

This chapter presents a comprehensive review of the current medical evidence in this debate. We focus particularly on risk stratification and the identification of patients most likely to benefit from each approach. Lastly, using the results of registries, we also examine what happens in the real world, when the results of clinical trials are translated into routine practice.

Early invasive or conservative therapy in randomized trials: the evidence so far

Revascularization, including percutaneous coronary intervention (PCI) or coronary artery bypass grafting (CABG), in NSTE-ACS patients is performed to treat ongoing myocardial ischemia and to prevent recurrent ischemia, progression to myocardial infarction (MI), or death. The indications for myocardial revascularization and the preferred approach depend on clinical characteristics, and the extent and angiographic characteristics of the lesions identified by coronary angiography.

Results from different randomized trials are conflicting. Findings from the FRISC II, the TACTICS-TIMI 18, and the RITA 3 trials suggested that an early invasive strategy was indicated in patients with electrocardiographic evidence of myocardial ischemia or elevation of biochemical markers of myocardial damage [4,6,8]. However, these results diverged from the neutral or negative findings of the previously published VANQWISH, TIMI IIIB, and MATE trials [1–3].

When comparing different trials of intervention versus conservative treatment, several factors must be taken into account. The Veterans Affairs study of unstable angina compared CABG surgery with medical treatment, and showed no survival benefit, except in patients with poor left ventricular function [1]. TIMI IIIB, published in 1994 when stent procedures and adjunctive medical therapy were not routinely used, reported shorter hospital stays, fewer readmissions, and less ischemia, but no significant decrease in death and MI in invasively treated patients [2]. The VANQWISH trial showed an increase in mortality that was sustained for more than a year in patients assigned early to invasive approach after NSTE-ACS. However, many of the deaths occurred among patients assigned to the early invasive group, but who never actually underwent any intervention [1]. In addition, in both of these trials there was only a modest difference in the frequency of interventional strategies between the invasive and conservative groups (61% versus 49% at 42 days in TIMI IIIB and 44% versus 33% after 1 year in VANQWISH). In contrast, in the FRISC II and RITA 3 trials, the groups were more clearly distinguished [4,8].

In the FRISC II trial, intervention led to a reduction in deaths that was not apparent until after 3 months and was sustained at 24 months [risk ratio (RR) = 0.68; CI, 0.47–0.98]. In addition, there was a significant reduction in MI (RR = 0.72; CI, 0.57–0.91) at 2 years in the invasive compared with the noninvasive group [9]. The greatest advantages were seen in patients most at risk, namely older men, with longer duration of angina, chest pain at rest, ST-segment depression, and elevated biochemical markers of myocardial damage. Furthermore, invasive strategy also leads to substantially better and more rapid symptom relief, and fewer readmissions than a noninvasive approach. Actually, FRISC II was the only study that showed a significant decrease in mortality from invasive therapy. The differences between previous studies and the FRISC II trial could be explained by the timing of the invasive procedures, which, in FRISC, included an initial period of stabilization with an intense antithrombotic medication. There was a significant relative decrease of 22% in death and MI in the invasive group compared with the noninvasive group after 6 months. But the lower event rate observed at 6 months in invasively treated patients was the result of a significant decrease in MI, with a nonsignificant decrease in total mortality.

The relative risks for mortality from the remaining studies were all nonsignificant and sometimes conflicting. In the TACTICS-TIMI 18 trial, the early invasive strategy was associated with a reduction in the combined endpoint of death/MI/repeat hospital admission [6]. However, there was no difference in death alone: 3.3% versus 3.5%, respectively in the invasive and conservative groups at 6 months. The benefit of an early invasive approach in the TACTICS-TIMI 18 trial was mainly seen in the first months, whereas in the FRISC II trial there was a continuous increase in benefit during the 2-year follow-up period. In addition, TACTICS-TIMI 18 reported an excess of early deaths with intervention (2.2% versus 1.6%), but these proportions were balanced at 6 months (3.3% versus 3.5%) [4,6]. Based on risk stratification concepts from FRISC II and TACTICS-TIMI 18, the largest benefit was observed in higher-risk and no gains in lower-risk patients.

More recently, RITA 3 showed a 34% reduction in the risk of death, reinfarction, or refractory angina in the invasive group at 4 months, mainly due to a 50% reduction in the rise of refractory angina (RR 0.47; 95% CI, 0.32–0.68), but without any survival benefit [8]. The heterogeneity in outcomes between these different trials might be related to the differences in proportions and timing of revascularization [10]. In FRISC II, TACTICS-TIMI 18, and RITA 3, early revascularization was performed in 85%, 73%, and 66% of patients, respectively, with significant coronary lesions [4,6,8]. In RITA 3, the benefits of an early invasive strategy could also have been diluted by events in invasive strategy patients with significant lesions without or awaiting revascularization, and by early crossover to the invasive strategy, as in 36% of the noninvasive group in TACTICS-TIMI 18. (The ICTUS trial, reported at the annual congress of the European Society of Cardiology in Munich, August 2004, did not show any difference between early invasive and conservative treatment. The data are not incorporated in this review, since they are not yet published.)

Data from metaanalyses

A composite analysis of all of the trials reveals that significant heterogeneity does exist with respect to the risk ratios of death or MI at 1 year (Figure 13.1) [8]. This composite analysis performed by Fox and colleagues, suggests a RR of 0.88 (95% CI, 0.78–0.99), on the borderline of significance, thus not providing conclusive evidence for a benefit with respect to death or MI.

A recently published metaanalysis [11] combined data from five studies in 6766 NSTE-ACS patients who were randomized to either routine invasive or conservative strategy in the era of GP IIb/IIIa inhibitors and intracoronary stents. Compared with conservative strategy, an invasive approach suggested a 20% reduction in mortality at 6–12 months (RR = 0.80; 95% CI, 0.60–0.99). There was no significant change in mortality at 1 month follow-up, although

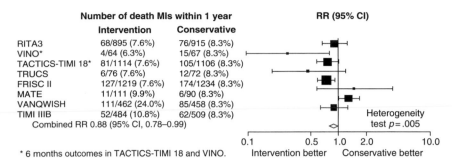

Figure 13.1 Reported incidence of MI and/or death in eight trials of intervention versus conservative management for NSTE-ACSs. Reproduced from Ref. 8, with permission.

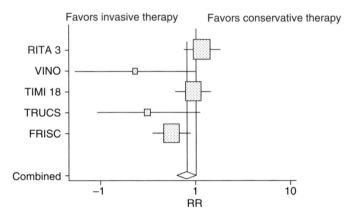

Figure 13.2 Plot for mortality at 6–12 months for invasive versus conservative strategies. Summary estimate: RR = 0.80; 95% CI, 0.63–1.03. Reproduced from Ref. 8, with permission.

the composite endpoint of death or MI was significantly reduced throughout all periods of follow-up (Figure 13.2).

However, the authors reported some heterogeneity in these outcomes. The relative risk for death was subsequently reduced by removing the two studies – TRUCS and RITA 3 – with a low proportion of troponin-positive patients, supposed to be at lower risk (RR = 0.70; CI 95%, 0.52–0.96) [5,8]. Invasive therapy reduced the relative risk of death or MI at 6–12 months to 0.74 (95% CI, 0.59–0.94) in the 2322 troponin-positive patients of this metaanalysis. Conversely, the relative risk for death assessed from studies conducted before the GP IIb/IIIa inhibitor and stent era suggested increased mortality at 6–12 months (RR = 1.31; 95% CI, 0.98–1.75) [1–3].

The need for risk stratification

The benefit of an early invasive strategy appears to be greater with increasing baseline risk. In different trials, the benefit of an early invasive strategy was consistent among the major subgroups, with a significantly greater benefit in patients with ST-segment changes at baseline, in diabetic patients, or in those with positive troponin on admission [4,6].

ST-segment depression

Patients with ST-segment depression on the electrocardiogram (ECG) at admission have a markedly increased risk for future cardiac events compared with those without ST-segment depression [12]. ST-segment depression occurred in 45.5% of patients in FRISC II and was associated with three-vessel disease or left main stenosis in 45% of the patients treated invasively. Thus, almost half of the patients with three-vessel or left main disease and ST-segment depression would not be identified with the noninvasive approach. Therefore, in NSTE-ACS with ST-segment depression, an early invasive approach has a very high priority. In FRISC II, an early invasive strategy had a remarkable effect in patients with ST-segment depression at entry: death or MI after 12 months was reduced from 18.2% to 12% ($p = .004$), while mortality was reduced from 5.8% to 3.3% ($p = .05$). In patients without ST-segment depression the corresponding rates concerning death/MI were 10.4% and 8.9%, and for mortality 2.0% and 1.2% (NS). Hence, there is an almost doubled risk of future cardiac events in patients with ST-segment depression, and a relative reduction of 42% in mortality when treated invasively.

In contrast, new T-wave inversion was associated with significantly lower mortality than was ST-segment depression or no ECG changes, even though a vast majority of the patients with T-wave inversion had elevated troponin levels and multivessel disease. T-wave inversion seems to identify a subgroup of patients with NSTE-ACS who have a favorable long-term outcome if revascularized very early [13].

Cardiac biomarkers

The value of cardiac troponin levels as a means of identifying high-risk patients has been well documented [14–16]. Elevations in troponin T and I levels have been found to identify patients who could most benefit from more intensive antithrombotic therapy, including low molecular weight heparin and inhibition of GP IIb/IIIa [17–20]. Furthermore, patients with elevated troponin levels at baseline derived a greater benefit from the early invasive strategy than those with no troponin elevation. Indeed, there is a 39% relative risk reduction of death, nonfatal MI, or rehospitalization for an ACS, with the use of the invasive strategy rather than the conservative strategy, in patients with positive troponin at admission in TACTICS-TIMI 18 trial. Similarly, invasive therapy was associated with a 26% reduction in death or MI at 6–12 months in 2322 troponin-positive patients in a recently published metaanalysis [11].

Conversely, patients with negative troponin have similar outcomes with either strategy. Interestingly, troponin T remains a strong predictor of mortality, even at low levels, in patients with NSTE-ACS who are treated with early revascularization [21]. Thus, assessment of troponin T or I at the time of presentation must be incorporated into management approaches for the triage of patients with respect to the optimal treatment strategy.

Brain-type natriuretic peptide or C-reactive protein (CRP) are other potential biomarkers to further stratify risk. Several recent prospective cohorts have shown that patients with a negative troponin and elevated brain natriuretic peptide levels have a six- to sevenfold increase in the odds of death [22,23]. A recent subanalysis from the TACTICS-TIMI 18 trial also revealed a trend toward improvement in patients with high brain natriuretic peptide who underwent a routine invasive approach [22]. In addition, a CRP level >10 mg/L has been shown to be a strong independent predictor of short- and long-term mortality after NSTE-ACS treated with early revascularization [24]. In the near future, risk stratification using these markers may help to guide troponin-negative patients toward the most appropriate therapy.

TIMI risk score

The TIMI risk score combines seven variables in an evenly weighted scale, and helps to identify patients that benefit most from GP IIb/IIIa inhibitors [25] and an early invasive strategy [4,6]. Analysis of combined data from the TIMI IIIB and TACTICS-TIMI 18 trials found that the efficacy of an early invasive strategy was strongly related to a patient's baseline risk, based on the TIMI risk score for NSTE-ACS [2,6,25]. Patients were risk stratified on the basis of the seven following baseline characteristics: age $\geq$ 65 years, $\geq$3 risk factors for coronary artery disease, known coronary artery disease, use of aspirin in the last 7 days, $\geq$2 episodes of angina in the previous 24 h, ST deviation $\geq$ 0.5 mm and elevated cardiac biomarkers of necrosis. Patients were assigned 1 point for each risk factor that was present, and were categorized on the basis of their TIMI risk score as low risk (0–2 points), intermediate risk (3–4 points), or high risk (5–7 points). The odds ration (OR) for the composite endpoint of death, MI, or rehospitalization for ACS at 6 months with an early invasive versus a conservative strategy was 1.39 (95% CI, 1.02–1.88; $p = .03$) in low-risk patients, 0.80 (95% CI, 0.64–0.99; $p = .04$) in intermediate-risk patients, and 0.57 (95% CI, 0.38–0.87; $p = .0083$) in high-risk patients. In a multivariate analysis, these differences in the efficacy of an invasive strategy based on risk group were highly statistically significant (Table 13.1). Interestingly, intermediate- or high-risk patients made up 75% of the TACTICS-TIMI 18 population. For the 25% of patients who were deemed to be at low risk for death and ischemic events, the outcomes were similar with the use of either strategy. Thus, using event rates stratified by the TIMI risk score reveals no benefit in low-risk patients, but approximately 20% and 40% reductions in death and ischemic complications in intermediate- and high-risk patients, respectively.

Table 13.1 Rates of death, MI, or rehospitalization for ACS stratified by TIMI risk score, trial, and treatment strategy, in combined data from TIMI IIIB and TACTICS-TIMI 18 [25].

TIMI risk score	Event rate %		OR	95% CI
	Invasive	Conservative		
Low (0–2)	19.8	15.1	1.39	1.02–1.88
Intermediate (3–4)	18.2	21.8	0.80	0.64–0.99
High (5–7)	22.7	34	0.57	0.38–0.87

Risk stratification according to guidelines

In their definition of high-risk patients who should benefit from early invasive strategy, the ESC guidelines [26] also include:

- Patients who develop hemodynamic instability within the observation period
- Patients with major arrhythmias
- Diabetics
- Patients with an ECG pattern that precludes assessment of ST-segment changes.

The updated ACC/AHA guidelines added patients with chronic heart failure symptoms, depressed left ventricular function, high-risk findings on non-invasive stress testing, prior CABG, or who underwent PCI within the last 6 months [27].

Invasive strategy in women

For NSTE-ACS, reports have been disparate about whether different outcomes exist for women when a routine invasive management strategy is used [4,8,28–33]. Women were noted to have less frequent elevations in cardiac markers and lower prevalence of severe coronary artery disease, as compared to men [4,6]. Indeed, in TACTICS-TIMI 18, the benefit of invasive management is primarily confined to women with markers of increased risk, namely those with ST-segment changes and elevated troponin levels [8,34], thus explaining why women in RITA 3, who were at low risk of death and MI, did not benefit from an invasive approach [8]. Similarly, in the metaanalysis by Boersma *et al.* the authors showed a benefit in women with elevated troponin who underwent PCI (OR = 0.80; 95% CI, 0.53–1.21) [35].

A recent prospective cohort study conducted in 1450 consecutive NSTE-ACS patients reported that women treated with very early aggressive revascularization have a better long-term outcome as compared with men [34]. In this study, women were noted to be older and have less frequent prior MI or CABG, as well as lower prevalence of severe coronary artery disease, compared with men. The PCI : CABG ratio was 4 : 1 in men and 5 : 1 in women. The combined endpoint of death or nonfatal MI was significantly reduced to 20 months in women compared to men (OR = 0.65; 95% CI, 0.28–0.92). In fact, with PCI-based very early revascularization, female gender was found to be a significant independent predictor of event-free survival. Thus, both the timing and the PCI : CABG ratio of the revascularization strategy may be important contributors to gender differences in the outcome of patients with NSTE-ACS. Indeed, with coronary angiography performed within the first 7 days and a PCI : CABG ratio of 1 : 1, women randomized to the invasive strategy in the FRISC II trial had a worse outcome than men.

Percutaneous coronary interventions

Advances such as intracoronary stenting and GP IIb/IIIa inhibitors gained clinical acceptance and were used to varying degrees in the FRISC II, TACTICS-TIMI 18, RITA 3, and ISAR-COOL trials [2,6,8,36]. These new therapeutic modalities for the care of patients with NSTE-ACS have been associated with lower rates of adverse cardiac events and a trend toward greater benefit of an early invasive strategy [25]. Overall, 65% of PCI patients were treated with a stent in FRISC II, 83% in TACTICS-TIMI 18 and 88% in RITA 3. Among patients who underwent PCI, 10% were treated with GP IIb/IIIb in FRISC II, 25% in RITA 3, and 94% (by design) in TACTICS-TIMI 18.

A metaanalysis of six major trials of patients with ACS undergoing PCI who were randomized to either a GP IIb/IIIa inhibitor or placebo found a significant reduction in death or MI at 30 days among the active treatment group (RR = 0.91; 95% CI, 0.84–0.98) [34].

By multivariable analysis, there was a trend for an early invasive strategy to be more beneficial in TACTICS-TIMI 18 than in TIMI IIIB (OR = 0.79; 95% CI, 0.56–1.11) [2,6]. These studies had virtually identical enrollment criteria and designs, except that upstream GP IIb/IIIa inhibition was mandated and coronary artery stenting was routinely used in TACTICS-TIMI 18 [25].

The explanations for this difference are likely multifactorial. In TACTICS-TIMI 18, 85% of patients who underwent PCI received an intracoronary stent, whereas no patient in TIMI IIIB received a stent. Stenting has been shown in multiple interventional studies to prevent restenosis and hence the need for target vessel revascularization. The safety and success of PCI in ACS have been markedly improved with the use of stents and administration of GP IIb/IIIa inhibitors. In this setting, stent implantation helps to mechanically stabilize the disrupted plaque at the lesion site [37]. Thus, the use of stents might partially explain the lower rate of rehospitalization for ACS, especially since patients who underwent stenting very likely also received a thienopyridine for 2–4 weeks. Results obtained with drug eluting stents are even more promising, since no restenosis occurred in the 220 patients with unstable angina in the RAVEL study [38].

Conversely, the use of GP IIb/IIIa inhibitors might be responsible for the reduction in the rate of death or MI. Indeed, treatment with tirofiban was associated with a 20% reduction in the rate of death or MI through

6 months in the PRISM-PLUS trial, and this benefit was seen as early as 48 h [39]. Moreover, a subanalysis of unstable angina patients from the EPIC, EPILOG, and CAPTURE trials convincingly demonstrated that intravenous abciximab significantly reduced the complication rate during balloon angioplasty, and that this initial benefit was sustained at 6 months and beyond [40–42].

In TACTICS-TIMI 18, treatment included the GP IIb/IIIa antagonist tirofiban, which was administered for an average of 22 h before coronary angiography. The routine use of the GP IIb/IIIa antagonists in this trial may have eliminated the excess risk of early (within 7 days) acute MI in the invasive arm, an excess risk that was observed in FRISC II and others trials in which there was no routine "upstream" use of a GP IIb/IIIa antagonist [2,3,4,6]. Although an early invasive approach is more efficacious in reducing adverse cardiac events when used in the setting of GP IIb/IIIa inhibition and intracoronary stenting, the optimum time of commencing these drugs – "upstream" as in TACTICS or just before the PCI – is not fully established. Recently published data from the ISAR-COOL randomized trial reported better clinical outcomes in patients receiving antithrombotic pretreatment for less then 6 h compared with patients receiving the same treatment for 3–5 days [36].

Coronary artery bypass surgery

In the VANQWISII trial, there was a weak trend toward lower mortality in the surgical group in the beginning, but this trend disappeared during the 10-year follow-up period [1]. The initial advantage in favor of the conservative strategy was related to a 30-day mortality rate of 11.6% after CABG in the invasive group, which was much higher than the corresponding mortality rate of 2.1% observed in the FRISC II trial. Thus, provided that the early procedure-related hazards of CABG can be kept at a low rate, an early strategy may lead to improved survival and a reduced risk of MI.

Among patients randomized to the invasive strategy, CABG surgery was performed in 35.2% of patients in FRISC II [4], 20% in TACTICS-TIMI 18 [6], and 22% in RITA 3 [8]. At 1 month, the mortality rate of the surgically treated patients was 2% in FRISC II, 1.7% in TACTICS, and 3.0% in RITA 3. These very low operative mortality may result from modern surgical techniques, since operative mortality rates and perioperative MI rates are known to be higher in patients with postinfarction unstable angina (6.8% and 5.9%, respectively) [26]. In the FRISC II trial, the proportion of patients who had CABG in triple and left main artery disease was 83%, while the 30-day mortality after surgery was very low at about 2%. It is known from previous trials that surgical revascularization is associated with a significant reduction in long-term mortality in patients with triple and left main artery disease. Therefore, this could explain the superior outcome observed in the invasive group of the FRISC II trial.

The risk of bleeding complications has to be taken into account in patients who undergo surgery and who are initially treated with aggressive antiplatelet therapy, including aspirin, clopidogrel, and GP IIb/IIIa inhibitors. However, pretreatment with aggressive antiplatelet therapy regimens should be considered as only a relative contraindication to early CABG, but may require cessation of GP IIb/IIIa inhibitors 2 h prior to surgery and platelet transfusions in some instances [26]. In the PURSUIT trial, major bleeding rates among patients who underwent immediate CABG, did not differ between patients receiving placebo and those receiving eptifibatide (64% versus 63%, respectively), with similar rate of blood transfusion (57% versus 59%, respectively) [43]. Ideally, in order to minimize the risk of hemorrhagic complications, clopidogrel should be stopped 5 days before surgery, and low molecular weight heparin 12 hours before surgery [44,45].

Respective indications for PCI or bypass surgery

The respective indications for PCI or CABG in ACS patients are well documented in the ESC guidelines on the management of ACS [26]. Patients with single-vessel disease and indication for revascularization are usually treated by PCI with stent implantation and adjunctive treatment with GP IIb/IIIa inhibitors. In these patients, surgical revascularization is only considered if unsuitable anatomy precludes safe PCI. In patients with left main or triple-vessel disease, CABG is the recommended procedure, particularly in patients with left ventricular dysfunction, except in cases of serious comorbidity contraindicating surgery. In this situation, CABG is well documented to prolong survival, improve quality of life, and reduce rehospitalizations [26]. In patients with multivessel disease and lesions suitable for stenting, either PCI or CABG may be appropriate. Subanalyses of different trials comparing the efficacy of stenting versus CABG, in this setting, reported similar success rates, with no significant difference in in-hospital mortality or MI, but with a significantly higher rate of repeat revascularization procedures for the PCI strategy compared with CABG [46–48]. In some patients, a staged procedure may be considered, with immediate stenting of the culprit lesion and subsequent reassessment of the need for treatment of other lesions, either by PCI or CABG. In any case, if PCI is the selected procedure, it may be performed immediately after angiography in the same session.

Complications and procedure-related complications

Despite the potential benefits of an early invasive strategy, the risk associated with PCI or CABG is increased in patients with unstable coronary syndromes [6,49–51].

The mortality associated with PCI was almost negligible in all trials comparing invasive versus noninvasive strategy. However, in the FRISC II trial, there was a higher early risk of MI in the invasive group (RR = 1.99; 95% CI, 1.31–3.02) that was mainly caused by procedure-related MI with elevations of cardiac markers and without any other signs of MI or any immediate or long-term clinical consequences [4]. In addition, this early increased risk was compensated by a reduction in spontaneous MI. More frequent use of GP IIb/IIIa inhibitors is likely to result in a lower rate of early procedure-related MI in invasively treated patients, as reported in the TACTICS-TIMI 18 trial [4,6].

The definition used for MI and the criteria for procedure-related infarctions are important issues to bear in mind when comparing invasive and conservative strategies in ACS patients. The criteria used for the diagnosis of MI among patients undergoing PCI are not appropriately defined. The threshold for the diagnosis of MI differed between patients undergoing revascularization (PCI or CABG) and those treated conservatively in FRISC II, RITA 3, and TACTICS-TIMI 18 [4,6,8]. In these three studies, the threshold defined as being an infarction varied from anything above the normal level, to three times the upper limit of normal, and even up to greater than or equal to 5 times the upper limit of normal in the setting of CABG.

The prognostic significance of PCI-related increases in enzyme concentrations as distinct from spontaneous MI is controversial. However, a report based on 8838 patients undergoing PCI concluded that the adverse prognostic implications (risk of death) from periprocedural myocardial necrosis should be considered as similar to spontaneous necrosis [52].

In the TIMI IIIB, MATE, and FRISC II trials, the rate of MI tended to be higher in the invasive-strategy group during the first several weeks, a finding that is consistent with the initially increased risk of cardiac events associated with coronary interventions [2–4]. In contrast, a lower rate of MI was observed during this period in TACTICS-TIMI 18, an effect that may be attributable to the well-documented protection afforded by the inhibition of GP IIb/IIIa [6]. This benefit is even observed in elderly patients, despite a higher risk of major bleeding events [53]. Data from the Global Registry of Acute Coronary Events reported that patients admitted first to hospitals with catheterization facilities had a significantly higher rate of major bleeding and a borderline significantly higher rate of stroke. This excess of major bleedings in hospitals with catheterization facilities is probably related to the higher rate of invasive procedures (Table 13.2) [54].

Timing of angiography and revascularization in ACS

The optimal timing of revascularization is still uncertain. The timing of PCI was similar in the FRISC II and RITA 3 trials (median 4 versus 3 days, respectively) but CABG was done later in RITA 3 (median 22 versus 7 days, respectively) [4,8]. In TACTICS-TIMI 18, cardiac procedures were carried out approximately 2–3 days earlier in the invasive group than in the conservative group, which may have averted events that would otherwise have occurred [6].

Table 13.2 Adjusted ORs (95% CI) for patients first admitted to hospitals with or without catheterization facilities according to final diagnosis of ACS [54].

	OR NSTE-MI	OR Unstable angina
In-hospital death	1.04 [0.74–1.31]	0.98 [0.40–1.31]
Death at 30 days	0.98 [0.80–1.20]	0.88 [0.68–1.13]
Death at 6 months	1.15 [0.97–1.37]	1.03 [0.84–1.36]
MI (up to 6 months after discharge)	0.72 [0.52–0.99]	0.85 [0.52–1.36]
Stroke in hospital	1.80 [0.92–3.55]	1.75 [0.81–3.80]
Major bleeding in hospital	1.65 [1.20–2.26]	1.69 [1.08–2.64]

Notes NSTE-MI = non-ST-elevation myocardial infarction, MI = myocardial infarction.

A subanalysis of TACTICS-TIMI 18 did not identify a clear benefit of early intervention in terms of death, MI, or rehospitalization between patients who underwent catheterization less than or greater than 48 h after randomization. Nonetheless, "watchful waiting" is probably not the best strategy, even in patients treated with a platelet GP IIb/IIIa receptor blocker.

The role of very early coronary angioplasty and carefully timed early bypass surgery in the treatment of NSTE-ACS were evaluated in the VINO randomized trial, which compared first day angiography/angioplasty with an early conservative approach [7]. All patients in the invasive group underwent coronary angiography on the day of admission (mean randomization-angiography time 6.2 h). Immediate angioplasty of the infarct-related artery (or carefully timed early bypass surgery in patients not suitable for angioplasty) was performed whenever possible. No GP IIb/IIIa inhibitors were used in the study. The composite endpoint of death or reinfarction at 6 months occurred in 6.2% of patients in the invasive group versus 22.3% in the conservative group ($p < .001$). Similarly, the 6-month mortality was significantly lower in the invasive group compared with the conservative group (3.1% versus 13.4%, respectively; $p < .03$).

Post hoc analysis of data from the PURSUIT trial indicates that outcome is favorable in patients with NSTE-ACS undergoing PCI when the procedure is performed within 24 h of admission under GP IIb/IIIa inhibitor protection [55]. Thirty-day rates of death or MI were only 9.5% for those undergoing PCI within 24 h, and treated with eptifibatide, compared with 14.3–16.5% for later PCI, or 12.2–13.2% for no PCI. Thus, there is an increased risk of death or MI under medical therapy. This risk is particularly high early after admission but diminishes gradually after admission under GP IIb/IIIa inhibitors and other antithrombotic therapy. In patients scheduled for PCI, the risk of preprocedural complications clearly increased with time, both in patients receiving placebo and those receiving eptifibatide.

Recently published data from the ISAR-COOL randomized trial confirmed that deferral of intervention for prolonged antithrombotic pretreatment did not improve outcome compared with immediate intervention accompanied by intense antiplatelet treatment in patients with unstable coronary syndromes [36]. Patients were randomly allocated to antithrombotic pretreatment for 3–5 days or to early intervention after pretreatment for less than 6 h. In both groups, antithrombotic pretreatment consisted of intravenous unfractionated heparin, oral aspirin, oral clopidogrel, and intravenous tirofiban. A significant increase in the cumulative 30-day incidence of large MI or death from any cause was observed in patients who underwent prolonged antithrombotic pretreatment compared with those submitted to immediate intervention (11.6% versus 5.9%, respectively; RR = 1.96; 95% CI, 1.01–3.82). Thus, a high loading dose of clopidogrel in combination with tirofiban affords strong platelet inhibition at the time of intervention that might help to achieve plaque passivation. During the pretreatment phase (median duration, 3.6 days), 6.3% of the patients receiving prolonged antithrombic therapy experienced an event. The authors concluded that antithrombotic pretreatment should be kept to the minimum duration required to organize early catheterization and revascularization in patients with unstable coronary syndromes.

Registries: a different picture

It is well known that discrepancies exist between randomized trials and registries, but the reasons for this are not fully understood. In clinical practice, early revascularization is only applied to a minority of patients. In large-scale international registries of NSTE-ACS, only 18–28% of patients underwent PCI or CABG during the initial hospitalization [56,57].

Recently published data from the Global Registry of Acute Coronary Events reported that early and late mortality in patients with NSTE-ACS who were first admitted to hospitals without catheterization facilities were similar to those in patients first admitted to hospitals with PCI facilities, despite fewer invasive interventions, but with a significantly higher risk of reinfarction after discharge (Table 13.2) [54]. Thus, a systematic invasive strategy does not result in a clear survival benefit. Similar results were reported in NSTE-ACS patients studied by the Organization to Assess Strategies for Ischemic Syndromes [56] and in those from the RESCATE study [57]. Van de Werf and colleagues suggest that these discrepancies between randomized trials and registries result from the reluctance of investigators to include high-risk patients in randomized studies [54]. A more selective use of invasive procedures in the high-risk patients of the GRACE registry may explain the favorable outcomes observed in those first admitted to hospitals without catheterization facilities.

This hypothesis is conflicting with results from the CRUSADE study, in which patients undergoing early catheterization were younger, and more commonly cared for by cardiologists, whereas older patients with comorbidities including cardiac heart failure or renal insufficiency were less likely to undergo early invasive management [58]. Thus, patients at higher risk of mortality were more frequently treated conservatively, even though they derived

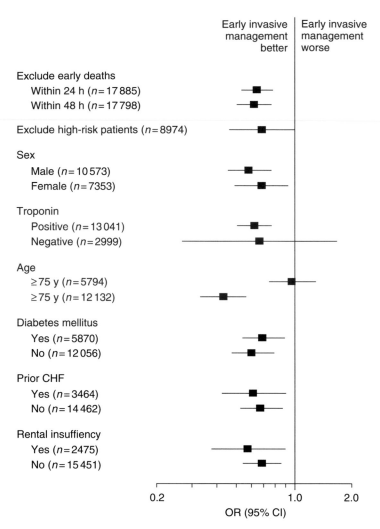

Figure 13.3 Sensitivity and subgroup analyses for adjusted in-hospital mortality by utilization of an early invasive management strategy ($n = 17\,926$). Reproduced from Ref. 58, with permission.

greater absolute benefit from aggressive management (Figure 13.3). However, despite the underutilization of early invasive management strategies, patients from the CRUSADE cohort who underwent early catheterization had a significantly lower in-hospital mortality rate, regardless of the risk score category. Indeed, in all three risk categories, patients undergoing early invasive management had a significantly lower risk of in-hospital mortality, although the highest-risk patients appeared to derive the greatest absolute benefit from early invasive management. In addition, the survival benefit occurred during the initial hospitalization, whereas the mortality benefit with early invasive strategy in FRISC II was not apparent until after 3 months [4].

Concluding remarks

Based on randomized trials and observational data, an early invasive strategy compared with a noninvasive strategy improves survival without recurrence of MI, readmission or urgent revascularization for severe angina in NSTE-ACS. This benefit is greatest in intermediate-risk and high-risk patients based on noninvasive risk indicators. This benefit concerns mainly the reduction in recurrent ischemic events rather than mortality. However, early invasive strategy is still largely underused in routine clinical practice and future efforts should focus on applying guidelines recommendations in this setting, especially in high-risk NSTE-ACS patients.

References

1. Boden WE, O'Rourke RA, Crawford MH *et al.* The veterans affairs non-Q-wave infarction strategy: outcomes in patients with acute non-Q-wave myocardial infarction randomly assigned to an invasive as compared with a conservative management strategy. *N Engl J Med* 1998; **338**: 1785–1792.
2. TIMI IIIB Investigators. Effects of tissue plasminogen activator and a comparison of early invasive and conservative strategies in unstable angina and non-Q-wave myocardial infarction: results of the TIMI IIIB Trial. *Circulation* 1994; **89**: 1545–1556.
3. McCullough PA, O'Neil WW, Graham M *et al.* A prospective randomized trial of triage angiography in acute coronary syndromes ineligible for thrombolytic therapy. Results of the Medicine versus Angiography in Thrombolytic Exclusion (MATE) trial. *J Am Coll Cardiol* 1998; **32**: 596–605.
4. Wallentin L, Lagerqvist B, Husted S *et al.* FRISC II Investigators. Outcome at 1 year after an invasive compared with a non-invasive strategy in unstable coronary-artery disease: the FRISC II invasive randomised trial. *Lancet* 2000; **356**: 9–16.
5. Michalis LK, Stroumbis CS, Pappas K *et al.* Treatment of refractory unstable angina in geographically isolated areas without cardiac surgery. Invasive versus conservative strategy (TRUCS study). *Eur Heart J* 2000; **21**: 1954–1959.
6. Cannon CP, Weintraub WS, Demopoulos LA *et al.* Comparison of early invasive and conservative strategies in patients with unstable coronary syndromes treated with the GP IIb/IIIa inhibitor tirofiban. *N Engl J Med* 2001; **344**: 1879–1887.
7. Spacek R, Widimsky P, Straka E *et al.* Value of first day angiography/angioplasty in evolving non-ST segment elevation myocardial infarction: an open multicentre randomized trial: the VINO study. *Eur Heart J* 2002; **23**: 230–238.
8. Fox KA, Poole-Wilson PA, Henderson RA *et al.* Interventional versus conservative treatment for patients with unstable angina or non-ST-elevation myocardial infarction: the British Heart Foundation RITA 3 randomised trial. Randomized Intervention Trial of unstable Angina Investigators. *Lancet* 2002; **360**: 743–751.
9. Lagerqvist B, Husted S, Kontny F *et al.* A long-term perspective on the protective effects of an early invasive strategy in unstable coronary artery disease: two-year

follow-up of the FRISC-II invasive study. Fast Revascularization during InStability in Coronary artery disease-II Investigators. *J Am Coll Cardiol* 2002; **40**: 1902–1914.

10. Wallentin L. Non-ST-elevation acute coronary syndrome: fuel for the invasive strategy. *Lancet* 2002; **360**: 738–739.

11. Bavry AA, Kumbhani DJ, Quiroz R *et al.* Invasive therapy along with GP IIb/IIIa inhibitors and intracoronary stents improves survival in non-ST-segment elevation acute coronary syndromes: a meta-analysis and review of the literature. *Am J Cardiol* 2004; **93**: 830–835.

12. Diderholm E, Andren B, Frostfeldt G *et al.* ST depression in ECG at entry indicates severe coronary lesions and large benefits of an early invasive treatment strategy in unstable coronary artery disease; the FRISC II ECG substudy. The Fast Revascularisation during InStability in Coronary artery disease Investigators. *Eur Heart J* 2002; **23**: 41–49.

13. Mueller C, Neumann FJ, Perach W *et al.* Prognostic value of the admission electrocardiogram in patients with unstable angina/non-ST-segment elevation myocardial infarction treated with very early revascularization. *Am J Med* 2004; **117**: 145–150.

14. Hamm CW, Ravkilde J, Gerhardt W *et al.* The prognostic value of serum troponin T in unstable angina. *N Engl J Med* 1992; **327**: 146–150.

15. Atman EM, Tanasijevic MJ, Thompson B *et al.* Cardiac-specific troponin I levels to predict the risk of mortality in patients with acute coronary syndromes. *N Engl J Med* 1996; **335**: 1342–1349.

16. Ohman EM, Armstrong PW, Christenson RH *et al.* Cardiac troponin T levels for risk stratification in acute myocardial ischemia. *N Engl J Med* 1996; **335**: 1333–1341.

17. Lindhal B, Venge P, Wallentin L. Troponin T identifies patients with unstable coronary artery disease who benefit from long-term antithrombotic protection. *J Am Coll Cardiol* 1997; **29**: 43–48.

18. Morrow DA, Antman EM, Tanasijevic M *et al.* Cardiac troponin I for stratification of early outcomes and the efficacy of enoxaparin in unstable angina: a TIMI-11B substudy. *J Am Coll Cardiol* 2000; **36**: 1812–1817.

19. Hamm CW, Heeschen C, Goldmann B *et al.* Benefit of abciximab in patients with refractory unstable angina in relation to serum troponin T levels. *N Engl J Med* 1999; **340**: 1623–1629. [Erratum, *N Engl J Med* 1999; **341**: 548].

20. Heeschen C, Hamm CW, Goldmann B *et al.* Troponin concentrations for stratification of patients with acute coronary syndromes in relation to therapeutic efficacy of tirofiban. *Lancet* 1999; **354**: 1757–1762.

21. Mueller C, Neumann FJ, Perruchoud AP *et al.* Prognostic value of quantitative troponin T measurements in unstable angina/non-ST-segment elevation acute myocardial infarction treated early and predominantly with percutaneous coronary intervention. *Am J Med* 2004; **117**: 897–902.

22. Morrow DA, de Lemos JA, Sabatine MS *et al.* Evaluation of B-type natriuretic peptide for risk assessment in unstable angina/non-ST-elevation myocardial infarction: B-type natriuretic peptide and prognosis in TACTICS-TIMI 18. *J Am Coll Cardiol* 2003; **41**: 1264–1272.

23. Jernberg T, Lindahl B, Siegbahn A *et al.* N-terminal pro-brain natriuretic peptide in relation to inflammation, myocardial necrosis, and the effect of an invasive strategy in unstable coronary artery disease. *J Am Coll Cardiol* 2003; **42**: 1909–1916.

24. Mueller C, Buettner HJ, Hodgson JM *et al.* Inflammation and long-term mortality after non-ST elevation acute coronary syndrome treated with a very early invasive strategy in 1042 consecutive patients. *Circulation* 2002; **105**: 1412–1415.

25. Sabatine MS, Morrow DA, Giugliano RP *et al.* Implications of upstream glycoprotein IIb/IIIa inhibition and coronary artery stenting in the invasive management of unstable angina/non-ST-elevation myocardial infarction: a comparison of the Thrombolysis In Myocardial Infarction (TIMI) IIIB trial and the Treat angina with Aggrastat and determine Cost of Therapy with Invasive or Conservative Strategy (TACTICS)-TIMI 18 trial. *Circulation* 2004; **109**: 874–880.

26. Bertrand ME, Simoons ML, Fox KA *et al.*; Task force on the management of acute coronary syndromes of the European Society of Cardiology. Management of acute coronary syndromes in patients presenting without persistent ST-segment elevation. *Eur Heart J* 2002; **23**: 1809–1840.

27. Braunwald E, Antman EM, Beasley JW *et al.* ACC/AHA guideline update for the management of patients with unstable angina and non-ST-segment elevation myocardial infarction – 2002: summary article. A report of the American College of Cardiology/American Heart Association task force on practice guidelines (Committee on the Management of Patients With Unstable Angina). *Circulation* 2002; **106**: 1893–1900.

28. Hochman JS, McCabe CH, Stone PH *et al.* Outcome and profile of women and men presenting with acute coronary syndromes: a report from TIMI IIIB. *J Am Coll Cardiol* 1997; **30**: 141–148.

29. Hochman JS, Tamis JE, Thompson TD *et al.* Sex, clinical presentation, and outcome in patients with acute coronary syndromes. *N Engl J Med* 1999; **341**: 226–232.

30. Stone P, Thompson B, Anderson H *et al.* Influence of race, sex, and age on management of unstable angina and non-Q-wave myocardial infarction: the TIMI III Registry. *JAMA* 1996; **275**: 1104–1112.

31. Lagerqvist B, Safstrom K, Stahle E, Wallentin L, Swahn E (for the FRISC II Study Group Investigators). Is early invasive treatment of unstable coronary artery disease equally effective for both women and men? *J Am Coll Cardiol* 2001; **38**: 41–48.

32. Malenka DJ, O'Connor GT, Quinton H. Differences in outcomes between women and men associated with percutaneous transluminal coronary angioplasty: a regional prospective study of 13,061 procedures. *Circulation* 1996; **94**(Suppl. 2): II99–II104.

33. Glaser R, Herrmann HC, Murphy SA *et al.* Benefit of an early invasive management strategy in women with acute coronary syndromes. *JAMA* 2002; **288**: 3124–3129.

34. Mueller C, Neumann FJ, Roskamm H *et al.* Women do have an improved long-term outcome after non-ST-elevation acute coronary syndromes treated very early and predominantly with percutaneous coronary intervention: a prospective study in 1,450 consecutive patients. *J Am Coll Cardiol* 2002; **40**: 245–250.

35. Boersma E, Harrington RA, Moliterno DJ *et al.* Platelet GP IIb/IIIa inhibitors in acute coronary syndromes: a meta-analysis of all major randomised clinical trials. *Lancet* 2002; **359**: 189–198.

36. Neumann FJ, Kastrati A, Pogatsa-Murray G *et al.* Evaluation of prolonged antithrombotic pretreatment ("cooling-off" strategy) before intervention in patients with unstable coronary syndromes: a randomized controlled trial. *JAMA* 2003; **290**: 1593–1599.

37. Serruys PW, van Hout B, Bonnier H *et al.* Randomised comparison of implantation of heparin-coated stents with balloon angioplasty in selected patients with coronary artery disease (Benestent II). *Lancet* 1998; **352**: 673–681.

38. Morice MC, Serruys PW, Sousa JE *et al.* Randomized study with the sirolimus-coated Bx velocity balloon-expandable stent in the treatment of patients with

de novo native coronary artery lesions. A randomized comparison of a sirolimus-eluting stent with a standard stent for coronary revascularization. *N Engl J Med* 2002; **346**: 1773–1780.

39. The PRISM-PLUS Study Investigators. Inhibition of the platelet GP IIb/IIIa receptor with tirofiban in unstable angina and non-Q-wave myocardial infarction. Platelet Receptor Inhibition in Ischemic Syndrome Management in Patients Limited by Unstable Signs and Symptoms. *N Engl J Med* 1998; **338**: 1488–1497.

40. Lincoff AM, Califf RM, Anderson KM. Evidence for prevention of death and myocardial infarction with platelet membrane glycoprotein IIb/IIIa receptor blockade by abciximab (c7E3 Fab) among patients with unstable angina undergoing percutaneous coronary revascularization. EPIC Investigators. Evaluation of 7E3 in Preventing Ischemic Complications. *J Am Coll Cardiol* 1997; **30**: 149–156.

41. The CAPTURE Investigators. Randomised placebo-controlled trial of abciximab before and during coronary intervention in refractory unstable angina: the CAPTURE Study. *Lancet* 1997; **349**: 1429–1435.

42. Lincoff AM. Trials of platelet glycoprotein IIb/IIIa receptor antagonists during percutaneous coronary revascularization. *Am J Cardiol* 1998; **82**: 36P–42P.

43. The PURSUIT Trial Investigators. Inhibition of platelet GP IIb/IIIa with eptifibatide in patients with acute coronary syndromes. *N Engl J Med* 1998; **339**: 436–443.

44. Clark SC, Vitale N, Zacharias J, Forty J. Effect of low molecular weight heparin (fragmin) on bleeding after cardiac surgery. *Ann Thorac Surg* 2000; **69**: 762–764.

45. Yusuf S, Zhao F, Mehta SR *et al.* Effects of clopidogrel in addition to aspirin in patients with acute coronary syndromes without ST-segment elevation. Clopidogrel in Unstable Angina to Prevent Recurrent Events Trial Investigators. *N Engl J Med* 2001; **345**: 494–502.

46. King SB 3rd, Lembo NJ, Weintraub WS. A randomized trial comparing coronary angioplasty with coronary bypass surgery. Emory Angioplasty versus Surgery Trial (EAST). *N Engl J Med* 1994; **331**: 1044–1050.

47. Hamm CW, Reimers J, Ischinger T *et al.* A randomized study of coronary angioplasty compared with bypass surgery in patients with symptomatic multivessel coronary disease. German Angioplasty Bypass Surgery Investigation (GABI). *N Engl J Med* 1994; **331**: 1037–1043.

48. Serruys PW, Unger F, Sousa JE *et al.* Comparison of coronary-artery bypass surgery and stenting for the treatment of multivessel disease. *N Engl J Med* 2001; **344**: 1117–1124.

49. Bjessmo S, Ivert T, Flink H, Hammar N. Early and late mortality after surgery for unstable angina in relation to Braunwald class. *Am Heart J* 2001; **141**: 9–14.

50. de Feyter PJ, van den Brand M, Laarman GJ *et al.* Acute coronary artery occlusion during and after percutaneous transluminal coronary angioplasty: frequency, prediction, clinical course, management, and follow-up. *Circulation* 1991; **83**: 927–936.

51. Schuhlen H, Kastrati A, Dirschinger J *et al.* Intracoronary stenting and risk for major adverse cardiac events during the first month. *Circulation* 1998; **98**: 104–111.

52. Antman EM, McCabe, CH, Gurfinkel EP *et al.* Enoxaparin prevents death and cardiac ischaemic events in unstable angina/non-Q-wave myocardial infarction: results of the thrombolysis in myocardial infarction (TIMI) 11B trial. *Circulation* 1999; **100**: 1593–1601.

53. Bach RG, Cannon CP, Weintraub WS *et al.* The effect of routine, early invasive management on outcome for elderly patients with non-ST-segment elevation acute coronary syndromes. *Ann Intern Med* 2004; **141**: 186–195.

54. Van de Werf F, Gore JM, Avezum A *et al.* Access to catheterisation facilities in patients admitted with acute coronary syndrome: multinational registry study. *BMJ* 2005; **330**: 441.

55. Ronner E, Boersma E, Akkerhuis KM *et al.* Patients with acute coronary syndromes without persistent ST elevation undergoing percutaneous coronary intervention benefit most from early intervention with protection by a glycoprotein IIb/IIIa receptor blocker. *Eur Heart J* 2002; **23**: 239–246.

56. Yusuf S, Flather M, Pogue J *et al.* Variations between countries in invasive cardiac procedures and outcomes in patients with suspected unstable angina or myocardial infarction without initial ST elevation. OASIS (Organisation to Assess Strategies for Ischaemic Syndromes) Registry Investigators. *Lancet* 1998; **352**: 507–514.

57. Lupon J, Valle V, Marrugat J *et al.* Six-month outcome in unstable angina patients without previous myocardial infarction according to the use of tertiary cardiologic resources. RESCATE Investigators. Recursos Empleados en el Sindrome Coronario Agudo y Tiempos de Espera. *J Am Coll Cardiol* 1999; **34**: 1947–1953.

58. Bhatt DL, Roe MT, Peterson ED *et al.* Utilization of early invasive management strategies for high-risk patients with non-ST-segment elevation acute coronary syndromes: results from the CRUSADE Quality Improvement Initiative. *JAMA* 2004; **292**: 2096–2104.

Section eight:
Therapeutic strategy

CHAPTER 14

Risk stratification and therapeutic strategy

Christian W. Hamm

Physicians taking care of acute chest pain patients are constantly challenged by unnecessary admissions or unqualified discharges. Up to 26% of patients are inappropriately hospitalized and 5% of myocardial infarctions are missed [1]. Acute coronary syndrome (ACS) without ST elevation is clinically defined and therefore encompasses a heterogeneous group of patients with widely variable symptoms and prognosis. Early and reliable risk stratification is mandatory for an effective therapeutic concept, thus improving patient care and reducing costs. Traditional coronary risk factors, such as hypertension, hyperlipidemia, smoking, or family history, correlate only weakly with the likelihood of acute ischemia and are therefore less important than symptoms, electrocardiogram (ECG) abnormalities, and biomarkers in the acute phase.

The basic treatment with the aim to relieve angina pain includes nitrates and β-blockers as well as antiplatelet therapy, such as aspirin. In recent years considerable achievements have been made with respect to improving the outcome by linking the better diagnostic tools to therapeutic strategies that target the underlying pathophysiology. These include more potent antithrombin and antiplatelet therapies as well as invasive means. The benefit is particularly evident in defined high-risk patients and results in a stratified management of ACS patients that also considers cost-efficacy calculations.

Classification and risk scores

Because of the need for simplified and widely applicable risk stratification tools facilitating the triage and management of ACS patients, classifications and risk scores have been developed. The Braunwald classification was empirically developed and is based on symptoms with respect to pain severity and duration as well as the pathogenesis of myocardial ischemia [2]. It was shown prospectively to be linked to risk, for example, patients with unstable angina at rest within the last 48 h (Class IIIB) have the highest risk of adverse cardiac events (11% in-hospital event rate) [3]. In addition, sophisticated scores based on large unselected registries resp. clinical trials have been developed. The GRACE and the TIMI score provide relatively simple methods to estimate the risk of death and myocardial infarction, and hence can be used to decide if a patient

Table 14.1 Parameters of acute risk.

Recurrent ischemia/ chest pain
Dynamic ST-segment changes
Elevated biomarkers: troponin
Hemodynamic instability
Major arrhythmias (Ventricular fibrillation, Ventricular tachycardia)
Diabetes

---

can be discharged [4,5]. However, they are only slowly accepted, because they cannot completely replace the complex decision-making involved with therapeutic strategies.

The guidelines of the European Society of Cardiology (ESC) on ACS provide a simple list (Table 14.1) of high-risk features [6]. These are meant to serve as decision criteria for drug treatment and invasive management. This list is evidence-based and is derived from studies as presented below. As in the US guidelines, troponins play a central role in the acute decision process [7]. A similar risk assessment can be made for the long-term follow-up, which, however, is more determined by the underlying disease and concomitant disorders (e.g. renal insufficiency, diabetes) than by acute disorders.

Electrocardiograhic abnormalities

The resting electrocardiogram plays a central role in the early assessment of patients with suspected ACS. It is a readily available tool in identifying patients with ST-segment elevations who are likely to have myocardial infarctions and who should receive reperfusion treatment. It is also useful for risk stratification and planning the therapeutic strategy in the absence of ST elevation. Exercise testing is contraindicated in symptomatic patients and in patients with elevated troponins. Only after stabilization and lack of high-risk features is treadmill testing useful for risk assessment.

ST-segment shifts and T-wave changes are the most reliable electrocardiographic indicators of unstable coronary disease that are associated with elevated risk [8,9]. Dynamic changes particularly during episodes of chest pain have a very high diagnostic value. ST-segment depression of >1 mm in two or more contiguous leads, in the appropriate clinical context, are highly suggestive of ACS. Inverted T-waves (>1 mm) in leads with predominant R-waves are also suggestive, although the latter finding is less specific. Continuous ST-segment monitoring was shown to provide the better electrocardiographic prediction, but should not delay the invasive management in symptomatic patients.

The risk for death and myocardial infarction in patients with ST depression is reduced by early invasive management, probably supported by glycoprotein (GP) IIb/IIIa antagonists [10,11]. In a conservative treatment strategy the risk is not reduced in this subgroup by GP IIb/IIIa inhibitors and low molecular weight heparins as compared with heparin alone [12,13]. The benefit of clopidogrel is similar in patients with and without ST abnormalities [14].

Troponins

Histopathological and angioscopic studies in patients with unstable angina revealed local thrombus formation at the sites of ruptured plaques followed by repetitive downstream embolization of platelet aggregates [15–17]. This results in about one-third of patients presenting with unstable angina in the release of troponin T and troponin I, but only rarely in a rise of creatine kinase. Numerous studies confirmed that in "troponin positive" patients the risk of myocardial infarction and death in 30 days is approximately 20% [18–22]. The best independent prognostic information is provided by the peak value of troponins during the first 24 h. Troponin T and quantitative ST-segment depression offer complementary prognostic information in the risk stratification [23]. The combination of the troponin test with a predischarge exercise test further improves risk assessment for unstable coronary disease [24]. During a period of 5-months follow-up, death and myocardial infarction occurred at a rate of only 1%, if both were normal, and reached 50% when both were abnormal.

If troponins are regarded as surrogate markers of ongoing thromboembolic events, a more effective antithrombotic treatment or more potent antiplatelet therapy should be a promising approach (Figure 14.1). Consequently, a superior treatment benefit was documented in the FRISC trial for troponin T positive patients receiving the low molecular weight heparin, dalteparin, in comparison to the placebo group [25]. Similarly, the benefit of the GP IIb/IIIa antagonist abciximab in the CAPTURE trial, enrolling patients suffering from refractory unstable angina was achieved by a profound effect in those patients with elevated troponin T levels at study entry [26]. CK-MB was not of predictive value for the therapeutic efficacy of abciximab. Similar to the CAPTURE results, a post hoc analysis of the PRISM study using the GP IIb/IIIa antagonist

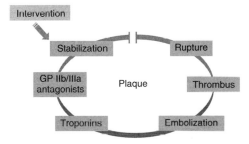

Figure 14.1 Troponin as surrogate marker for thrombosis and treatment consequences.

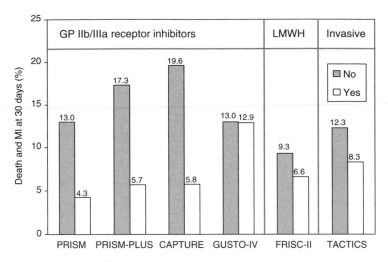

Figure 14.2 Treatment effects in troponin T/I positive patients.

tirofiban demonstrated that the benefit of treatment is limited to patients with elevated troponin T or troponin I [27]. Furthermore, this benefit was evident in the invasively as well as noninvasively treated group and resulted in a reduction in duration of hospitalization from 15 to 8 days.

The highly beneficial effect of GP IIb/IIIa antagonists in troponin positive patients as opposed to patients with negative troponins has been confirmed in several studies by retrospective analyses (Figure 14.2). Short-term (30 days) risk may be reduced absolutely by up to 10%, and relatively up to 75%. Only in the GUSTO IV trial where troponin was used as one entry criteria was it associated with increased risk, but abciximab used in a conservative management was not predictive of benefit [28]. The low rate of acute interventions may be responsible for the lack of effectiveness of abciximab.

First evidence that an invasive management results over long term in decreased mortality and myocardial infarction rate was provided by the FRISC II study [10]. There was already a trend that patients with elevated troponin T levels had a higher benefit. In the TACTICS – TIMI 18 study it was demonstrated that an early invasive strategy results in a lower event rate including rehospitalization [11]. This was, however, limited to troponin T positive patients, whereas in troponin negative patients the invasive strategy resulted in an even harmful trend. The 9.9% absolute risk reduction at 6 months in the troponin T positive subgroup was achieved without an early hazard, possibly because of routine GP IIb/IIIa pretreatment (tirofiban).

A special benefit of antiplatelet treatment with clopidogrel in patients with elevated biomarkers could not be evidenced [14]. Accordingly, guidelines recommend to give clopidogrel independent of the troponin status and invasive strategy to all patients presenting with ACS.

Inflammatory markers

Convincing evidence has been generated that inflammatory mechanisms are involved in the pathogenesis of ACS by promoting plaque fissuring or erosion, which exposes thrombogenic contents such as collagen to the circulation. Of the numerous inflammatory markers that have been investigated over the past decade, C-reactive protein (CRP) is the most widely studied. The exact source of elevated CRP levels among patients with unstable coronary syndromes remains unclear. Given that myocardial damage is also a major inflammatory stimulus, it is important to note that in a combined analysis of FRISC II and GUSTO IV, CRP elevation over a period of up to 120 h was only found in patients with elevated troponin levels [29]. Similarly, in the CAPTURE study, CRP levels were significantly higher in troponin-positive patients [30]. This suggests that an acute inflammatory process induced by myocardial damage is superimposed on a chronic inflammatory condition, both of which might influence long-term outcome in ACS.

There is robust evidence that even among patients with troponin negative ACS, elevated levels of CRP are predictive of future risk. In the CAPTURE trial, only troponin T was predictive for the initial 72 h period, but both CRP and troponin T were independent predictors of risk at 6 months [30]. The FRISC study confirmed that mortality is associated with elevated CRP levels at the time of the index event and continues to increase for several years [31]. However, in a prospective population study, CRP added little to the predictive value provided by the assessment of traditional risk factors, including LDL-cholesterol [32].

Only recently, it was demonstrated that the long-term risk in patients with ACS and elevated CRP levels can be positively modified dose-dependently by statins, which not only lower LDL-cholesterol but also exert anti-inflammatory properties [33]. CRP as well as LDL levels appear to be independent predictors for the benefit achieved by statins. Other antiinflammatory drugs, such as COX-2 inhibitors, have not yet been clinically investigated in this scenario and have questionable effects after the experience with rofecoxib. Whether antiinflammatory effects of angiotensin converting enzyme (ACE) inhibitors play a role in ACS, has also not yet been clearly defined in ACS patients [34].

Markers of neurohumoral activation

Neurohumoral activation of the heart can be monitored by measuring the systemic levels of natriuretic peptides secreted from the heart due to increased stretch or wall-tension. Brain (B-type) natriuretic peptides are mainly synthesized in the ventricular myocardium as prohormones (proBNP), which upon secretion are cleaved into biologically active peptides (BNP) and N-terminal prohormone fragments (NT-proBNP). Both BNP and NT-proBNP are highly sensitive and fairly specific markers for the detection of left ventricular dysfunction in patients with congestive heart failure. Similarly, it was demonstrated in patients with ACS that elevated NT-proBNP and BNP levels have a three- to five-fold increased mortality compared to those with lower levels. In addition, the level of NT-proBNP was strongly associated to mortality even when adjusted for age, Killip class, and left ventricular ejection fraction [35,36]. The NT-proBNP level measured at 72 h after presentation seems to correlate even better with outcome than the measurement on admission [37]. However, there is currently no conclusive answer about what this means for the therapeutic management, except that patients pretreated with ACE-inhibitors seem to have a more favorable outcome in the presence of elevated NT-proBNP levels.

New biochemical markers

The elevation of troponins is considered to indicate irreversible myocardial cell damage [38]. Naturally, the aim should be to find biomarkers that are earlier elevated in the pathophysiological cascade. Promising markers under investigation are soluble CD40 ligand, myeloperoxidase (MPO), placental growth factor (PlGF), and pregnancy-associated plasma protein A (PAPP-A) that have already been linked to treatment outcome.

Soluble CD40 ligand is a powerful biochemical marker of thrombotic inflammatory activation in patients with ACS, supporting the close relationship between inflammation and thrombotic activation. Plaque rupture induces platelet activation resulting in increased surface expression of sCD40 ligand that is subsequently cleaved from the membrane surface. The released sCD40 ligand can activate CD40 receptors on endothelial cells and, thereby, induce a proinflammatory cascade in the vessel wall. Moreover, sCD40 ligand can activate CD40 that is also expressed on inflammatory cells, such as monocytes and T cells. The subsequent activation of these inflammatory cells and their invasion into the ruptured or eroded plaque results in a further inflammatory perturbation of the vessel wall. Importantly, blockade of the glycoprotein IIb/IIIa receptor on platelets inhibits the release of sCD40 ligand through inhibition of platelet aggregation via fibrinogen. It has been shown that levels of soluble sCD40 ligand not only identifies patients with ACS that are at highest risk for ischemic events, but also predicts which patient will derive major benefit from antiplatelet treatment with the GP IIb/IIIa receptor antagonist abciximab [39,40].

There is growing evidence that myocardial cell injury is not only related to platelet activation but also preceded by recruitment and activation of leukocytes, most notably polymorphonuclear neutrophils. These undergo degranulation within the coronary circulation in ACS. One of the principal mediators secreted upon degranulation is MPO. There is accumulating evidence that MPO displays potent proatherogenic properties. For example,

MPO can oxidise LDL-cholesterol, thereby propagating uptake by macrophages and perpetuating foam cell formation. Furthermore, MPO has been shown to activate metalloproteinases and promote destabilization and rupture of the atherosclerotic plaque surface. Also, MPO catalytically consumes endothelial derived nitric oxide, thereby reducing nitric oxide bioavailability and impairing its vasodilatory and antiinflammatory functions. Two studies have revealed that MPO is a powerful predictor of adverse outcome in patients with ACS [41,42]. Particularly in individuals with low troponin levels, MPO identified patients at increased risk for early cardiovascular events that occur within days after the onset of symptoms [41]. This suggests that MPO unmasks states of acute inflammation in the coronary circulation indicative of increased neutrophil activation, which ultimately precedes myocardial injury. In contrast to CRP, MPO is predictive of cardiac events within 72 h itself and may be used to identify patients undergoing coronary angioplasty that benefit from abciximab [41]. In patients with MPO levels above the median, relative risk reduction was 78% at 72 h, 76% at 30 days, and 61% at 6 months. However, in a multivariate model that including troponin T, sCD40L, and MPO only sCD40L remained an independent predictor of the effect of abciximab [41]. While future prospective studies are warranted to confirm these results, the current findings support the rationale to further evaluate MPO for risk stratification in patients with ACS and encourage the development of pharmacologic strategies to modulate the catalytic activity of this enzyme.

Current research activities focus on the identification of more upstream markers of the inflammatory cascade that may be more representative of vascular inflammation as opposed to systemic inflammation. Experimental data suggest that PlGF, a member of the vascular endothelial growth factor family, acts as primary inflammatory instigator of atherosclerotic plaque instability and thus may be useful for risk prediction in patients presenting with ACS. In the first combined retrospective and prospective study it was shown that PlGF levels appear to extend the predictive and prognostic information gained from traditional inflammatory markers, particularly to early follow-up and mortality [43]. Accordingly, PlGF provided independent prognostic information on top of troponin T and sCD40L. The combination of PlGF and sCD40L appeared particularly interesting in patients negative for troponins, but the link to therapeutic strategies has not yet been established.

Pregnancy-associated plasma protein A is a zinc-binding matrix metalloproteinase abundantly expressed in eroded and ruptured plaques and may, thereby, serve as a marker of plaque destabilization. A clinical study suggests that measurement of plasma PAPP-A is an independent predictor of ischemic cardiac events and need of revascularization in patients who present with suspected myocardial infarction but remain troponin negative [44]. These data require validation in larger cohorts and need to be linked to treatment effects before they can enter routine use.

Special subgroups

Among special subgroups that are of increased risk resulting in therapeutic consequences are females, diabetics, and elderly patients.

Female patients with ACS have atypical pain more frequently, have less specific ECG changes, respond differently to treatment, and have higher complication rates. Accordingly, females have less or no benefit from the early invasive strategy and clopidogrel, but GP IIb/IIIa antagonists seem to be even harmful [10,12,14]. In contrast, the effect of statins was comparable [45]. One explanation might be that females represent only around 30% of most study populations and therefore studies are not powered to show a difference in this subgroup. However, too little attention has so far been paid to gender-specific drug doses and cutoff levels for laboratory parameters. Accordingly, the treatment recommendations may be extrapolated more critically to females.

Diabetic patients have an enormously high risk when presenting with ACS. This risk is most effectively reduced by an early invasive management and GP IIb/IIIa antagonists [46]. The evidence for statins and clopidogrel is less well established in this high-risk subgroup, but may be extrapolated from other studies.

There is an increasing number of elderly patients. Although complications increase with age, the benefit of an invasive strategy tends to be even more pronounced, at least with respect to quality of life, but also depending on the age cutoff with respect to mortality and myocardial infarction [10]. The effect of the antiplatelet therapy has to be considered similar despite higher bleeding rates [12,14].

Markers of long-term risk

Patients with ACS continue to be at increased risk even after stabilization of the clinical condition. Markers of long-term risk play no role for acute decision-making, but should be evaluated before the patient is discharged (Table 14.2). Biochemical markers associated with long-term outcome, such as CRP and BNP (NT-proBNP), and the consequences for treatment have already been addressed (see above). Renal function, for example, creatine clearance, has not yet found adequate attention as very potent marker of long-term

Table 14.2 Parameters of long-term risk.

Risk factors (smoking, hypertension, cholesterol, diabetes)
Renal insufficiency
C-reactive protein
BNP/NT-proBNP
Reduced left ventricular function
Angiographic findings (three-vessel disease, main stem)

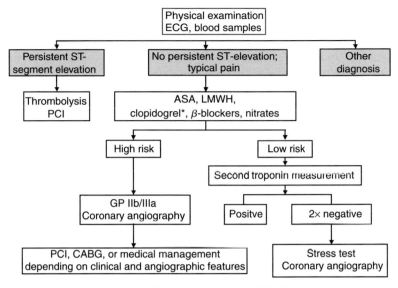

*Omit clopidogrel if the patient is likely to go to CABG within 5 days.

Figure 14.3 Treatment algorithm according to ESC guidelines.

mortality [29,47]. However, there is currently no concept established, by which means the outcome can be positively influenced.

More information on risk is derived from imaging techniques, for example, left ventricular function and angiographic findings, such as main stem lesions. These patients benefit from revascularization as this has been established for stable angina.

Conclusions

The electrocardiogram remains the most useful and cost-effective tool in the first evaluation of patients with chest pain. After exclusion of myocardial infarction, repeat troponin measurements provide valuable diagnostic tools for improving efficacy and safety in acute decision-making in patients presenting with acute chest pain (Figure 14.3). The risk in troponin positive patients is effectively reduced by early invasive management and glycoprotein IIb/IIIa antagonists. BNP (NT-proBNP) in combination with creatinine clearance are powerful predictors of mortality, but specific therapeutic strategies are not yet developed. The long-term risk is assessed by inflammatory markers, such as CRP and LDL-cholesterol, which can be modified by statins.

References

1. Pope JH, Aufderheide TP, Ruthazer R *et al*. Missed diagnoses of acute cardiac ischemia in the emergency department. *N Engl J Med* 2000; **342**: 1163–1170

2. Braunwald E. Unstable angina: an etiologic approach to management. *Circulation* 1998; **98**: 2219–2222.

3. v Miltenburg-van Zijl AJ, Simoons ML, Veerhoek RJ, Bossuyt PM. Incidence and follow-up of Braunwald subgroups in unstable angina pectoris. *J Am Coll Cardiol* 1995; **25**: 1286–1292.

4. Morrow DA, Antman EM, Parsons L *et al*. Application of the TIMI risk score for ST-elevation MI in the National Registry of Myocardial Infarction 3. *JAMA* 2001; **286**: 1356–1359.

5. Eagle KA, Lim MJ, Dabbous OH *et al*. A validated prediction model for all forms of acute coronary syndrome: estimating the risk of 6-month postdischarge death in an international registry. *JAMA* 2004; **291**: 2727–2733.

6. Bertrand ME, Simoons ML, Fox KAA *et al*. Management of acute coronary syndromes in patients presenting without persistent ST-segment elevation. *Eur Heart J* 2002; **23**: 1809–1840.

7. Braunwald E, Antman EM, Beasley JW *et al*. ACC/AHA guideline update for the management of patients with unstable angina and non-ST-segment elevation myocardial infarction—2002. *Circulation* 2002; **106**: 1893–1900.

8. Cannon CP, McCabe CH, Stone PH *et al*. The electrocardiogram predicts one-year outcome of patients with unstable angina and non-Q-wave myocardial infarction: results of the TIMI III Registry ECG Ancillary Study. Thrombolysis in Myocardial Ischemia. *J Am Coll Cardiol* 1997; **30**: 133–140.

9. Savonitto S, Ardissino D, Granger CB *et al*. Prognostic value of the admission electrocardiogram in acute coronary syndromes. *JAMA* 1999; **281**: 707–713

10. Wallentin L, Lagerqvist B, Husted S *et al*. Outcome at 1 year after an invasive compared with a non-invasive strategy in unstable coronary-artery disease: the FRISC II invasive randomised trial. *Lancet* 2000; **356**: 9–16.

11. Cannon CP, Weintraub WS, Demopoulos LA *et al*. Comparison of early invasive and conservative strategies in patients with unstable coronary syndromes treated with the glycoprotein IIb/IIIa inhibitor tirofiban. *N Engl J Med* 2001; **344**: 1879–1887.

12. Boersma E, Harrington R, Moliterno D *et al*. Platelet glycoprotein IIb/IIIa inhibitors in acute coronary syndromes: a meta-analysis of all major randomised clinical trials. *Lancet* 2002; **359**: 189–198.

13. The SYNERGY Trial Investigators. Enoxaparin vs unfractionated heparin in high-risk patients with non-ST-segment elevation acute coronary syndromes managed with an intended early invasive strategy. *JAMA* 2004; **292**: 45–54.

14. Yusuf S, Zhao F, Mehta SR *et al*. Effects of clopidogrel in addition to aspirin in patients with acute coronary syndromes without ST-segment elevation. Clopidogrel in Unstable Angina to Prevent Recurrent Events Trial Investigators. *N Engl J Med* 2001; **345**: 494–502.

15. Davies MJ, Thomas AC, Knapman PA, Hangartner JR. Intramyocardial platelet aggregation in patients with unstable angina suffering sudden ischemic cardiac death. *Circulation* 1986; **73**: 418–427.

16. Falk E. Unstable angina with fatal outcome: dynamic coronary thrombosis leading to infarction and/or sudden death: autopsy evidence of recurrent mural thrombosis with peripheral embolization culminating in total vascular occlusion. *Circulation* 1985; **71**: 699–708.

17. Okamatsu K, M Takano, S Sakai *et al*. Elevated troponin T levels and lesion characteristics in non-ST-elevation acute coronary syndromes. *Circulation* 2004; **109**: 465–470.

18. Hamm CW, Ravkilde J, Gerhardt W *et al*. The prognostic value of serum troponin T in unstable angina. *N Engl J Med* 1992; **327**: 146–150.
19. Antman EM, Braunwald E, Wybenga D *et al*. Cardiac-specific troponin I levels to predict the risk of mortality in patients with acute coronary syndromes. *N Engl J Med* 1996; **335**(18): 1342–1349.
20. Hamm CW, Goldmann BU, Heeschen C *et al*. Emergency room triage of patients with acute chest pain by means of rapid testing for cardiac troponin T or troponin I. *N Engl J Med* 1997; **337**: 1648–1653.
21. Ottani F, Galvani M, Nicolini FA *et al*. Elevated cardiac troponin levels predict the risk of adverse outcome in patients with acute coronary syndromes. *Am Heart J* 2000; **140**: 917–927.
22. Olatidoye AG, Wu AH, Feng YJ, Waters D. Prognostic role of troponin T versus troponin I in unstable angina pectoris for cardiac events with meta-analysis comparing published studies. *Am J Cardiol* 1998; **81**: 1405–1410.
23. Kaul P, Newby K, Fu Y *et al*. (for the PARAGON-B Investigators). Troponin T and quantitative ST-segment depression offer complementary prognostic information in the risk stratification of acute coronary syndrome patients. *J Am Coll Cardiol* 2003; **41**: 371–380.
24. Lindahl B, Andren B, Ohlsson J, Venge P, Wallentin L (and the FRISK Study Group). Risk stratification in unstable coronary artery disease. Additive value of troponin T determinations and pre-discharge exercise tests. *Eur Heart J* 1997; **18**: 762–770.
25. Lindahl B, Venge P, Wallentin L (for the FRISC Study Group). Troponin T identifies patients with unstable coronary artery disease who benefit from long-term antithrombotic protection. *J Am Coll Cardiol* 1997; **29**: 43–48.
26. Hamm CW, Heeschen C, Goldmann BU *et al*. Benefit of abciximab in patients with refractory unstable angina in relation to serum troponin T levels. *N Engl J Med* 1998; **347**: 1623–1629.
27. Heeschen C, Hamm CW, Goldmann B *et al*. Troponin concentrations for risk stratification of patients with acute coronary syndromes in relation to therapeutic efficacy of tirofiban. *Lancet* 1999; **354**: 1757–1762.
28. GUSTO IV-ACS investigators. Effect of glycoprotein IIb/IIIa receptor blocker abciximab on outcome in patients with acute coronary syndromes without early coronary revascularisation: the GUSTO IV-ACS randomised trial. *Lancet* 2002; **357**: 1915–1924.
29. James SK, Lindahl B, Siegbahn A *et al*. N-terminal pro-brain natriuretic peptide and other risk markers for the separate prediction of mortality and subsequent myocardial infarction in patients with unstable coronary artery disease: a Global Utilization of Strategies To Open occluded arteries (GUSTO)-IV substudy. *Circulation* 2003; **108**: 275–281.
30. Heeschen C, Hamm CW, Bruemmer J, Simoons ML. Predictive value of C-reactive protein and troponin T in patients with unstable angina: a comparative analysis. *J Am Coll Cardiol* 2000; **35**: 1535–1542.
31. Lindahl B, Toss H, Siegbahn A, Venge P, Wallentin L (for the FRISC Study Group). Markers of myocardial damage and inflammation in relation to long-term mortality in unstable coronary artery disease. *N Engl J Med* 2000; **343**: 1139–1147.
32. Danesh J, Wheeler JG, Hirschfield GM *et al*. C-reactive protein and other circulating markers of inflammation in the prediction of coronary heart disease. *N Engl J Med* 2004; **350**: 1387–1397.

33. Ridker PM, Cannon CP, Morrow D *et al.* (for the PROVE IT-TIMI 22 Investigators). C-reactive protein levels and outcomes after statin therapy. *N Engl J Med* 2005; **352**: 20–28

34. Mitrovic V, Klein HH, Krekel N *et al.* Influence of the angiotensin converting enzyme inhibitor ramipril on high-sensitivity C-reactive protein (hs-CRP) in patients with documented atherosclerosis. *Z Kardiol* 2005; **94**: 336–342.

35. Jernberg T, Stridsberg M, Venge P, Lindahl B. N-terminal pro brain natriuretic peptide on admission for early risk stratification of patients with chest pain and no ST-segment elevation. *J Am Coll Cardiol* 2002; **40**: 437–445

36. de Lemos JA, Morrow DA, Bentley JH *et al.* The prognostic value of B-type natriuretic peptide in patients with acute coronary syndromes. *N Engl J Med* 2001; **345**: 1014–1021.

37. Heeschen C, Hamm CW, Mitrovic V, Nicte-Ha L, White HD (for the Platelet Receptor Inhibition in Ischemic Syndrome Management (PRISM) Investigators). N-terminal pro-B-type natriuretic peptide levels for dynamic risk stratification of patients with acute coronary syndromes. *Circulation* 2004; **110**: 3206–3212.

38. Myocardial infarction redefined-a consensus document of The Joint European Society of Cardiology/American College of Cardiology Committee for the redefinition of myocardial infarction. *Eur Heart J* 2000; **21**: 1502–1513.

39. Heeschen C, Dimmeler St, Hamm CW *et al.* for the CAPTURE Study Investigators Soluble CD40 ligand in acute coronary syndromes. *N Engl J Med* 2003; **348**: 1104–1111.

40. Varo N, de Lemos JA, Libby P *et al.* Soluble CD40L: risk prediction after acute coronary syndromes. *Circulation* 2003; **108**: 1049–1052.

41. Baldus S, Heeschen C, Meinertz T *et al.* Myeloperoxidase serum levels predict risk in patients with acute coronary syndromes. *Circulation* 2003; **108**: 1440–1445.

42. Brennan ML, Penn MS, Van Lente F *et al.* Prognostic value of myeloperoxidase in patients with chest pain. *N Engl J Med* 2003; **349**: 1595–1604.

43. Heeschen C, Dimmeler S, Fichtlscherer S *et al.* (for the CAPTURE Investigators). Prognostic value of placental growth factor in patients with acute chest pain. *JAMA* 2004; **291**: 435–441.

44. Heeschen C, Dimmeler S, Hamm CW, Fichtlscherer S, Simoons ML, Zeiher AM (for the CAPTURE Study Investigators). Pregnancy-associated plasma protein-A levels in patients with acute coronary syndromes. *J Am Coll Cardiol* 2005; **45**: 229–237.

45. Cannon C, Braunwald E, McCabe C *et al.* Intensive versus moderate lipid lowering with statins after acute coronary syndromes. *N Engl J Med* 2004; **350**: 1495–1504.

46. Roffi M, Chew DP, Mukherjee D *et al.* Platelet glycoprotein IIb/IIIa inhibitors reduce mortality in diabetic patients with non-ST-segment-elevation acute coronary syndromes. *Circulation* 2001; **104**: 2767–2771.

47. Masoudi FA, Plomondon ME, Magid DJ *et al.* Renal insufficiency and mortality from acute coronary syndromes. *Am Heart J* 2004; **147**: 623–629.

CHAPTER 15

Indication for revascularization in non-ST-elevation acute coronary syndrome

Lars Wallentin

Introduction – the rationale of revascularization

The manifestations of ischemia in non-ST-elevation acute coronary syndrome (NSTE-ACS), are caused by a severe flow-limiting stenosis or occlusion of a coronary artery. In the majority of cases there are also signs of myocardial infarction, which might be related to thrombotic occlusion of the culprit coronary lesion as well as to downstream embolization of thrombotic material from the lesion. The thrombotic component of the disease can be influenced by the modern treatment with platelet and thrombin inhibitors [1,2]. Despite such treatment, most often there remain severe coronary stenoses [3–4] leading to a risk of recurrences at the withdrawal of the initially intense antithrombotic treatment [5–7]. Therefore, there is a rationale for the early use of coronary angiography and revascularization. Elimination of the flow-limiting lesions by percutaneous coronary intervention (PCI) or coronary artery bypass grafting (CABG) might be the ideal solution for rapid as well as long-term stabilization of the condition.

Evidence for the benefit of an early invasive strategy

Recently three large-scale prospective randomized trials have convincingly demonstrated the superiority of an early strategy invasive compared with a primarily noninvasive strategy [8–12]. A recent metaanalysis [13] confirms the overall superiority of the early invasive regimen, when taking into account the more equivocal results of the older TIMI (Thrombolysis in Myocardial Ischemia) IIIb [14–15], VANQWISH (Veterans Affairs Non-Q-Wave Infarction Strategies in Hospital) [16], MATE (Medicine versus Angiography in Thrombolytic Exclusion) [17], and VINO [18] trials – Figures 15.1 and 15.2. Much of the differences in outcome among these trials are explained by the different managements that are finally used in the different arms. In some trials,

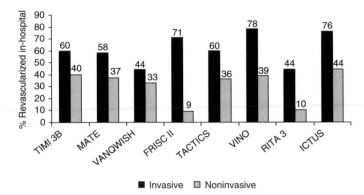

Figure 15.1 Proportion revascularized in hospital in prospective randomized trials of an early invasive compared with a noninvasive approach in NSTE-ACS.

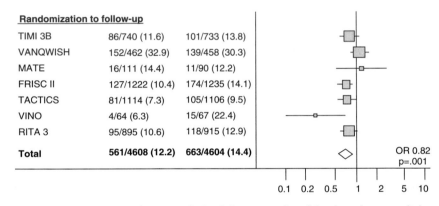

Figure 15.2 Summary and metaanalysis of the composite of death and myocardial infarction during long-term follow-up of the prospective randomized trials comparing invasive versus a noninvanvasive strategy in NSTE-ACS (8–18).

patients' in the invasive arm had less than 50% early revascularization procedure and/or 35–45% early revascularization rate in the noninvasive arm – Figure 15.1. Therefore, it is impressive that the overall results show 18% relative reduction in the composite of death and myocardial infarction after 1 year – Figure 15.2. In the study with the largest contrast (62% in hospital difference) in revascularization procedures, there was an improved survival by the early invasive approach [9–10]. Furthermore, there was, especially in the trials with a larger contrast in procedure rates between the treatment arms, a substantial reduction in anginal symptoms [8–10,12,13], exercise tolerance, exercise induced ischemia [19], readmissions to hospital [8–10,12], and an improved quality of life [20]. Several health economy analyses have also consistently shown that the higher initial costs for the early invasive treatment was compensated later by lower costs for rehospitalization, outpatient visits,

Table 15.1 Risk indicators of use for selection of patients for early invasive treatment in ACS.

- Age (>65 years)
- Coronary risk factors – diabetes mellitus, hyperlipidemia, hypertension, smoking
- Renal dysfunction – reduced GFR (<95 mL/min, even higher risk at <60 mL/min)
- Previous myocardial infarction, previous angina pectoris
- Cardiac dysfunction – elevated NT-proBNP (>240 ng/L, even higher risk at >2000 ng/L)
- History of chest pain at rest or during last 24 h or recurrences despite treatment
- Myocardial ischemia – ST-segment depression ($\geq$0.1 mV, even higher risk at $\geq$0.2 mV)
- Coronary thrombosis elevated troponin (Troponin-T $\geq$ 0.01, even higher risk at $\geq$0.5μg/L)
- Inflammation – elevation of CRP (>10 mg/L)
- Severe coronary artery lesion at coronary angiography

---

and medical treatment during long-term follow-up [21–23]. Thus, compared with a primarily noninvasive approach, an early invasive strategy in ACS is associated with improved survival, lower morbidity, and improved quality of life at no increased cost for the healthcare system.

Risk stratification for selection of patients for early invasive procedures

As with most other treatments, the risk reduction of an early invasive treatment is larger in patients at higher risk and the symptom relief better in patients with more severe symptoms. Many clinical and laboratory observations are related to the subsequent risk of new events in ACS as summarized in Table 15.1 and presented in previous chapters. Thus, much prognostic information is already available in the patient's history, that is, the risk is raised by age, male gender, diabetes, renal failure, previous myocardial infarction, previous severe angina, congestive heart failure, or medication for any of these conditions. The severity of the manifestations of the disease, for example, episodes of chest pain during the last 12–24 h and/or recurrent episodes of pain despite pharmacological treatment is associated with higher risk. Signs of ischemia (ST-segment depression) in electrocardiogram (ECG) at entry and/or episodes of ST-depression during continuous monitoring are also related to a worse prognosis. Left ventricular dysfunction, for example, as evaluated by elevation of NT-proBNP or echocardiography, are other observations associated with guarded prognosis [24]. Recently, a moderate renal dysfunction, for example, glomerular filtration rate (GFR) <95 mL/min, has also been associated with worse outcomes. The occurrence of elevated biochemical markers of myocardial infarction, that is, troponins, is a well-established marker of raised risk for subsequent myocardial infarction as well as for mortality. Finally in the recent past, biochemical markers of inflammatory activity, for example,

C-reactive protein (CRP) and Interleukin-6, have been shown to be associated with worse prognosis. The combination of several of these risk indicators provides a better risk stratification than any marker alone. Thus, the combination of ST-segment depression as a probable indicator of severe coronary stenosis, elevation of troponin as a marker of coronary thrombosis and/or myocardial infarction, elevation of NT-proBNP as a marker of reduced cardiac performance, reduced GFR as an indicator of renal dysfunction, and elevated CRP as an indicator of inflammatory activity provide better prognostic information than any of these factors alone [24,25]. The multivariate analyses of the combination of the patient history, clinical presentation, and these laboratory markers have allowed the presentation of risk scores of key factors containing the most important prognostic information [25–27]. As most of these variables are easily and rapidly available within a short timespan after arrival, they can also be widely applied as a support for the selection of patients for early invasive treatment in clinical practice.

Risk stratification in relation to the effects of invasive treatment

The two largest trials FRISC II and TACTICS/TIMI 18 – (FRISC, Fast Revascularization during instability in coronary artery disease; TACTICS, Treat Angina with aggrastat and determine Cost of Therapy with an Invasive or Conservative Strategy) – randomizing patients to an early invasive versus a selected invasive strategy [8–11] have provided a wealth of information on the outcome of an invasive strategy in relation to risk stratification. Therefore, the present chapter will mainly use the results from these two trials when recommending the most appropriate indications currently for early revascularization.

Both the FRISC II [8–10] and the TACTICS [11] trials showed that the absolute risk reduction concerning subsequent coronary events were larger in patients at higher risk according to most of these risk indicators – Figures 15.3 and 15.4 [11,27]. The invasive treatment was associated with a larger risk in older patients. Still, there were substantially larger relative benefits as well as absolute benefits in patients above 65 years of age [10–12]. Corresponding findings have also been reported from observational trials [28,29]. Still, real-life experiences show that early revascularization procedures are less often used in the elderly [28–31]. Likewise, patients with diabetes mellitus have a considerably increased risk at ACS. However, the proportional risk reduction by early revascularization was similar in patients with or without diabetes [32]. Thereby, the absolute risk reduction concerning death as well as myocardial infarction was larger in patients with diabetes. Despite these successful results, there is an underutilization of early revascularization procedures in patients with diabetes [33]. Also, patients with previous myocardial infarction, left ventricular dysfunction, or renal dysfunction had a larger risk reduction by the early invasive approach [34]. Patients with signs of severe ischemia as indicated by the degree of ST-segment depression or T-wave changes in ECG

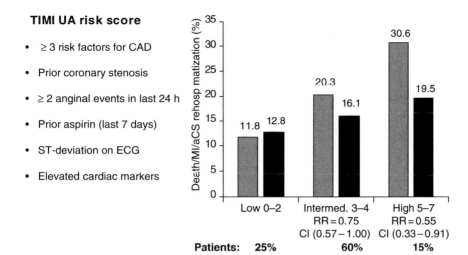

Figure 15.3 Outcome of an early invasive strategy in relation to the TIMI UA risk score in the TIMI-18/TACTICS trial [11,26].

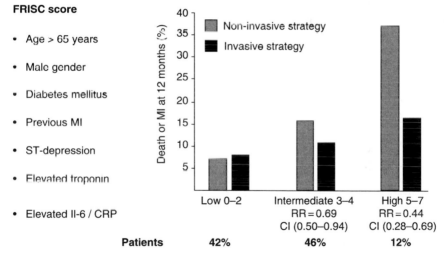

Figure 15.4 Outcome of an early invasive strategy in relation to the FRISC II score in the FRISC II trial [27].

at rest had a considerably larger benefit of early invasive procedures than patients without these findings [35–37]. Both the FRISC II and the TACTICS trial indicated that almost all the benefits from the invasive strategy were seen in patients with detectable troponin in serum samples at entry [11,38]. The risk of a subsequent infarction is similar in all patients with any elevation of troponin, while there is a linear relation between the level of troponin

and mortality [24]. Thus, in the prioritization of patients for invasive procedures any detectable troponin would suggest an invasive approach, while the
urgency of the procedure is raised at higher troponin levels. Patients without
any detectable troponin are at very low risk and have little to gain from invasive procedures unless indicated by incapacitating symptoms of angina or other
risk indicators [38]. In relation to the levels of CRP the relative effects of the
invasive approach were similar at all levels and, thereby, the absolute effects
larger in patients with higher levels of these inflammation markers. However,
according to the FRISC II study results, the initial level of Interleukin-6 seemed
to be a more specific marker of both raised mortality and the effects of early
invasive treatment [39].

Risk scores in relation to the effects of early invasive treatment

Using combinations of several markers both the FRISC II and the TACTICS
trial demonstrated that the benefits of the invasive strategy seemed confined
to patients with a combination of elevated troponin level and ST-segment
depression [11,38]. However, the outcome based on troponin and ST-segment
depression was modulated by the other factors, for example, age, diabetes,
renal dysfunction, previous myocardial infarction, left ventricular dysfunction, severity of previous and current symptoms of angina, and inflammatory
activity. The multivariate approach made it possible to identify the key risk
factors that are needed for introduction in a risk score for evaluation of prognosis and selection of invasive treatment [26,27]. According to these risk
scores the largest benefit of an early invasive treatment was seen at higher
scores, that is, in patients with several of these risk indicators – Figures 15.3 and
15.4. Patients with a high risk score (≥5 risk indicators) had as well improved
survival chances as a lower risk of (re)infarction. At an intermediate risk score
(3–4 risk indicators) there was mainly a reduction in (re)infarction. Finally
the early invasive treatment, with its inherent risk for peri-procedural complications, did not reduce the risk of death or myocardial infarction in the low
risk score patients (0–2 risk indicators). However, it needs to be emphasized
that low as well as high-risk patients with incapacitating symptoms obtain the
same symptom relief and improvement in quality of life from the invasive procedures (8–13,20]. Thus, in many cases there might, because of symptoms, be
reasons to consider invasive procedures even in lower-risk patients. However,
the urgency of the procedures is less in such patients because of their lower
risk for coronary events while awaiting the procedures.

Stress tests for risk stratification

In low-risk patients a stress test will allow further risk stratification. At these
tests a new high-risk category is constituted by either large or multiple areas
of exercise-induced myocardial ischemia or low exercise tolerance. A low-risk
category is defined by an adequate exercise tolerance without any signs of

ischemia. In the high-risk category early catheterization and revascularization is indicated. In the low-risk category no early invasive procedures should be performed, as the periprocedural risks are greater than the potential benefits in this patient category [19]. A strategy with an initial evaluation based on clinical presentation and signs of ischemia followed by a predischarge exercise test, and taking all patients with ischemia to early invasive procedures, were recently found to provide similar long-term outcome as a direct invasive approach in a troponin positive population [40].

Coronary angiography for early risk stratification and selection of treatment

In many instances, the performance of a coronary angiography might provide the most reliable information concerning risk stratification and selection of treatment for an individual patient. By catheterization not only the culprit lesion and its characteristics are identified but also the extent of coronary artery disease, the existence of collaterals, the myocardial area at risk, and the left ventricular function are elucidated by the catheterization. In patients with a clinical diagnosis of ACS there is around 10% with left main, 25% with three-vessel, 25% with two-vessel, 25% with 1-vessel, and 15% with no significant coronary artery disease at coronary angiography. Most of the above outlined risk indicators, that is, age, male gender, diabetes, previous myocardial infarction, previous severe angina, renal dysfunction, left ventricular dysfunction, ST-segment depression, elevated troponin, elevated CRP, and higher risk response at a stress test, are associated with a raised occurrence of multivessel or left main coronary artery disease [41]. However, the relations between these risk indicators and the extent of coronary artery disease is far from perfect. Thus, from the individual patient's perspective it might be preferable to obtain results both from a coronary angiography and from the noninvasive risk indicators as a basis for a decision of early revascularization. The possible disadvantage of such an approach is that all lesions identified at a coronary angiography tend to be dilated and stented at the same session regardless of other risk indicators. In the invasive arm of the FRISC II trial there was no relation between the extent of initial coronary artery disease and subsequent coronary events, indicating that the early invasive procedures will eliminate the risk for new events associated with severe coronary lesions. These findings support the recommendation of early coronary angiography in the majority of ACS patients in order to identify all severe coronary lesions, the risk of which can be reduced by early revascularization.

Gender and selection of invasive treatment

In the FRISC II and the RITA 3 (Randomized Intervention Trial of unstable Angina) trials there was a significantly better effect of the invasive strategy in men than in women [42,44]. This was partly explained by the lower proportion of women revascularized in the invasive group because of the lower rate of significant lesions in females than males. Another reason was that in women with coronary artery by-pass surgery, there was a raised risk for periprocedural complications, especially at diabetes mellitus and higher age [42,44]. However, these gender-related differences in the effects of early invasive treatment were neither observed in the TACTICS or the ICTUS (Invasive versus Conservative Treatment in Unstable coronary Syndromes) trial [40,43], nor in reports from observational materials [28]. In order to properly evaluate women with ACSs it seems, therefore, preferable to use the same indications for diagnostic coronary angiography as in men. However, in the selection of the most appropriate treatment, the higher risk of women at coronary by-pass surgery should be taken into consideration [42,44].

Strategy for selections of patients for early invasive procedures

Patients with suspected or definite ACSs should immediately on admission receive a combination treatment with antithrombotic medications. The risk stratification process, based on history, clinical presentation, response to treatment, ECG-findings and biochemical markers, will also start on admission. At persistent symptoms or signs of ischemia despite medication or at other indicators of high risk, the antithrombotic treatment should be intensified, usually by the addition of glycoprotein IIb/IIIa inhibitor, and the patient taken immediately to the catheterization laboratory for invasive procedures (Figure 15.5). If the symptoms and signs of ischemia subside but there still are several risk

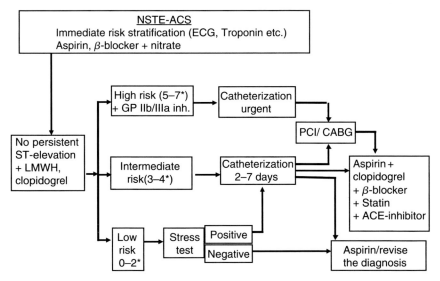

* **Number of risk indicators according to the TIMI or FRISC II scores**

Figure 15.5 Selection and timing of invasive coronary procedures in relation to early risk stratification by the TIMI UA or FRISC II scores.

indicators corresponding to an intermediate risk, there should be planning for an early catheterization although the patient might safely wait for a few days if invasive facilities are not immediately available. Finally in patients without persisting or previous symptoms of ischemia and who are in the low-risk category, further diagnostic procedures with stress testing are needed as the risk of complications might outweigh the potential benefits of invasive procedures. Using this strategy will optimize the utilization and timing of invasive procedures to the benefit of the patient and cost-effectiveness of the healthcare system.

References

1. Bertrand ME, Simoons ML, Fox KA *et al*. Management of acute coronary syndromes: acute coronary syndromes without persistent ST segment elevation; recommendations of the Task Force of the European Society of Cardiology. *Eur Heart J* 2000; **21**: 1406–1432.
2. Braunwald E, Antman EM, Beasley JW *et al*. ACC/AHA guideline update for the management of patients with unstable angina and non-ST-segment elevation myocardial infarction – 2002: summary article. A report of the American College of Cardiology/American Heart Association Task Force on Practice Guidelines (Committee on the Management of Patients With Unstable Angina). *Circulation* 2002; **106**: 1893–1900
3. CAPTURE Investigators. Randomised placebo-controlled trial of abciximab before and during coronary intervention in refractory unstable angina – the CAPTURE Study. *Lancet* 1997; **349**: 1429–1435.
4. Lindahl B, Diderholm E, Lagerqvist B, Venge P, Wallentin L. Mechanisms behind the prognostic value of troponin T in unstable coronary artery disease: a FRISC II substudy. *J Am Coll Cardiol* 2001; **38**(4): 979–986.
5. Theroux P, Waters D, Lam J, Juneau M, McCans J. Reactivation of unstable angina after the discontinuation of heparin. *N Engl J Med* 1992; **327**(3): 141–145.
6. FRISC study group. Low-molecular-weight heparin during instability in coronary artery disease, Fragmin during Instability in Coronary artery disease (FRISC) study group. *Lancet* 1996; **347**: 561–568.
7. TRIM study group. A low molecular weight, selective thrombin inhibitor, inogatran, vs heparin, in unstable coronary artery disease in 1209 patients. A double-blind, randomized, dose-finding study. *Eur Heart J* 1997; **18**: 1416–1425.
8. FRISC-II Investigators. Invasive compared with non-invasive treatment in unstable coronary-artery disease: FRISC II prospective randomised multicentre study. Fragmin and Fast Revascularisation during InStability in Coronary artery disease Investigators. *Lancet* 1999; **354**: 708–715.
9. Wallentin L, Lagerqvist B, Husted S, Kontny F, Stahle E, Swahn E. Outcome at 1 year after an invasive compared with a non-invasive strategy in unstable coronary-artery disease: the FRISC II invasive randomised trial. FRISC II Investigators. *Lancet* 2000; **356**: 9–16.
10. Lagerqvist B, Husted S, Kontny F *et al*. A long-term perspective on the protective effects of an early invasive strategy in unstable coronary artery disease: two-year follow-up of the FRISC-II invasive study. Fast Revascularization during InStability in Coronary artery disease-II Investigators. *J Am Coll Cardiol* 2002; **40**: 1902–1914

11. Cannon CP, Weintraub WS, Demopoulos LA *et al.* Comparison of early invasive and conservative strategies in patients with unstable coronary syndromes treated with the glycoprotein IIb/IIIa inhibitor tirofiban. *N Engl J Med* 2001; **344**: 1879–1887.

12. Fox KA, Poole-Wilson PA, Henderson RA *et al.* Interventional versus conservative treatment for patients with unstable angina or non-ST-elevation myocardial infarction: the British Heart Foundation RITA 3 randomised trial. Randomized Intervention Trial of unstable Angina Investigators. *Lancet* 2002; **360**: 743–751.

13. Mehta SR, Cannon CP, Fox KA *et al.* Routine versus selective invasive strategies in patients with acute coronary syndromes: a collaborative meta-analysis of the randomized trials. *JAMA* 2005; **293**: 2908–2917.

14. TIMI IIIB Investigators. Effects of tissue plasminogen activator and a comparison of early invasive and conservative strategies in unstable angina and non-Q-wave myocardial infarction. Results of the TIMI IIIB Trial. *Circulation* 1994; **89**: 1545–1556.

15. Anderson HV, Cannon CP, Stone PH *et al.* One-year results of the Thrombolysis in Myocardial Infarction (TIMI) IIIB clinical trial. A randomized comparison of tissue-type plasminogen activator versus placebo and early invasive versus early conservative strategies in unstable angina and non-Q wave myocardial infarction. *J Am Coll Cardiol* 1995; **26**: 1643–1650.

16. Boden WE, O'Rourke RA, Crawford MH *et al.* Outcomes in patients with acute non-Q-wave myocardial infarction randomly assigned to an invasive as compared with a conservative management strategy. Veterans Affairs Non-Q-Wave Infarction Strategies in Hospital (VANQWISH) Trial Investigators [see comments]. *N Engl J Med* 1998; **338**: 1785–1792.

17. Spacek R, Widimsky P, Straka Z *et al.* Value of first day angiography/angioplasty in evolving non-ST segment elevation myocardial infarction: an open multicenter randomized trial. The VINO Study. *Eur Heart J* 2002; **23**: 230–238

18. McCullough PA, O'Neill WW, Graham M *et al.* A prospective randomized trial of triage angiography in acute coronary syndromes ineligible for thrombolytic therapy. *J Am Coll Cardiol* 1998; **32**: 596–605.

19. Diderholm E, Andren B, Frostfeldt G *et al.* Effects of an early invasive strategy on ischemia and exercise tolerance among patients with unstable coronary artery disease. *Am J Med* 2003; **115**: 606–612.

20. Janzon M, Levin LA, Swahn E. Invasive treatment in unstable coronary artery disease promotes health-related quality of life: results from the FRISC II trial. *Am Heart J* 2004; **148**: 5–6.

21. Janzon M, Levin L-Å, Swahn E, FRISCII Investigators. Cost-effectiveness of early invasive treatment in unstable coronary artery disease: a one year follow-up from the FRISCII invasive trial. *J Am Coll Cardiol* 2001; **37**: 376A.

22. Janzon M, Levin LA, Swahn E. Cost-effectiveness of an invasive strategy in unstable coronary artery disease; results from the FRISC II invasive trial. *Eur Heart J* 2002; **23**: 31–40.

23. Mahoney EM, Jurkovitz C, Chu H *et al.* Length of stay for the treatment of acute coronary syndromes: international experience from the TACTICS-TIMI18 trial. *Eur Heart J* 2001; **22**: 223.

24. James SK, Lindahl B, Siegbahn A *et al.* N-terminal pro-brain natriuretic peptide and other risk markers for the separate prediction of mortality and subsequent myocardial infarction in patients with unstable coronary artery disease: a Global

Utilization of Strategies To Open occluded arteries (GUSTO)-IV substudy. *Circulation* 2003; **108**: 275–281.

25. Holmvang L, Clemmensen P, Lindahl B *et al.* Quantitative analysis of the admission electrocardiogram identifies patients with unstable coronary artery disease who benefit the most from early invasive treatment. *J Am Coll Cardiol.* 2003; **41**: 905–915.

26. Antman EM, Cohen M, Bernink PJ *et al.* The TIMI risk score for unstable angina/non-ST elevation MI: a method for prognostication and therapeutic decision making. *JAMA* 2000; **284**: 835–842.

27. Lagerqvist B, Diderholm E, Lindahl B, *et al.* FRISC-score for selection of patients for an early invasive treatment strategy in unstable coronary artery disease. *Heart* 2005; **91**: 1047–1052.

28. Stenestrand U, Wallentin L. Early revascularisation and 1-year survival in 14-day survivors of acute myocardial infarction: a prospective cohort study. *Lancet* 2002; **359**: 1805–1811.

29. Bach RG, Cannon CP, Weintraub WS *et al.* The effect of routine, early invasive management on outcome for elderly patients with non-ST-segment elevation acute coronary syndromes. *Ann Intern Med* 2004; **141**: 186–195.

30. Avezum A, Makdisse M, Spencer F *et al.* Impact of age on management and outcome of acute coronary syndrome: observations from the Global Registry of Acute Coronary Events (GRACE). *Am Heart J* 2005; **149**: 67–73.

31. Bhatt DL, Roe MT, Peterson ED *et al.* Utilization of early invasive management strategies for high-risk patients with non-ST-segment elevation acute coronary syndromes: results from the CRUSADE Quality Improvement Initiative. *JAMA* 2004; **292**: 2096–2104.

32. Norhammar A, Malmberg K, Diderholm E *et al.* Diabetes mellitus: the major risk factor in unstable coronary artery disease even after consideration of the extent of coronary artery disease and benefits of revascularization. *J Am Coll Cardiol* 2004; **43**: 585–591.

33. Norhammar A, Malmberg K, Ryden L, Tornvall P, Stenestrand U, Wallentin L, (Register of Information and Knowledge about Swedish Heart Intensive Care Admission (RIKS-HIA)). Under utilisation of evidence-based treatment partially explains for the unfavourable prognosis in diabetic patients with acute myocardial infarction. *Eur Heart J* 2003; **24**: 838–844.

34. Jernberg T, Lindahl B, Siegbahn A *et al.* N-terminal pro-brain natriuretic peptide in relation to inflammation, myocardial necrosis, and the effect of an invasive strategy in unstable coronary artery disease. *J Am Coll Cardiol* 2003; **42**: 1909–1916.

35. Diderholm E, Andren B, Frostfeldt G *et al.* ST depression in ECG at entry indicates severe coronary lesions and large benefits of an early invasive treatment strategy in unstable coronary artery disease. The FRISC II ECG substudy. *Eur Heart J* 2002; **23**: 41–49.

36. Jacobsen MD, Wagner GS, Holmvang L *et al.* Quantitative T-wave analysis predicts 1 year prognosis and benefit from early invasive treatment in the FRISC II study population. *Eur Heart J* 2005; **26**: 112–118.

37. Holmvang L, Clemmensen P, Lindahl B *et al.* Quantitative analysis of the admission electrocardiogram identifies patients with unstable coronary artery disease who benefit the most from early invasive treatment. *J Am Coll Cardiol* 2003; **41**: 905–915.

38. Diderholm E, Andren B, Frostfeldt G *et al.* The prognostic and therapeutic implications of increased troponin levels and ST-depression in unstable coronary artery disease. *Am Heart J* 2002; **143**: 760–767.

39. Lindmark E, Diderholm E, Wallentin L, Siegbahn A. Relationship between interleukin 6 and mortality in patients with unstable coronary artery disease: effects of an early invasive or noninvasive strategy. *JAMA* 2001; **286**: 2107–2113.

40. de Winter RJ (on behalf of the Invasive versus Conservative Treatment in Unstable coronary Syndromes (ICTUS) Investigators). Invasive versus conservative treatment in troponin positive patients with acute coronary syndrome. European Society of Cardiology Congress, August 29, 2004, Munich, Germany.

41. Wallentin L. Revascularization in acute coronary syndromes – which patients and why. In: Theroux P, ed. *Acute Coronary Syndrome – a companion to Braunwalds Heart Disease* Saunders, New York, 2002.

42. Lagerqvist B, Safstrom K, Stahle E, Wallentin L, Swahn E. Is early invasive treatment of unstable coronary artery disease equally effective for both women and men? FRISC II Study Group Investigators. *J Am Coll Cardiol* 2001; **38**: 41–48.

43. Glaser R, Herrmann HC, Murphy SA *et al.* Benefit of an early invasive management strategy in women with acute coronary syndromes. *JAMA* 2002; **288**: 3124–3129.

44. Clayton TC, Pocock SJ, Henderson RA *et al.* Do men benefit more than women from an interventional strategy in patients with unstable angina or non-ST-elevation myocardial infarction? The impact of gender in the RITA 3 trial. *Eur Heart J* 2004; **25**: 1641–1650.

CHAPTER 16

Management of patients with nonamenable lesions for myocardial revascularization

Victor Legrand

Introduction

Current therapy of acute coronary syndromes (ACSs) is multifactorial, aiming first to control the acute pathophysiological process and the progression of atherothrombosis, then treating complications of atherosclerosis and cardiac dysfunction as well as preventing plaque progression. It has been very clearly shown that an early invasive approach in all patients with non-ST-elevation ACS (nonSTE-ACS) or ST-elevation ACS (STE-ACS) is beneficial [1,2]. The invasive strategy includes cardiac catheterization and revascularization. Combined with the use of high-dose clopidogrel or glycoprotein IIb/IIIa inhibitors, aspirin, (low molecular weight) heparin, and (drug eluting) stents, early revascularization of the culprit lesion by angioplasty or immediate surgery, whenever possible, is nowadays the recommended strategy [3,4]. This approach significantly reduces death, myocardial infarction (MI), or recurrent ischemia.

However, based on GRACE and EuroHeart Survey registries, among patients catheterized for nonSTE-ACS, only 43–53% had a percutaneous revascularization and only 10–12% underwent a surgical revascularization. For those admitted for STE-ACS, the respective figures were 72–73% for percutaneous coronary intervention (PCI) and 6–10% for surgery [5,6]. Thus, a substantial proportion of patients catheterized for ACS are not considered suitable for a revascularization. Reasons why these patients are not amenable for revascularization are numerous and are listed on Table 16.1. Management of these patients is closely related to the underlying cause that precluded the revascularization approach.

ACS associated with nonobstructive coronary lesion

Acute coronary syndrome represents a heterogeneous spectrum of conditions and it has long been recognized that acute myocardial ischemia and/or necrosis may occur in the absence of obstructive coronary lesion of the

Table 16.1 Clinical situations nonamenable for myocardial revascularization.

No epicardial stenosis
Myocardial stunning
Spasm
Embolization
Toxic substance
Coagulation disorder
Syndrome X
Pericarditis, myocarditis
Aortic dissection
Single-vessel disease
Lesion not suitable for angioplasty
Procedural risk outweighting clinical benefit
No residual ischemia
Multivessel disease
Excessive risk of major cardiac and
cerebrovascular events
Severe diffuse atherosclerosis
Poor distal run-off/distal bed not visualized
No residual ischemia

---

epicardial vessel. The overall prevalence rate of MI with a normal coronary angiogram, although low, is 3–5% and the incidence of normal arteries in nonSTE-ACS is 5–10% [7–9]. Patients with normal coronary arteries are most often young females. Various mechanisms have been recognized including coronary spasm [10–12], embolization [13] , toxic conditions, such as drug abuse (cocaine, metamphetamine, smoking, alcohol) [14–17], or inherited coagulation disorders [18–20].

A screening survey for these conditions includes a provocative test for coronary spasm (either ergonovine or the more specific acetylcholine), search for embolic sources (including paradoxal embolism through a patent foramen ovale) and clinical signs of systemic embolizations, exclusion of an intoxication, as well as evaluation of the hemostasis.

Results of this etiologic research might influence the management of these patients. Notably, provocation of a coronary spasm represents a relative contraindication for the use of β-blockers in these patients. However, despite a systematic search, etiological factors are found in only one-third of these patients.

The transient left ventricular apical ballooning syndrome is another peculiar presentation of ACS with normal coronary arteries that mimics acute MI. This syndrome was first recognized in Japan in 1991 [21]. It more often affects postmenopausal women and is characterized by chest pain, ST-segment elevation in the precordial leads, minor elevation of cardiac enzymes, and transient apical systolic dysfunction. It may represent a cathecolamine-mediated myocardial stunning [22]. Management of these patients remains symptomatic with the use of β-blockers, angiotensin-converting enzyme inhibitors, aspirin, anticoagulation agents, and diuretics as needed. Prognosis is usually good, with complete recovery of systolic ventricular function within few weeks [23].

Similarly, diffuse microvascular dysfunction or myocardial metabolic disturbancies may explain occurrence of chest pain and ST–T wave changes in the absence of obstructive epicardial coronary disease. This syndrome, often referred to as cardiac syndrome X, most often occurs in middle-age women and may mimic unstable angina [24,25]. Likewise, for the apical ballooning syndrome, there is no specific treatment for this situation even if prognosis is good.

Normal coronary arteries with chest pain, electrocardiographic abnormalities, and troponin rise may also occur in the setting of pericarditis or myocarditis. Diagnosis is usually confirmed by serology, elevation of inflammatory markers, echographic findings, and electrocardiographic patterns. Other obvious causes that can mimic ACS include intracranial bleeding, pheochromocytoma, hypertrophic cardiomyopathy, hyperthyroidism, aortic dissection, etc.

One notable finding, with diagnostic and etiologic considerations aside, is that patients presenting with ACS having normal coronary arteries have a significantly better prognosis than do those with identified coronary artery disease.

ACS in patients with coronary artery disease

Atherosclerosis is the most frequent cause of ACSs, accounting for more than 90% of the cases. Coronary angiography confirms the diagnosis and allows an accurate evaluation of the severity and the extent of the disease that closely relates to the prognosis of the patient. According to the results of coronary angiography, revascularization is often recommended. Either coronary artery bypass surgery or angioplasty are proposed to bypass or open the occluded coronary segment(s) responsible for the clinical syndrome. However, in some instances, medical therapy may be preferred or other treatment strategies can be pursued when revascularization is deemed impossible.

Medical treatment
Individual risk assessment should be performed to select patients for coronary revascularization and a careful analysis of the risk and benefit ratio of revascularization is needed especially for older patients. On one hand, one must assess the extent and location of myocardial ischemia or viability, and the recurrence or the risk of ischemic symptoms. On the other hand, one must consider the risk related to early invasive percutaneous or surgical revascularization.

Specifically, the survival benefit of revascularization over medical management is not obvious in patients presenting with one-vessel coronary disease, except for the proximal LAD. In these situations, surgical revascularization is usually not recommended and percutaneous revascularization should be avoided when the operator considers that the probability of complications or technical failure is high. This is particularly relevant when the jeopardized territory is small. Anatomic situations usually associated with a higher incidence of failure or complication following angioplasty are usually referred as Type C lesions and include chronic total occlusion, extreme tortuosity, heavily calcified vessel, bifurcation lesion, presence of visible thrombus, or lesion in old saphenous venous graft. Although the use of new percutaneous intervention techniques has dramatically improved the success rate in these situations, medical treatment should always be considered as a valuable (if not the best) alternative, particularly in older patients and in those with severe comorbidities or short life expectancy.

Revascularization is usually recommended in patients with two or more vessel disease, left main stenosis, or proximal LAD lesion, provided that myocardial ischemia or viability is demonstrated. When surgery is considered, the operative risk must be evaluated. The EuroSCORE (www.euroscore.org) may be used to estimate the early mortality risk. The scoring system used for the EuroSCORE is given on Table 16.2. Those with a score of 6 or above carry an operative mortality risk higher than 12%.

Clearly, no scoring system will predict the specific outcome for every patient. Risk stratification, however, should form part of the basis on which the patient, surgeon, and interventionalist decide to proceed. In high surgical risk patients, coronary angioplasty may represent an attractive alternative to surgery. However, there are no guidelines defining the indications of PCI as an alternative treatment to surgery. Therefore, the method of revascularization in complex situations should always be discussed between the surgeon and the cardiologist and the most appropriate approach may differ from one center to the other according to local circumstances. In rare instances, the clinical and/or the anatomic situation is not suitable for either a percutaneous or a surgical revascularization. Such situations concern:

1 patients with multivessel disease and an extremely high risk of death or complications following surgery, who are also poor candidates for PCI because they are not amenable for adequate revascularization or are at similar high risk;

2 patients with severe diffuse coronary atherosclerosis and poor distal run-off who cannot be revascularized adequately.

Usually, these situations cannot be managed by conventional medical treatment alone and alternative approaches must be considered.

In any case, however, those patients nonamenable for revascularization therapy should be encouraged to adopt lifestyle changes, such as stopping smoking, diet modifications, weight control, and increased physical activity. Also, optimal medical management including β-blockers, nitrates, and calcium

Table 16.2 EuroSCORE scoring system.

	Score
Patient-related factors	
Age: (Per 5 years over 60 years)	1
Sex: Female	1
Chronic pulmonary disease:	1
Long-term use of bronchodilators or steroids	
Extracardiac arteriopathy:	2
Claudication, carotid >50% stenosis, previous or	
planned intervention on aorta,	
limb arteries, or carotids	
Neurological disease: Severely affecting ambulation	2
or day-to-day functioning	
Previous cardiac surgery: Requiring opening of the pericardium	3
Serum creatinine: >200μmol/L preoperatively	2
Active endocarditis: Patient still under antibiotics at the time of surgery	3
Critical preoperative state: Any of the following: ventricular tachycardia or	3
fibrillation or aborted sudden death, preoperative cardiac	
massage, ventilation, inotropic support,	
intaaortic balloon counterpulsation or acute renal failure	
Cardiac-related factors	
Unstable angina: Rest angina requiring IV nitrates	2
LV dysfunction: Moderate or LVEF 30–50%	1
Poor or LV < 30%	3
Recent myocardial infarct: <90 days	2
Pulmonary hypertension: Systolic PA pressure > 60 mm Hg	2
Operation-related factors	
Emergency: Carried out before beginning of the next day	2
Other than isolated CABG: Major cardiac procedure other than	2
or in addition to	
Surgery on thoracic aorta: CABG	3
Postinfarct septal rupture: For disorder of ascending, arch, or descending aorta	4

Notes: CABG – coronary artery bypass grafting; LV – left ventricular; LVEF – left ventricular ejection fraction.

antagonists should be considered as part of the routine standard therapy together with the control of dyslipidemia, hypertension, and diabetes. Basic medical management also includes prescription of statins and ACE-inhibitors as well as optimal antiagregant treatment [3,4].

Counterpulsation

Enhanced external counterpulsation (EECP) is a noninvasive technique to enhance diastolic filling and reduce cardiac afterload, similar to intraaortic balloon counterpulsation. Large pneumatic cuffs are wrapped around the legs and inflated during protodiastole to 300 mm Hg. The standard treatment regimen consists of sessions of 1 h duration. Cardiac output is increased by the Starling mechanism as venous return is increased upon inflation and afterload reduced by the sudden drop in diastolic pressure on deflation. The initial increase in diastolic pressure may also improve coronary blood flow and the left ventricular unloading theoretically decreases myocardial oxygen demand. In addition, other mechanisms such as the growth of new collateral vessels and a sustained coronary vasodilatation initiated by an increase in plasma nitric oxide and a reduction in endothelin may account for the benefit of this treatment [26,27].

Case series and the MUST-EECP trial have demonstrated that EECP can improve symptoms, exercise tolerance, and reduce myocardial ischemia [28]. Limitations of this technique include patient uncomfort (pain in the back and legs) as well as superficial skin lesions. Moreover, the EECP compressor is cumbersome and not widely available. In addition, this treatment is contraindicated in patients with severe aortic insufficiency, atrial fibrillation or frequent ectopy, and severe peripheral vascular disease.

As improvement achieves a plateau after 36 h of therapy [29], there is little evidence to confirm that this treatment should be considered for more than 4–7 weeks.

Despite these limitations, EECP deserves consideration in patients not amenable to revascularization and who are refractory to medical therapy.

Transmyocardial laser

Creation of ventricular channels mimicking vessels to deliver blood to the myocardium was the idea beyond the development of the laser revascularization technique. However, several histologic studies have demonstrated that these channels occlude shortly after their creation. To explain the symptomatic improvement observed in some patients, alternative mechanisms have been proposed such as sympathetic denervation of the left ventricle [30,31], promotion of angiogenesis [32,33], or a placebo effect. Since no increase in myocardial perfusion has been observed in multiple trials, the former mechanism is more likely.

Laser energy can be delivered by a carbon dioxide or a holmium : YAG laser system. The latter uses a fiber optic catheter enabling a percutaneous approach. The percutaneous approach needs retrograde left ventricular catheterization and orientation of the laser catheter toward the affected myocardium under electromechanical mapping guidance. The surgical transmyocardial laser approach allows a direct visualization of the myocardium and thus results in a more precise creation of channels. It has been used by some surgeons as an adjunct to CABG in areas not amenable for revascularization.

In clinical trials in patients not amenable to complete revascularization by surgery, a combination of laser revascularization plus CABG appears to have some symptomatic benefit [34–37] as do surgical laser revascularization without CABG [38–40]. Clear improvement in objective measurements, such as mortality or myocardial perfusion imaging, has never been reported, however. Results achieved by the percutaneous laser myocardial revascularization are also disappointing. Although two randomized trials (PACIFIC and BELIEF trials) reported some symptomatic improvement in laser-treated patients, the DIRECT trial failed to demonstrate any significant benefit with the laser therapy [39]. These findings thus suggest that the benefits seen are largely due to the placebo effect. Although myocardial laser revascularization is recommended as an alternative procedure for patients not amenable to conventional revascularization, the recent results of sham/placebo controlled trial have greatly diminished the enthusiasm for this therapeutic approach, which is no longer considered superior to medical therapy [41].

Angiogenesis

The transfer of proteins or genes of naturally occurring growth factors to develop neovascularization as well as the capacity of progenitor cells to increase vascularity have been proposed for the treatment of patients with intractable angina who are not candidates for conventional revascularization techniques [42–45].

Following research in animal models that showed promising results, therapeutic angiogenesis was first used for the treatment of critical limb ischemia [46], then applied for the treatment of myocardial ischemia [47]. Although proof of the principle has been established in animal models, the true efficacy of therapeutic angiogenesis is not yet established and many uncertainties persist on the optimal agent(s), its mode of administration, and the associated risks.

Fundamentally, angiogenesis should be distinguished from arteriogenesis that describes the process of development of new arteries with fully developed tunica media. Arteriogenesis correspond to blood vessel creation, and formation of visible collaterals – distal to a severe stenosis – is a prime example of this naturally occurring mechanism, probably from preexisting collaterals. Angiogenesis refers to the neoformation of vessels that lack tunica media, such as the development of the capillary network along the border zone of a myocardial infarction. This latter mechanism can be enhanced by vascular growth factors, by the introduction of genetic material that control the production of these proteins, or by myocardial homing of mesenchymal stem cells (MSCs). The advantages and disadvantages of each modality are listed in Table 16.3.

The angiogenic growth factors that have been studied most extensively are those in the vascular endothelial growth factor (VEGF) and fibroblast growth factor (FGF) families, as well as the granulocyte/macrophage colony-stimulating factor. Introduction of genetic material that control the production of these angiogenic growth factors can be performed using the adenoviral vector or plasmids (small, circular DNA pieces). Administration of viral vector has the potential for targeting specific cells (cardiac myocytes), while plasmids are less efficiently taken up by the target cell and more easily degraded. Protein

Table 16.3 Protein-, gene- and cell-based therapies for angiogenesis.

	Protein	Gene	Stem cell
Advantages	• Titratable dose • Easy repeat administration • Finite, temporary effect • No viral vectors	• Single administration • Cell-type specificity • Localized administration	• Titratable administration • Autologous cell • Myocardial regeneration • No viral vectors
Disadvantages	• Short half-life • Need for redosing • Lack of efficacy	• Foreign genetic material • Inflammatory response • Inefficient delivery • Untoward angiogenesis	• Indirect mechanism

therapy avoids introduction of foreign genetic material and adverse immune and inflammatory response, but is limited by its short half-life and need for repeated titration. In comparison, stem cell therapy is less specific involving heterogeneous group of cells and many controversies remain regarding the ideal subtype and exact mechanism of action [43,45].

There are also controversies about the mode of administration of viral agents, plasmid, proteins, or stem cells. Intramyocardial administration of adenovirus or plasmids tends to produce focal gene expression around the site of the needle tract. Therefore, intracoronary infusion by catheter appears to be the simplest and more promising approach although limited by the washout effect by coronary flow, the imprecise localization and consequently the unknown amount of therapeutic agent effectively adsorbed at the target site. Local, intracoronary, administration of stem cells has similar limitations and intravenous infusion may offer the same results [48].

Human trials in therapeutic angiogenesis have consistently shown encouraging results. Most of these trials have been performed to evaluate the safety and feasibility of therapeutic angiogenesis, however. The largest reported study is the AGENT trial that evaluated intracoronary administration of adenovirus containing FGF in 79 pts (placebo in 19 pts) [49]. It showed a significant increase in exercise duration and tolerance time in treated patients without serious adverse events during long-term follow-up (311 days). Because of the limited number of patients evaluated so far, the potential benefit of this approach is difficult to assess objectively. It is hoped that the larger ongoing AGENT 3 and 4 studies would produce more definitive results on safety and efficacy of angiogenic gene therapy.

Similarly, stem cell therapy is still in its infancy and is used mostly as a regeneration therapy aiming to improve cardiac function. The therapeutic potential of endothelial progenitor cell (EPC) and MSC for local vasculogenesis and tissue repair is well recognized [43,45]. These cells can be purified and

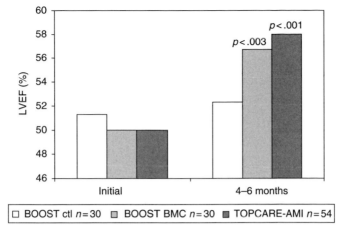

Figure 16.1 Global left ventricular ejection fraction at baseline and at control angiography in the BOOST randomized trial and in the TOPCARE-AMI efficacy trial assessing the effect of bone marrow cell (BMC) transfer after MI.

extracted from the bone marrow or simply mobilized by exogenous granulo-cyte colony stimulating factor (G-CSF) and different cytokines. However, the efficacy of this strategy to induce angiogenesis is difficult to estimate and the mechanisms by which EPCs and MSCs improve neovascularization and or myocardial regeneration remain unclear.

Initial results of safety/efficacy TOPCARE-AMI trial (50) and randomized BOOST trial [51] performed in acute MI demonstrated significant improve-ment of global left ventricular ejection fraction after 6 months in the group of patients receiving autologous bone marrow cells (Figure 16.1), together with a significant reduction of infarct size. Results of larger multicentric ongoing ran-domized trial are awaited to confirm these encouraging preliminary results, however. It is worth underlining that these trials were conducted in patients initially treated by angioplasty. Whether similar results can be reproduced in a population nonamenable for revascularization is yet unclear. Interestingly, circulating EPCs are significantly increased in patients with unstable angina, which could suggest that a natural triggering of these repair mechanisms already exists [52].

Although most angiogenic and stem cell therapy studies reported low rates of procedural related morbidity and mortality, hypotension, proteinuria, and angioma formation have been described. Also, there is concern about the risks of undesirable angiogenesis in diabetic retinopathy, worsening of atherosclerotic process, and potentiation of malignancies.

Currently, angiogenesis therapy and stem cell therapy for patients not amenable to conventional revascularization represent an exciting perspective that need further experimental and clinical evaluation before it can be accepted as a valuable treatment strategy.

Neurostimulation

Several adjunctive treatment have demonstrated efficacy on anginal symptoms when revascularization is contraindicated. Transcutaneous electrical nerve stimulation (TENS) and spinal cord stimulation (SCS) modifies the neurologic input and output of the heart by delivering a very low dose of electrical current. The former uses precordial electrodes connected to a portable stimulator, the latter involves implantation of an electrode at the level of the first or second thoracic vertebra connected to a permanent stimulator placed in the upper abdomen. Direct neurostimulation of the dorsal columns of the high thoracic spinal cord by the implantable system (SCS) appears to be the most effective method. Beside its modulating effect on pain sensation, SCS has been shown to improve myocardial perfusion in ischemic areas [53–58]. This may be favored by the recruitment of collateral vessels by the calcitonin gene-related peptide and other endogenous vasodilators release [59]. Benefit of SCS may be even larger after an acute coronary event, when sympathetic tone is increased in response to myocardial ischemia. SCS may indeed stop the reflex increase in sympathetic tone elicited by the ischemic tissue.

Small, open-label trials with SCS have shown clinical improvement [57]. However, a placebo effect cannot be ruled out. Complications of SCS include neurologic damage, electrode migration, infection, and cerebrospinal leak [53].

In acute situations, high thoracic epidural blockade with local anesthetic infusion into the epidural space produces a rapid and potent sympatholysis and coronary vasodilation, and reduces myocardial oxygen demand [60–62]. This technique is mostly used by anesthesiologists as a perioperative adjunct to coronary artery bypass grafting surgery and can also be used as a temporary treatment in refractory coronary disease.

Heart transplantation

For patients who have disabling ischemia, with or without heart failure, and in whom all conventional and alternative therapeutics have failed, heart transplantation should be discussed. This ultimate treatment modality must consider the risks of the surgical procedure and the survival probability of the patient after transplantation, as some patients may be expected to live longer with their symptoms.

Conclusion

Various situations may account to carry on with medical management and lifestyle modifications among patients presenting with ACS. This includes mostly those patients without significant narrowing of the epicardial arteries as well as those with single-vessel coronary disease not suitable or relevant for angioplasty. More difficult are situations where patients present with severe multivessel disease nonamenable for revascularization. Beside optimal medical and lifestyle management, alternate methods for reducing ischemia have been proposed such as EECP, neurostimulation, transmyocardial laser therapy, and angiogenesis. Although some clinical benefit may be expected, none of these strategies have demonstrated a pronounced effect in reducing ischemia and/or in preventing future coronary events. Angiogenesis appears to be the most promising approach, but the optimum treatment modalities still have to be established.

References

1. Cannon CP, Turpie AGG. Unstable angina and no-ST-elevation myocardial infarction. Initial antithrombotic therapy and early invasive strategy. *Circulation* 2003; **107**: 2640–2645.
2. Antman EM, Van de Werf F. Pharmacoinvasive therapy: the future of treatment for ST elevation myocardial infarction. *Circulation* 2004; **109**: 2480–2486.
3. Bertrand ME, Simoons ML, Fox KA *et al.* Task force on the management of acute coronary syndromes of the European Society of Cardiology. Management of acute coronary syndromes in patients presenting without persistent ST-segment elevation. *Eur Heart J* 2002; **23**: 1809–1840.
4. Van de Werf F, Ardissino D, Betriu A *et al.* Task force on the management of acute myocardial infarction of the European Society of Cardiology. Management of acute myocardial infarction in patients presenting with ST-segment elevation. *Eur Heart J* 2003; **24**: 28–66.
5. Fox KAA, Goodman SG, Klein W *et al.* (for the GRACE Investigators). Management of acute coronary syndromes. Variations in practice and outcome; findings from the Global Registry of Acute Coronary Events (GRACE) *Eur Heart J* 2002; **23**: 1177–1189.
6. Hasdai D, Behar S, Wallentin L *et al.* A prospective survey of the characteristics, treatments and outcomes of patients with acute coronary syndromes in Europe and the Mediterranean basin; the Euro Heart Survey of acute coronary syndromes (Euro Heart Survey ACS) *Eur Heart J* 2002; **23**: 1190–1201.
7. Da Costa A, Isaaz K, Faure E, Mourot S, Cerisier A, Lamaud M. Clinical characteristics, aetiologic factors and long-term prognosis of myocardial infarction with an absolutely normal coronary angiogram. A 3-year follow-up study of 91 patients. *Eur Heart J* 2001; **22**: 1459–1465.
8. Legrand V, Deliege M, Henrard L, Boland J, Kulbertus H. Patients with myocardial infarction and normal coronary arteriogram. *Chest* 1982; **6**: 678–685.
9. Zimmerman FH, Cameron A, Fisher LD, Grace NG. Myocardial infarction in young adults: angiographic characterization, risk factors and prognosis (coronary artery surgery registry). *J Am Coll Cardiol* 1995; **26**: 654–661.
10. Bott-Silverman C, Heupler FA. Natural history of pure coronary artery spasm in patients treated medically. *J Am Coll Cardiol* 1983; **2**: 200–205.
11. Vincent GM, Anderson JE, Marshall HW. Coronary spasm producing coronary thrombosis and myocardial infarction. *N Engl J Med* 1983; **309**: 220–223.
12. Conti CR. Myocardial infarction: thoughts about pathogenesis and the role of coronary spasm. *Am Heart J* 1985; **110**: 187–193.
13. Gonzales M, Herandez E, Aranda JM, Linares E, Cortes F, Contron G. Acute myocardial infarction due to intracoronary occlusion after elective cardioversion

for atrial fibrillation in a patient with angiographically nearly normal coronary arteries. *Am Heart J* 1981; **102**: 932–934.

14. Isner JM, Estes NAM, Thompson PD *et al.* Acute cardiac events temporally related to cocaine abuse. *N Engl J Med* 1986; **315**: 1438–1443.

15. Minor RL, Scott BD, Brown DI, Winniford MD. Cocaine induced myocardial infarction in patients with normal coronary arteries. *Ann Intern Med* 1991; **115**: 797–806.

16. Regan TJ, Wu CF, Weisse AB, Moschos CB, Ahme SS, Lyons MM. Acute myocardial infarction in toxic cardiomyopathy without coronary obstruction. *Circulation* 1975; **51**: 453–461.

17. Williams MJA, Restieaux NJ, Low CJS. Myocardial infarction in young people with normal coronary arteries. *Heart* 1998; **79**: 191–194.

18. Holm, J, Zöller B, Svensson PJ *et al.* Myocardial infarction associated with homozygous resistance to activated protein C. *Lancet* 1994; **344**: 952–953.

19. Kyriakidis M, Androulakis A, Triposkiadis F *et al.* Lack of a thrombotic tendency in patients with acute myocardial infarction and angiographically normal coronary arteries. *Circulation* 1995; **86**: 22–24.

20. Da Costa A, Tardy BR, ls-aaz K *et al.* Prevalence of factor V Leiden and other inherited thrombophilias in young patients with myocardial infarction and normal coronary arteries. *Heart* 1998; **80**: 338–340.

21. Kurisu S, Sato H, Kawagoe T *et al.* Tako-tsubo-like left ventricular dysfunction with ST-segment elevation: a novel cardiac syndrome mimicking acute myocardial infarction. *Am Heart J* 2002; **143**: 448–455.

22. Wittstein IS, Thiemann DR, Lima JAC *et al.* Neurohumoral features of myocardial stunning due to sudden emotional stress. *N Engl J Med* 2005; **352**: 539–548.

23. Bybee KA, Kara T, Prasad A *et al.* Systematic review : Transient left ventricular apical ballooning. A syndrome that mimics ST-segment elevation myocardial infarction. *Ann Intern Med* 2004; **141**: 858–865.

24. Legrand V, Hodgson JM, Bates ER *et al.* Abnormal coronary flow reserve and abnormal radionuclide exercise test results in patients with normal coronary angiograms. *J Am Coll Cardiol* 1985; **6**: 1245–1253.

25. Maseri A, Crea F, Kaski JC, Crake T, Mechanisms of angina pectoris in syndrome X. *J Am Coll Cardiol* 1991; **17**: 499–506.

26. Soran O, Crawford LE, Schneider VM *et al.* Enhanced external counterpulsation in the management of patients with cardiovascular disease. *Clin Cardiol* 1999; **22**: 173–178.

27. Urano H, Ikeda H, Ueno T *et al.* Enhanced external counterpulsation improves exercise tolerance, reduces exercise-induced myocardial ischemia and improves left ventricular diastolic filling in patients with coronarv artery disease. *J Am Coll Cardiol* 2001; **37**: 93–99.

28. Arora R, Chou T, Jam D *et al.* The Multicenter Study of Enhanced External Counter-Pulsation (MUST-EECP): effect of EECP on exercise-induced myocardial ischemia and anginal episodes. *J Am Coll Cardiol* l999; **33**: l33–140.

29. Lawson WE. Current use of enhanced external counterpulsation and patient selection. *Clin Cardiol* 2002; **25** (Suppl. II): II-16–II-21.

30. Kwong KF, Kanellopoulos GK, Nickols JC *et al.* Transmyocardial laser treatment denervates canine myocardium. *J Thorac Cardiovasc Surg* 1997; **114**: 883–889.

31. AI-Sheikh T, Allen KB, Straka SP *et al.* Cardiac sympathetic denervation after transmyocardial laser revascularization. *Circulation* 1999; **100**: 135–140.

32. Yamamoto N, Kohmoto T, Gu A, DeRosa C, Smith CR, Burkhoff D. Angiogenesis is enhanced in ischemic canine myocardium by transmyocardial laser revascularization. *J Am Coll Cordiol* 1998; **31**: 1426–1433.

33. Hughes GC, Kypson AP, Annex BH *et al.* Induction of angiogenesis after TMR: a comparison of holmium: YAG, CO, and excimer lasers. *Ann Thorac Surg* 2000; **70**: 504–509.

34. Schofield PM, Sharples LD, Caine N *et al.* Transmyocardial laser revascularisation in patients with refractory angina: a randomised controlled trial. *Lancet* 1999; **353**: 519–524.

35. Frazier OH, March RJ, Horvath KA. Transmyocardial revascularization with a carbon dioxide laser in patients with end-stage coronary artery disease. *N Engl J Med* 1999; **341**: 1021–1028.

36. Burkhoff D, Schmidt S, Schulman SP *et al.* (for the ATLANTIC Investigators). Transmyocardial laser revascularisation compared with continued medical therapy for treatment of refractory angina pectoris: a prospective randomised trial. *Lancet* 1999; **354**: 885–890.

37. Allen KB, Dowling RD, Fudge TL *et al.* Comparison of transmyocardial revascularization with medical therapy in patients with refractory angina. *N Engl J Med* 1999; **341**: 1029–1036.

38. Oesterle SN, Sanborn TA, Ali N *et al.* Percutaneous transmyocardial laser revascularisation for severe angina: the Potential Class Improvement From Intramyocardial Channels (PACIFIC) randomized trial. *Lancet* 2000; **356**: 1705–1710.

39. Leon MB. DIRECT trial. Presented at late breaking trials, Transcatheter Cardiovascular Therapeutics, October 20, 2000, Washington, DC.

40. Salem M, Rotevatn S, Stavnes S *et al.* Blinded Evaluation of Laser Intervention Electively For angina pectoris (BELIEF). *Circulation* 2001; **104** Suppl. II: II144.

41. Saririan M, Eisenberg MJ Myocardial laser revascularization for the treatment of end-stage coronary artery disease. *J Am Coll Cardiol* 2003; **41**: 173–183.

42. Melo LG, Gnecchi M, Pachori AS, Wang K, Dzau VJ. Gene and cell-based therapies for cardiovascular disease: current status and future directions. *Eur Heart J* 2004; **6** (Suppl. E): E24–E35.

43. Melo LG, Pachori AS, Kong D *et al.* Molecular and cell-based therapies for protection, rescue and repair of ischemic myocardium. Reasons for cautious optimism. *Circulation* 2004; **109**: 2386–2393.

44. Losordo DW, Dimmeler S. Therapeutic angiogenesis and vasculogenesis for ischemic disease. Part I: Angiogenic cytokines. *Circulation* 2004; **109**: 2487–2491.

45. Losordo DW, Dimmeler S. Therapeutic angiogenesis and vasculogenesis for ischemic disease. Part II: Cell-based therapies. *Circulation* 2004; **109**: 2692–2697.

46. Isner JM, Pieczek A, Schainfeld R *et al.* Clinical evidence of angiogenesis after arterial gene transfer of ph VEGF 165 in patient with ischemic limb. *Lancet* 1996; **348**: 370–374.

47. Losordo DW, Vale PR, Symes JF *et al.* Gene therapy for myocardial angiogenesis: initial clinical results with direct myocardial injection of ph VEGF 165 as sole therapy for myocardial ischemia. *Circulation* 1998; **98**: 2800–2804.

48. Kleiman NS, Patel NC, Allen KB *et al.* Evolving revascularization approaches for myocardial ischemia. *Am J Cardiol* 2003; **92** (Suppl.): 9N–17N.

49. Grines CL, Watkins MW, Helmer G *et al.* Angiogenic Gene Therapy (AGENT) trial in patients with stable angina pectoris. *Circulation* 2002; **105**: 1291–1297.

50. Schächinger V, Assmus B, Britten MB *et al*. Transplantation of progenitor cells and regeneration enhancement in acute myocardial infarction. Final one-year results of the TOPCARE-AMI Trial. *J Am Coll Cardiol* 2004; **44**: 1690–1699.

51. Wollert KC, Meyer GP, Lotz J *et al*. Intracoronary autologous bone-marrow cell transfer after myocardial infarction: the BOOST randomised controlled clinical trial. *Lancet* 2004; **364**: 141–148.

52. George J, Goldstein E, Abashidze S *et al*. Ciculating endothelial progenitor cells in patients with unstable angina: association with systemic inflammation. *Eur Heart J* 2004; **25**: 1003–1008.

53. Svorkdal N. Treatment of inoperable coronary disease and refractory angina: spinal stimulators, epidurals, gene therapy, transmyocardial laser and counterpulsation. *Seminars Cardiothorac Vasc Anesth* 2004; **8**: 43–58.

54. Mannheimer C, Carlsson CA, Emanuelson H *et al*. The effects of transcutaneous electrical stimulation in patients with severe angina pectoris. *Circulation* 1985; **71**: 308–316.

55. Hautvast RWM, Brouwer J, deJonste MJL, Lie KI. Effect of spinal cord stimulation on heart rate variability and myocardial ischemia in patients with chronic intractable angina pectoris: a prospective ambulatory electrocardiographic study. *Clin Cardiol* 1998; **21**: 33–38.

56. Latif OA, Nedeljkovic SS, Stevenson LW. Spinal cord stimulation for chronic intractable angina pectoris: a unified theory on its mechanism. *Clin Cardiol* 2001; **24**: 533–541.

57. deJongste MJ, Hautvast RW, Hillege HL, Lie KI. Efficacy of spinal cord stimulation as adjuvant therapy for intractable angina pectoris: a prospective randomized, clinical study-working group on neurocardiology. *J Am Coll Cardiol* 1994; **23**: 1592–1597.

58. Chauhan A, Mullins PA, Thuraisingham SI, Taylor G, Petch MC, Schofield PM. Effect of transcutaneous electrical nerve stimulation on coronary blood flow. *Circulation* 1994; **89**: 694–702.

59. Eliasson T, Mannheimer C, Waagstein F *et al*. Myocardial turnover of endogenous opioids and calcitonin-gene-related peptide in the human heart and the effects of spinal cord stimulation on pacing induced angina pectoris. *Cardiology* 1998; **89**: 170–177.

60. Olausson K, Magnusdotrir H, Lurje L *et al*. Anti-ischemic and anti-anginal effects of thoracic epidural anesthesia versus those of conventional medical therapy in the treatment of severe refractory unstable angina pectoris. *Circulation* 1997; **96**: 2178–2182.

61. Gramling-Babb PM, Zile MR, Reeves ST. Preliminary report on high thoracic epidural analgesia: relationship between its therapeutic effects and myocardial blood flow as assessed by thallium distribution. *J Cardiothorac Vasc Anesth* 2000; **14**: 657–661.

62. Richter A, Cederholm I, Jonasson L *et al*. Effect of thoracic epidural analgesia on refractory angina pectoris: long term home self assessment. *J Cardiothorac Vasc Anesth* 2002; **16**: 679–684.

CHAPTER 17

Non-ST-segment elevation coronary syndromes: European Society of Cardiology guidelines

Michel E. Bertrand

Clinical expression of coronary artery disease has markedly changed over the last 15 years. Nowadays, acute coronary syndromes (ACSs) represent the most frequent clinical aspect of coronary artery disease. In Europe and the United States more than 2.5 million patients are admitted to hospital every year with the working diagnosis of ACS.

A European survey conducted in only 103 centers of 25 European countries has recorded 10 484 patients within an 8-month period in 2000 [1]. Of them, 52% had non-ST-segment elevation ACSs.

Acute coronary syndromes, share a common anatomic substrate: pathological, angioscopic, and biological observations have demonstrated that they have different clinical presentations that result from a common underlying pathophysiological mechanism, namely, atherosclerotic plaque rupture or erosion, with differing degrees of superimposed thrombosis and distal embolization [2–5].

In practice, two categories of patients may be encountered

Patients with a presumed ACS with ongoing chest discomfort and persistent ST-segment elevation [or new-onset left bundle branch block (LBBB)]. Persistent ST-segment elevation generally reflects acute total coronary occlusion. The therapeutic objective is either rapid, complete, and sustained recanalization by primary angioplasty (if technically feasible) or fibrinolytic treatment (if not contraindicated). European Society of Cardiology (ESC) guidelines concerning the management of these patients have been published in 2003 [6].

Patients who present with chest pain with electrocardiogram (ECG) abnormalities suggesting acute ischemic heart disease. Persistent or transient ST-segment depression or T-wave inversion, flat T waves, pseudonormalization of T-waves, nonspecific ECG changes, or even a normal ECG at presentation.

The management of patients without persistent ST-segment elevation was addressed in the ESC guidelines published in 2000 [7] that were updated in 2002 [8].

Treatment options

The treatment options described in the guidelines are based on the evidence collected from numerous clinical trials or metaanalyses. Guidelines classified the therapeutic options according to the strength of evidence. Accordingly, in this document, the strength of evidence will be ranked according to three levels:

Level of evidence A: data derived from multiple randomized clinical trials or metaanalyses.

Level of evidence B: data derived from a single randomized trial or nonrandomized studies.

Level of evidence C: consensus opinion of the experts.

The strength of recommendations is presented using the following classification:

Class I: conditions for which there is evidence that a given therapy is useful and effective.

Class II: conditions for which there is conflicting evidence and/or divergence about the efficacy/usefulness of a given treatment. There is no Class III in the ESC guidelines since Class III represent contraindications that do not need to be recommended.

Five categories of treatment might be proposed: antiischemic agents, antithrombin therapy, antiplatelet agents, fibrinolytics, and coronary revascularization.

Table 17.1 summarizes the strength of recommendations and the levels of evidence. For this specific point, evidences concerning early benefit [reduction of ischemia and prevention of death and myocardial infarction (MI)] were considered, while sustained early benefits and even additional long-term reduction of death and MI were also mentioned.

1 Antiischemic agents decrease myocardial oxygen utilization (heart rate, blood pressure, contractility) or induce vasodilatation. The beneficial effects of β-blockers are based upon a limited number of randomized trials (level of evidence B). There is no randomized placebo-controlled trials to confirm the benefit of nitrates that are usually used to relieve chest pain (level of evidence C). There are no specific data on potassium channel activators. A metaanalysis of the effects of calcium channel blockers suggests no benefit to prevent death or MI (level of evidence C).

2 Antithrombin agents include indirect antithrombin agents [unfractionated heparin or low molecular weight heparin (LMWH)]. Heparin is certainly superior to placebo (Figure 17.1). All LMWH are not alike and a recent metaanalysis showed that enoxaparin is more efficient and equally safe than unfractionated heparin [9].

Table 17.1 Level of evidence of the different therapeutic options.

Treatment	Class	Strength of evidence			
		Early benefit reduction ischemia	Early benefit prevention, MI, death	Sustained effect of early benefit	Additional long-term reduction, death, MI
β-blockers	I	A	B	B	A
Nitrates	I	C	—	—	—
Calcium antagonists	II	B	B		
Aspirin	I	—	A	A	A
Thienopyridine	I	B	B	B	B
IIb–IIIa receptor blockers	II	A	A	A	A*
Unfractionated heparin	I	C	B	—	—
LMWH	I	A	A	A	C**
Specific antithrombins	I	—	A	A	—
Revascularization	1	A	A	A	B

*No additional benefit; in contrast indications for a negative effect.
**In selected patients.

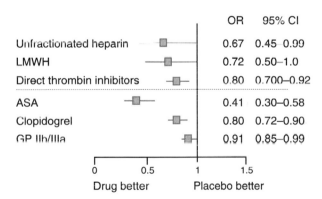

Figure 17.1 Comparison of the different antithrombotic drugs versus placebo.

3 It is mandatory to prescribe aspirin (evidence level A) and clopidogrel (evidence level B) in all patients with ACS. Glycoprotein (GP) IIb/IIIa are also very effective (evidence level A) but are mainly beneficial in high-risk patients with elevated troponins, diabetics, and all ACS patients undergoing interventions.
4 An invasive strategy including early coronary angiography followed by per-cutaneous coronary intervention (PCI) or coronary artery by-pass grafting (CABG) if the lesions are suitable for revascularization is superior to a conservative strategy including medical treatment followed by ischemic assessment

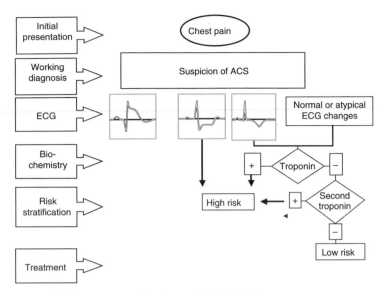

Figure 17.2 Initial assessment of patients with ACS in five steps.

by noninvasive stress tests (evidence level A). Three randomized trials have clearly shown the benefit of invasive strategies. More recently, the ICTUS (Invasive versus Conservative Treatment in Unstable Coronary Syndromes) trial failed to find significant differences in mortality rates in two groups of patients randomized to immediate invasive strategy or elective strategy. However, in most of the trials [except FRISC II (Fragmin and Fast Revascularization During Instability in Coronary Artery Disease)], the results of the conservative arm were spoiled by a number of patients who underwent interventions.

Strategy

Initial assessment at presentation

In most patients chest discomfort (chest pain) is the main clinical expression. Initial assessment includes the following five steps (Figure 17.2):

1 It is important to obtain a careful history and a precise description of the symptoms. A physical examination with particular attention to the possible presence of valvular heart disease (aortic stenosis), hypertrophic cardiomyopathy, heart failure, and pulmonary disease is required.

2 An electrocardiogram is recorded: comparison with a previous electrocardiogram (ECG), if available, is very valuable, particularly in patients with preexisting cardiac pathology, such as left ventricular hypertrophy or known coronary disease. The ECG allows differentiation of patients with a suspicion of ACS into three categories requiring different therapeutic approaches:

(a) ST-segment elevation signifies complete occlusion of a major coronary artery and immediate reperfusion therapy is usually indicated. This represented

42% of the cases in the European Heart Survey on ACS. Management of these patients falls outside the scope of the present guidelines.

(b) ST-segment changes but without persistent ST-segment elevation or a normal ECG (51% of cases).

(c) In a few cases (7%), there is no definite characterization and there are undetermined ECG changes such as bundle branch block or pacemaker rhythm.

3 In points (b) and (c), biochemical markers are required for further characterization. Laboratory assessments should include hemoglobin (to detect anemia), creatinine, glycemia, and markers of myocardial damage, preferably cardiac troponin T or I . Elevated troponins mean irreversible cell damage and these patients must be regarded as having had MI according to the definition of the consensus conference [10].

Troponin measurements are *diagnostic* tools in patients with normal ECG, atypical ECG changes, or ECG profiles precluding diagnostic assessment. They, are useful tools for risk stratification in patients with negative or flat T-waves, atypical ST–T-segment changes.

4 Then starts an observational period that includes a multilead ECG ischemia monitoring. If the patient experiences a new episode of chest pain, a 12-leads ECG should be obtained and compared with a tracing obtained when symptoms have resolved spontaneously or after nitrates. In addition, an ECG may be recorded to assess left ventricular function and eliminate other cardiovascular causes of chest pain. If the first troponin measurement is normal, a second troponin measurement should be obtained between 6 and 12 h.

5 Patients can then be classified as suffering from ACS, distinguishing MI (with elevated markers of necrosis), and unstable angina (ECG changes but no signs of necrosis) with a remaining group of other disease or as yet undetermined cause of their symptoms.

Once diagnosed, ACSs without persistent ST-segment elevation (ST-segment depression, negative T-waves, pseudonormalization of T waves, or normal ECG) require an initial medical treatment including aspirin (75–150 mg daily), clopidogrel, LMWH or unfractionated heparin, β-blockers, and oral or intravenous nitrates in case of persistent or recurrent chest pain. Clopidogrel should replace aspirin in patients with hypersensitivity or major gastrointestinal intolerance to aspirin. In the subsequent observation period (8–12 h) specific attention should be given to recurrence of chest pain during which an ECG will be recorded. Signs of hemodynamic instability should be carefully noted (hypotension, pulmonary rales) and treated.

Within this initial period, risk assessment can be performed based on the clinical, electrocardiographical, and biochemical data, and a further treatment strategy can be selected.

Risk assessment should be precise, reliable and, preferably, easily and rapidly available at low cost. Two types of risk should be considered:

Acute risk: this is the risk of progression to death or large MI, a risk of 13% at 30 days.

Long-term risk that is clearly depending on the extent of the lesions, left ventricular function, and inflammation.
(A) Markers of thrombotic risk, that is, acute risk

(a) Recurrence of chest pain
(b) ST-segment depression
(c) Dynamic ST-segment changes
(d) Elevated level of cardiac troponins
(e) Thrombus on angiography.

(B) Markers of underlying disease that is, long-term risk

(B1) Clinical markers

(a) Age
(b) History of previous MI, prior CABG, diabetes, congestive heart failure, hypertension.

(B2) Biological markers

(a) Renal dysfunction (elevated creatinine or reduced creatinine clearance)
(b) Inflammatory markers, CRP elevation, fibrinogen elevation, IL-6 elevation, BNP, soluble CD40 ligand.

(B3) Angiographical markers

(a) Left ventricular dysfunction
(b) Extent of coronary artery disease.

The level of evidence for all these markers is 1A.

Strategies according to risk stratification
Clinical examination, ECG records, and troponin measurements permit the identification of high-risk patients (Figure 17.3).

Patients judged to be at high risk for progression to MI or death
High-risk patients include those:
1 with recurrent ischemia (either recurrent chest pain) or dynamic ST-segment changes (in particular, ST-segment depression or transient ST-segment elevation): ST-segment depression alone allows the classification of patients as high risk (21% risk of death, MI, and refractory ischemia within 30 days) [11,12];
2 with elevated troponin levels (mortality risk × 7.7 in the short term and × 2.7 in the long term) [13];
3 who develop hemodynamic instability within the observation period;
4 with major arrhythmias (repetitive ventricular tachycardia, ventricular fibrillation);

Risk stratification
Risk of progression to death and MI

Baseline treatment:: Heparin (LMWH or Unfractionated heparin), ASA, Clopidogrel,
β-blockers, Nitrates

High-risk patients	**Low-risk patients**
Patients with recurrent ischemia Recurrent chest pain	✓ No recurrence of chest pain within observational period
Dynamic ST-segment changes (ST-segment depression or transient ST-segment elevation)	✓ No ST-segment depression negative T-waves , flat T-waves, normal ECG
Early postinfarction unstable angina Elevated troponin levels Diabetes	✓ No elevation of troponin or other biochemical markers ✓ **Troponin twice negative**
Hemodynamic instability Major arrhythmias (ventricular fibrillation, ventricular tuchy curdia)	**Conservative strategy**

Infusion of GP IIb/IIIa
Invasive strategy (< 24 h)

Figure 17.3 Risk stratification.

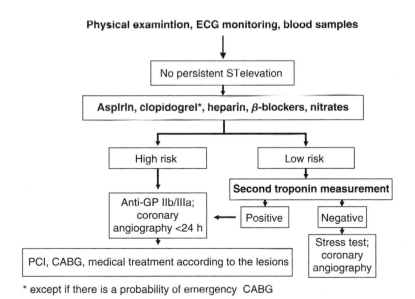

Physical examintion, ECG monitoring, blood samples

No persistent STelevation

Aspirin, clopidogrel*, heparin, β-blockers, nitrates

High risk   Low risk

Second troponin measurement

Anti-GP IIb/IIIa; coronary angiography <24 h ← Positive   Negative

Stress test; coronary angiography

PCI, CABG, medical treatment according to the lesions

* except if there is a probability of emergency CABG

Figure 17.4 Recommended strategy in ACS.

5 with diabetes mellitus: this condition is highly thrombogenic with a poorer prognosis than nondiabetics;

6 with an ECG pattern that precludes assessment of ST-segment changes.

In these patients the following strategy is recommended:

1 waiting and preparing for angiography, treatment with LMWH should be continued. Administration of GP IIb/IIIa receptor inhibitors will be started.

2 Coronary angiography should be planned as soon as possible, but without undue urgency. A very small group of patients with major arrhythmias (Ventricular tachycardia or Ventricular fibrillation) or hemodynamic instability (hypotension, pulmonary edema) will require a coronary angiogram within the first hours. In patients with lesions suitable for myocardial revascularization, the decision regarding the most suitable procedure will be made after careful evaluation of the extent and characteristics of the lesions, where appropriate, in consultation with surgical colleagues. In general, recommendations for the choice of a revascularization procedure in unstable angina are similar to those for elective revascularization procedures. In patients with single-vessel disease, percutaneous intervention of the culprit lesion is the first choice. In patients with left main or triple-vessel disease, CABG is the recommended procedure, particularly in patients with left ventricular dysfunction, except in cases of serious comorbidity, which contraindicates surgery. In double-vessel and in some cases of triple-vessel coronary disease, either percutaneous intervention or coronary bypass surgery may be appropriate. In some patients, a staged procedure may be considered, with immediate balloon angioplasty and stenting of the culprit lesion and subsequent reassessment of the need for treatment of other lesions, either by a percutaneous procedure or CABG. If percutaneous intervention is the selected procedure, it may be performed immediately after angiography in the same session.

Patients with suitable lesions for PCI will receive clopidogrel. In patients planned for CABG clopidogrel will be stopped, except if the operation is deferred. In that case, clopidogrel should be stopped about 5 days before operation.

If angiography shows no options for revascularization, owing to the extent of the lesions and/or poor distal run-off, or reveals no major coronary stenosis, patients will be referred for medical therapy. In case of completely normal coronary angiography an ergonovine test may be performed: if negative, the diagnosis of an ACS may need to be reconsidered and particular attention should be given to other possible reasons for presenting the symptoms.

Patients considered to be at low risk for rapid progression to MI or death

Low-risk patients include those:

1 who have no recurrence of chest pain within the observational period;

2 without ST-segment depression or elevation but rather negative T-waves, flat T-waves, or a normal ECG;

3 without elevation of troponin or other biochemical markers of myocardial necrosis on the initial and repeat measurement (performed between 6 and 12 h).

In these patients, oral treatment should be recommended, including aspirin, clopidogrel (loading dose of 300 mg followed by 75 mg daily), β-blockers, and possibly nitrates or calcium antagonists. Secondary preventive measures should be instituted. Low molecular weight heparin may be discontinued when, after the observational period, no ECG changes are apparent and a second troponin measurement is negative.

A stress test is recommended. The purpose of such a test is (1) to confirm or establish a diagnosis of coronary artery disease and when this is yet uncertain (2) to assess the risk for future events in patients with coronary artery disease.

In patients with significant ischemia during the stress test, coronary angiography and subsequent revascularization should be considered, particularly when this occurs at a low workload on the bicycle or treadmill. It should be appreciated that a standard exercise test may be inconclusive (no abnormalities at a relatively low workload). In such patients, an additional stress echocardiogram or stress myocardial perfusion scintigram may be appropriate.

In some patients, the diagnosis may remain uncertain, particularly in patients with a normal ECG throughout the observation period, without elevated markers of myocardial necrosis, and with a normal stress test and good exercise tolerance. The symptoms resulting in presentation to the hospital were probably not caused by myocardial ischemia, and additional investigations of other organ systems may be appropriate. In any case, the risk for cardiac events in such patients is very low. Therefore, additional tests can usually be performed at a later time, at the outpatient clinic.

Comparison with the ACC/AHA guidelines

The ACC/AHA guidelines have been published in 2000 and 2002 [14,15]. On average, ESC and American guidelines are very similar. They differ only with the risk assessment that separates three types of risk in ACC/AHA guidelines low, intermediate, and high risk . The European guidelines consider two categories of patients: low- and high-risk patients. The latter is characterized by acute thrombotic risk, namely, the major cardiac events, death, or large MI. In addition, the European guidelines include diabetics in the high-risk patients. This is consistent with the recognized high thrombogenicity of diabetic patients and thereby, their classification in the high-risk group of patients.

As far as the strategy is concerned, both guidelines are almost similar. Nevertheless, ACC/AHA guidelines recommend enoxaparin as first-line treatment. The European guidelines acknowledge the pharmacologic advantages of LWMH over unfractionated heparin and particularly, the greater bioavailability, the convenient administration, the decreased risk of thrombocytopenia of

LMWH, and that they require no special monitoring but do not recommend a special compound.

In spite of these minor differences, both guidelines are based on risk stratification and recognize that an aggressive antiplatelet treatment associated with antithrombins are necessary in high-risk patients who benefit from an invasive strategy if they have suitable lesions for myocardial revascularization.

Conclusions

Acute coronary syndromes represent an important segment of cardiovascular medicine and a very rapidly evolving field.

In the near future, we will have more information concerning several important points such as biological markers for risk stratification, role of assessment of antiplatelet drugs at bedside, antiplatelet resistance, importance of renal dysfunction, role of new antithrombotic drugs (new thienopyridins, GP IIb/IIIA with higher bolus dose, new antithrombins), upstream treatment with GP IIb/IIIa, or very high loading dose of clopidogrel, which will be considered or revisited. For these reasons, an update of both ESC and ACC/AHA guidelines is ongoing.

References

1. Hasdai D, Behar S, Wallentin L, *et al.* A related prospective survey of the characteristics, treatments and outcomes of patients with acute coronary syndromes in Europe and the Mediterranean basin; the Euro Heart Survey of Acute Coronary Syndromes (Euro Heart Survey ACS). *Eur Heart J* 2002; **15**: 1190–1201.
2. Davies M. Acute coronary thrombosis: the role of plaque disruption and its initiation and prevention. *Eur Heart J* 1995; **16**(Suppl. L): 3–7.
3. Davies MJ. Stability and instability: two faces of coronary atherosclerosis. The Paul Dudley White Lecture 1995. *Circulation* 1996; **94**: 2013–2020.
4. Davies M. The composition of coronary artery plaque. *N Engl J Med* 1997; **336**: 1312–1313.
5. Davies MJ, Woolf N, Katz DR, Mann J. Risk of thrombosis in human atherosclerotic plaques: role of extracellular lipid, macrophage, and smooth muscle cell content. *Br Heart J* 1993; **69**: 377–381.
6. Van de Werf F, Ardissino D, Betriu A *et al.* Management of acute myocardial infarction in patients presenting with ST-segment elevation. The Task Force on the Management of Acute Myocardial Infarction of the European Society of Cardiology. *Eur Heart J* 2003; **24**: 28–66.
7. Bertrand ME, Simoons ML, Fox KA *et al.* Management of acute coronary syndromes: acute coronary syndromes without persistent ST segment elevation; recommendations of the Task Force of the European Society of Cardiology. *Eur Heart J* 2000; **21**: 1406–1432.
8. Bertrand ME, Simoons ML, Fox KA *et al.* Management of acute coronary syndromes in patients presenting without persistent ST-segment elevation. *Eur Heart J* 2002; **23**: 1809–1840.

9. Petersen JL, Mahaffey KW, Hasselblad V *et al*. Efficacy and bleeding complications among patients randomized to enoxaparin or unfractionated heparin for antithrombin therapy in non-ST-segment elevation acute coronary syndromes: a systematic overview. *JAMA* 2004; **292**: 89–96.

10. Myocardial infarction redefined – a consensus document of The Joint European Society of Cardiology/American College of Cardiology Committee for the redefinition of myocardial infarction. *J Am Coll Cardiol* 2000; **36**: 959–969.

11. Nyman I, Areskog M, Areskog NH, Swahn E, Wallentin L. Very early risk stratification by electrocardiogram at rest in men with suspected unstable coronary heart disease. The RISC Study Group. *J Intern Med* 1993; **234**: 293–301.

12. Diderholm E, Andren B, Frostfeldt G *et al*. ST depression in ECG at entry indicates severe coronary lesions and large benefits of an early invasive treatment strategy in unstable coronary artery disease. The FRISC II ECG substudy. *Eur Heart J* 2002; **23**: 41–49.

13. Ottani F, Galvani M, Nicolini FA *et al*. Elevated cardiac troponin levels predict the risk of adverse outcome in patients with acute coronary syndromes. *Am Heart J* 2000; **140**: 917–927.

14. Braunwald E, Antman EM, Beasley JW *et al*. ACC/AHA guideline update for the management of patients with unstable angina and non-ST-segment elevation myocardial infarction – 2002: summary article. A report of the American College of Cardiology/American Heart Association Task Force on Practice Guidelines (Committee on the Management of Patients With Unstable Angina). *Circulation* 2002; **106**: 1893–1900.

15. Braunwald E, Antman EM, Beasley JW *et al*. ACC/AHA guidelines for the management of patients with unstable angina and non-ST-segment elevation myocardial infarction. A report of the American College of Cardiology/American Heart Association Task Force on Practice Guidelines (Committee on the Management of Patients With Unstable Angina). *J Am Coll Cardiol* 2000; **36**: 970–1062.

CHAPTER 18

Non-ST-segment elevation acute coronary syndromes: ACC/AHA guidelines

Pierre Théroux

The term acute coronary syndrome (ACS) was introduced in the late 1980s in order to link pathophysiological mechanisms and manifestations of acute myocardial ischemia to clinical diagnosis and treatment application. ACS is a working diagnosis that helps rapid screening, orientation, and treatment of patients consulting for chest pain. A more definitive diagnosis is usually reached rapidly; it can be nonspecific pain, an extracardiac pain, or a cardiac pain but not coronary, unstable angina (UA), non-ST-segment elevation myocardial infarction (NSTEMI), or ST-segment elevation myocardial infarction (STEMI).

Such a large spectrum of diagnoses associated with a prognosis varying from benign to life threatening, combined with the development of highly case-specific effective therapies has driven the development of guidelines for clinical management. The European Society of Cardiology and the American College of Cardiology and American Heart Association have independently developed two sets of guidelines, one addressing the management of STEMI [1,2] and the other the management of UA and NSTEMI [3,4]. The latter were first published in 1999 and updated in 2002. Keeping pace with the widespread emergence of new effective therapies and with the objective of facilitating their prompt incorporation into clinical practice, the working groups of these three organizations are preparing a new update to be published in early 2006. In parallel, huge efforts are being invested to promote awareness to these guidelines and measure their implementation and effectiveness through large registries, such as the Can Rapid Risk Stratification of Unstable Angina Patients Suppress Adverse Outcomes With Early Implementation of the ACC/AHA Guidelines? (CRUSADE) [5] registry and through different initiatives such as the ACC's Guidelines Applied in Practice (GAP) Program [6].

The intent of this manuscript is to provide an overview of the recommendations put forth by the ACC/AHA 2002 guidelines on risk stratification, patient orientation, and early treatment emphasizing the strongest Class 1 recommendations. A rapid scan of some of the most recent evidence that has emerged since the guidelines were last published will also be provided.

Priorities considered in the STEMI and NSTEMI guidelines

Since the immediate treatment priorities for STEMI and of NSTEMI are basically different, separate sets of guidelines have been produced for the two entities. Otherwise, both guidelines share much in common. STEMI is usually the consequence of an acute thrombotic occlusion of a major coronary artery resulting in a focal area of severely ischemic myocardium, progressing exponentially within minutes and hours to cell necrosis and irreversible left ventricular damage. In NSTEMI, an unstable plaque loaded with a thrombus that is usually not completely occlusive creates ischemia by obstructing flow and/or by distal microembolizations of plaque debris creating small foci of necrosis. As only flow restoration can effectively interrupt the exponential growth in the area of necrosis, STEMI mandates immediate reperfusion therapy without compromising on delays. The sooner reperfusion is achieved, the lesser the extent of necrosis, resulting in better left ventricular function and patient survival. Reperfusion can occur spontaneously, or can be mechanically or medically induced. Although timely percutaneous reperfusion and stenting is the preferred treatment, fibrinolysis is also a highly effective therapy; the choice between the two are influenced by many factors such as time of consultation after onset of pain, delays associated with treatment application, contraindications and indications for each approach, and local prehospital and hospital facilities. The ACC/AHA guidelines for the management of STEMI were updated in 2004 [7]. In NSTEMI, the priority of treatment is to prevent progression to myocardial infarction and eventually death, and of recurrent ischemia. This is achieved by controlling or "passivating" the unstable plaque.

As the various therapeutic strategies are associated with different risk/benefit and cost/effectiveness ratios, risk stratification schemes are required for determining the best orientation and treatment of patients.

Risk stratification

In practice, risk stratification starts with the patient who has to decide when to consult and how to access the healthcare system, often following the advice of relatives or friends. He can consult his physician, in a clinic or in an emergency department, or call 911 for assistance. Part of the effort of the guidelines and of the GAP programs pertains to patient education and participation, and to approaches for behavioral change and measures of effectiveness [6]. Recommendations following the initial contact with health professionals and the subsequent progression in intensity of care have been extensively elaborated in the guidelines, with tables, diagnostic and treatment algorithms, and gauged priority grades I, II, III inspired both by the evidence and expert opinions following the definitions:

- Class I: Conditions for which there is evidence and/or general agreement that a given procedure or treatment is useful and effective.
- Class II: Conditions for which there is conflicting evidence and/or a divergence of opinion about the usefulness/efficacy of a procedure or treatment.

  Class IIa: Weight of evidence/opinion is in favor of usefulness/efficacy.

  Class IIb: Usefulness/efficacy is less well established by evidence/opinion.

- Class III: Conditions for which there is evidence and/or general agreement that the procedure/treatment is not useful/effective and in some cases may be harmful.

Triage starts by a medical questionnaire and physical examination. The likelihood of the presence of coronary artery disease (CAD), of unstable CAD, or of an alternative cause for the pain is evaluated, taking into account that signs and symptoms may be atypical in many patients, especially women, the elderly, and the diabetic patients. When symptoms are consistent with CAD, a 12-lead (electrocardiogram) ECG is obtained as soon as possible – within 10 min if the chest pain is still evolving – and troponin T or troponin I levels are determined. Additional ECGs are required in these patients to rule out evolutionary changes or changes that occur at the times of recurrent symptoms. Cardiac markers are also reassessed after 6–8 h since blood elevation occurs many hours after the onset of pain. A prolonged chest pain accompanied with persistent ST–T changes usually indicate NSTEMI, a diagnosis that is confirmed by marker elevation.

The current class I recommendations for risk stratification are given below.

A rapid assessment on the likelihood that the acute ischemia is caused by CAD are high, intermediate, or low should be made in all patients with chest discomfort suggestive of an ACS.

1 Patients who present with chest discomfort should undergo early risk stratification that focuses on anginal symptoms, physical signs, ECG findings, and biomarkers of cardiac injury.

2 A 12-lead ECG should be obtained immediately (within 10 min) in patients with ongoing chest discomfort and as rapidly as possible in patients who have a history of chest discomfort consistent with ACS but whose discomfort has resolved by the time of evaluation.

3 Biomarkers of cardiac injury should be measured in all patients who present with chest discomfort consistent with ACS. A cardiac-specific troponin is the preferred marker, and if available, it should be measured in all patients. CK-MB by mass assay is also acceptable. In patients with negative cardiac markers within 6 h of the onset of pain, another sample should be drawn in the 6–12 h time frame.

By integrating all the above, the clinician can usually stratify the patients into one of the four diagnostic categories: a noncardiac diagnosis, chronic stable angina, possible ACS, and definite ACS. This evaluation allows for the appropriate orientation and treatment of patients. A provocative testing is useful for diagnosing patients with noncardiac chest pain or with a possible ACS, and for evaluating the severity of ischemia in patients with stable angina.

This risk stratification allows rapid orientation and treatment of patients according to the following schemes:

1 Patients with definite or possible ACS, but whose initial 12-lead ECG and cardiac marker levels are normal, should be observed in a facility with cardiac monitoring (e.g. chest pain unit), and a repeat ECG and cardiac marker measurement should be obtained 6–12 h after the onset of symptoms.

2 In patients in whom ischemic heart disease is present or suspected, if the follow-up 12-lead ECG and cardiac marker measurements are normal, a stress test (exercise or pharmacological) to provoke ischemia may be performed from the Emergency Department, a chest pain unit, or an outpatient basis shortly after discharge. Low-risk patients with a negative stress test can be managed as outpatients.

3 Patients with definite ACS and ongoing pain, positive cardiac markers, new ST-segment deviations, new deep T-wave inversions, hemodynamic abnormalities, or a positive stress test should be admitted to the hospital for further management.

4 Patients with possible ACS and negative cardiac markers who are unable to exercise or who have an abnormal resting ECG should undergo a pharmacological stress test.

5 Patients with definite ACS and ST-segment elevation should be evaluated for immediate reperfusion therapy (level of evidence: A).

Potential new options for risk stratification

The 12-lead ECG and the levels of CK-MB and troponin T or I values have been extensively validated as being highly effective and performing from a cost/benefit perspective, for identifying high-risk and low-risk patients, those who will benefit or not from a more aggressive medical management, and also from invasive procedures. Noteworthy, however this risk stratification focuses exclusively on the presence of acute focal ischemia related to a culprit lesion as suggested by symptoms, and is documented objectively by the presence of ST-segment shifts and/or marker elevation.

The pathology of ACS is not, however, restricted to the formation of an intracoronary thrombus on a plaque that has ruptured or fissured, the so-called culprit lesion. A close examination of the coronary arteries of patients with NSTEMI frequently unveils more than one culprit lesion, marking a diffuse disease. Inflammation and metabolic factors are important components of the disease and contribute to plaque instability and to an impaired prognosis. New options for risk stratification are therefore emerging. Thus, patients with elevated C-reactive protein and other inflammation markers and patients with diabetes or renal failure are at a higher risk of subsequent adverse events.

Numerous large database studies have further identified that the levels of the cardiac neurohormones, brain natriuretic peptide (BNP) and

N-terminal-proBNP (NT-proBNP) are also important risk stratifiers [7–9]. When stretched, the ventricular cardiomyocytes release pre-proBNP, which is enzymatically cleaved to the NT-proBNP and, subsequently, to BNP. From a pathophysiological perspective, the elevation in these neurohormones may pertain to the recently documented prognostic value of slight reductions in ejection fraction in patients with NSTEMI [10]. Clearly, subsets of patients, including the elderly and patients with diabetes, renal failure, or depressed left ventricular function, need more aggressive therapy.

Treatment

Currently available therapies address three important pathophysiological mechanisms of the disease: the thromboembolic process with anticoagulants and antiplatelet drugs; cell ischemia and cell protection with antiischemic drugs; and disease progression with secondary prevention drugs. Revascularization is key to rapid correction of the stenotic plaque, while likely facilitating the benefits derived from most drugs interventions.

Antithrombotic drugs

The complex interactions that exist between coagulant factors and platelets in the formation of the intracoronary thrombus are now best addressed by a combination of antiplatelet and anticoagulant drugs. Tissue factor expressed by monocytes and diseased endothelial cells is believed to act as the main trigger to thrombus formation by forming a complex with factor VIIa, whereas platelets facilitate the assembly of the coagulation factors on their surface while releasing a number of active proinflammatory compounds, and growth factors.

Anticoagulants

The recommended anticoagulants are unfractionated heparin (UFH) or low molecular weight heparins (LMWHs); among LMWHs, enoxaparin has been most studied and validated and is presented in the guidelines as a preferred anticoagulant over UFH. This does not appear to be supported by recent data from the Superior Yield of the new Strategy of Enoxaparin, Revascularization, and Glycoprotein IIb/IIIa inhibitors (SYNERGY) trial which compared enoxaparin versus unfractionated heparin in high-risk patients with NSTEMI managed with an intended early invasive strategy. The trial showed that enoxaparin was neither inferior nor superior to UFH while being associated with a significantly greater risk of bleeding [11]. The trial recruited a total 10 007 patients to be treated with an intended early invasive strategy. Percutaneous revascularization procedures were performed in 47% of patients and surgical revascularization in 19% of patients. Median time from randomization to angiography was 22 h. The lack of superiority of enoxaparin in this trial could be related to the short duration of administration of enoxaparin and the high rates of revascularization procedures compared with previous LMWH trials. In the meantime, a large trial performed of 15 570 STEMI patients documented a statistically significant mortality reduction with the LMWH raviparin compared with placebo [12].

Although additional benefits of recombinant hirudin over UFH have been observed [13], particularly r-hirudin, direct antithrombins are not included in current recommendations. The long-term benefits of r-hirudin were not consistently maintained while the dose range for benefit versus risk of bleeding was narrow. Bivalirudin with bail-out use of abciximab was compared with UFH plus routine abciximab in patients undergoing PCI [14], but no such results are available from a trial in NSTEMI.

Antiplatelet drugs

Aspirin and clopidogrel have consistently been associated with benefits in NSTEMI, independently of study designs, time of entry into trials, duration of follow-up, and partly of doses used [15–17]. This benefit was recently extended to patients with STEMI to cover the entire spectrum of ACSs. The Clopidogrel as Adjunctive Reperfusion TherapY TIMI 28 trial (CLARITY) trial randomized 3491 patients to a 300 mg loading of clopidogrel followed by 75 mg daily or to placebo [18]. The occurrence of the primary endpoint of an absence of reperfusion (TIMI grade flow 0 or 1) on an angiogram obtained 48 h to 192 after fibrinolysis, or of death or myocardial infarction (MI) through angiography, was reduced from 21.7% to 15.0% (odds reduction 36%, $p < .001$). In the COMMIT/CCS-2 trial of 45 851 patients, clopidogrel, administered without a loading dose, reduced the risk of death within 1 month by 7.0% ($p = .03$) compared with placebo [19].

Glycoprotein (GP) IIb/IIIa antagonists are generally recommended in NSTEMI. Based on metaanalyses that included various GP IIb/IIIa antagonists, a greater benefit was shown in patients undergoing PCI than in those treated medically. This led to a strong recommendation for their use in the former patients and a weaker recommendation in the latter. In most of these trials, the decision to proceed to angiography was, however, made after randomization. The recommendation was downgraded from 1a in 2000 to 2a in 2002 in patients receiving clopidogrel, due to the very positive results with the drug observed in the CURE trial [17], and the absence of a randomized trial that directly compared a GP IIb/IIIa antagonist with aspirin to the combination of clopidogrel to aspirin. Interestingly, two randomized trials that excluded all high-risk and NSTEMI patients showed no benefit of abciximab on the endpoints of death compared with placebo on a background therapy of clopidogrel and aspirin in [20,21]. Also of interest is a study of 3797 patients, which showed that the addition of aspirin to clopidogrel following a stroke or transient ischemic episode provided no significant benefits to clopidogrel over clopidogrel alone while increasing the risk of bleeding [22].

The current Class I, II, and III recommendations for antithrombotic therapy are as described below.

Class I

1 Antiplatelet therapy should be initiated promptly. ASA should be administered as soon as possible after presentation and continued indefinitely (level of evidence: A).

2 Clopidogrel should be administered to hospitalized patients who are unable to take ASA because of hypersensitivity or major gastrointestinal intolerance (level of evidence: A).

3 In hospitalized patients in whom an early noninterventional approach is planned, clopidogrel should be added to ASA as soon as possible on admission and administered for at least 1 month (level of evidence: A) and for up to 9 months (level of evidence: B).

4 In patients for whom a PCI is planned, clopidogrel should be started and continued for at least 1 month (level of evidence: A) and up to 9 months in patients who are not at high risk for bleeding (level of evidence: B).

5 In patients taking clopidogrel in whom elective CABG is planned, the drug should be withheld for 5–7 days. (level of evidence: B).

6 Anticoagulation with subcutaneous LMWH or intravenous UFH should be added to antiplatelet therapy with ASA and/or clopidogrel (level of evidence: A).

7 A platelet GP IIb/IIIa antagonist should be administered, in addition to ASA and heparin, to patients in whom catheterization and PCI are planned. The GP IIb/IIIa antagonist may also be administered just prior to PCI (level of evidence: A).

Class IIa

1 Eptifibatide or tirofiban should be administered, in addition to ASA and LMWH or UFH, to patients with continuing ischemia, an elevated troponin or with other high-risk features in whom an invasive management strategy is not planned (level of evidence: A).

2 Enoxaparin is preferable to UFH as an anticoagulant in patients with NSTEMI, unless CABG is planned within 24 h (level of evidence: A).

3 A platelet GP IIb/IIIa antagonist should be administered to patients already receiving heparin, ASA, and clopidogrel in whom catheterization and PCI are planned. The GP IIb/IIIa antagonist may also be administered just prior to PCI (level of evidence: B).

Class IIb

1 Eptifibatide or tirofiban, in addition to ASA and LMWH or UFH, to patients without continuing ischemia who have no other high-risk features and in whom PCI is not planned (level of evidence: A).

2 Contraindicated in NSTEMI is intravenous fibrinolytic therapy in patients without acute ST-segment elevation, a true posterior MI, or a presumed new left bundle branch block (LBBB), and abciximab administration in patients in whom PCI is not planned.

Antiischemic therapy

Class 1 recommendations for antiischemic therapy are:

1 Bed rest with continuous ECG monitoring for ischemia and arrhythmia detection in patients with ongoing rest pain (level of evidence: C).

2 Nitroglycerine (NTG), sublingual tablet or spray, followed by intravenous administration, for the immediate relief of ischemia and associated symptoms.

3 Supplemental oxygen for patients with cyanosis or respiratory distress; finger pulse oxymetry or arterial blood gas determination to confirm adequate arterial oxygen saturation (SaO_2 >90%) and continued need for supplemental oxygen in the presence of hypoxemia.

4 Morphine sulfate administered intravenously when symptoms are not immediately relieved with NTG or when acute pulmonary congestion and/or severe agitation is present.

5 A β-blocker, with the first dose administered intravenously if there is ongoing chest pain, followed by oral administration, in the absence of contraindications.

6 In patients with continuing or frequently recurring ischemia when β-blockers are contraindicated, a nondihydropyridine calcium antagonist (e.g. verapamil or diltiazem) as initial therapy in the absence of severe left ventricular dysfunction or other contraindications.

7 An angiotensin converting enzyme inhibitor (ACEI) when hypertension persists despite treatment with NTG and a β-blocker in patients with left ventricular systolic dysfunction or (CHF) and in ACS patients with diabetes.

Revascularization procedures

An invasive management strategy is the current standard in the management of high-risk patient with ischemic ST–T changes or elevation of blood markers. The Fragmin and Fast Revascularization During Instability in Coronary Artery Disease (FRISC II) study first showed a mortality reduction with routine angiography done within the first 7 days and revascularization within the first 10 days compared with a nonroutine invasive management strategy [23]; at 1 year the rates of death were reduced from 3.9% to 8.6% ($p = .016$) and of death or MI from 14.1% to 10.4% ($p = .005$). In the Treat angina with Aggrastat® and determine Costs of Therapy with Invasive or Conservative Strategies (TACTICS-TIMI-18) trial, the early invasive arm with interventions performed within 4–48 h showed a reduction in rates of death or MI at 6 months from 9.5% to 7.3% ($p < .05$). At 30 days, however, there was a nonstatistically significant increase in mortality in the invasive arm and, in patients with no ST-segment changes and troponin T levels less than or equal to 0.01 ng/mL, there were no differences between the invasive and conservative management strategy arms in the rates of composite primary endpoint of death, MI, or rehospitalization for recurrent acute coronary syndromes [24]. Although no trials have directly investigated whether a very early timing for the procedure was superior to a slightly delayed timing, the current trend is to proceed with the intervention within the first 24 or 48 h. The recommendations for an invasive procedure extend to various subsets of high-risk patients.

Class I
1 An early invasive strategy in patients with NSTEMI and any of the following high-risk indicators (level of evidence: A).

(a) Recurrent angina/ischemia at rest or with low-level activities despite intensive antiischemic therapy.
(b) Elevated TnT or TnI.
(c) New or presumably new ST-segment depression.
(d) Recurrent angina/ischemia with CHF symptoms, an S3 gallop, pulmonary edema, worsening rales, or new or worsening MR.
(e) High-risk findings on noninvasive stress testing.
(f) Depressed left ventricular systolic function (e.g. ejection fraction less than 0.40 on noninvasive study).
(g) Hemodynamic instability.
(h) Sustained ventricular tachycardia.
(i) PCI within 6 months.
(j) Prior CABG.

2 In the absence of these findings, either an early conservative or an early invasive strategy in hospitalized patients without contraindications for revascularization (level of evidence: B).

Class IIa
1 An early invasive strategy in patients with repeated presentations for ACS despite therapy and without evidence for ongoing ischemia or high risk (level of evidence: C).
2 An early invasive strategy in patients greater than 65 years old or patients who present with ST-segment depression or elevated cardiac markers and no contraindications to revascularization (level of evidence: C).
Coronary angiography is not indicated in patients with extensive comorbidities (e.g. liver or pulmonary failure, cancer), in whom the risks of revascularization are not likely to outweigh the benefits (level of evidence: C), in patients with acute chest pain and a low likelihood of ACS (level of evidence: C), and in patients who will not consent to revascularization regardless of the findings (level of evidence: C).

Options for the future

Although current therapy highly successfully addresses important mechanisms of the disease, other mechanisms that appear equally important are less well addressed. Thus, metabolic factors implicated in diabetes and renal failure have a negative impact on medium- and long-term prognosis; and inflammatory reactions trigger, entertain, and prevent healing of the plaque disease leading to plaque degeneration, necrosis, apoptosis, and rupture.

Proinflammatory cytokines, matrix metalloproteinases, and activated complement proteins are all important mediators of these processes. To date, no real benefit of drugs acting at various levels of the inflammation cascade could be demonstrated; most studies, however, were designed to test the hypothesis of an infarct size reduction in patients with STEMI, not explicitly addressing passivation of the culprit lesions associated with UA/NSTEMI. The benefit of statins, and of a magnified benefit with lower LDL-cholesterol, has been well documented in these patients but within the range and timing observed in other categories of patients at risk, suggesting there could be no special benefit during the acute phase of UA/NSTEMI [25–28]. The efficacy of ACEIs initiated past the acute phase has been demonstrated but the drugs have not been tested during the acute phase.

Nevertheless, strict control of risk factors helped with an appropriate pharmacotherapy composed of a statin, an ACEI, aspirin, and clopidogrel is strongly indicated in these UA/NSTEMI patients as they remain at high risk of recurrence in the following months and years.

References

1. Van de Werf F, Ardissino D, Betriu A *et al.* Management of acute myocardial infarction in patients presenting with ST-segment elevation. The Task Force on the Management of Acute Myocardial Infarction of the European Society of Cardiology. *Eur Heart J* 2003; **24**: 28–66.
2. Antman EM, Anbe DT, Armstrong PW *et al.* ACC/AHA guidelines for the management of patients with ST-elevation myocardial infarction. A report of the American College of Cardiology/American Heart Association task force on practice guidelines (Committee to Revise the 1999 Guidelines for the Management of patients with acute myocardial infarction). *J Am Coll Cardiol* 2004; **44**: E1–E211.
3. Bertrand ME, Simoons ML, Fox KA *et al.* Management of acute coronary syndromes in patients presenting without persistent ST-segment elevation. *Eur Heart J* 2002; **23**: 1809–1840.
4. Braunwald E, Antman EM, Beasley JW *et al.* ACC/AHA 2002 guideline update for the management of patients with unstable angina and non-ST-segment elevation myocardial infarction – summary article. A report of the American College of Cardiology/American Heart Association task force on practice guidelines (Committee on the Management of Patients With Unstable Angina). *J Am Coll Cardiol* 2002; **40**: 1366–1374.
5. Hoekstra JW, Pollack CV, Jr, Roe MT *et al.* Improving the care of patients with non-ST-elevation acute coronary syndromes in the emergency department: the CRUSADE initiative. *Acad Emerg Med* 2002; **9**: 1146–1155.
6. http://www.acc.org/gap/gap.htm
7. Sabatine MS, Morrow DA, de Lemos JA *et al.* Multimarker approach to risk stratification in non-ST elevation acute coronary syndromes: simultaneous assessment of troponin I, C-reactive protein, and B-type natriuretic peptide. *Circulation* 2002; **105**: 1760–1763.
8. James SK, Lindahl B, Siegbahn A *et al.* N-terminal pro-brain natriuretic peptide and other risk markers for the separate prediction of mortality and subsequent

myocardial infarction in patients with unstable coronary artery disease: a Global Utilization of Strategies To Open occluded arteries (GUSTO)-IV substudy. *Circulation* 2003; **108**: 275–281.

9. Galvani M, Ottani F, Oltrona L *et al*. N-terminal pro-brain natriuretic peptide on admission has prognostic value across the whole spectrum of acute coronary syndromes. *Circulation* 2004; **110**: 128–134.

10. Bosch X, Theroux P. Left ventricular ejection fraction to predict early mortality in patients with non-ST elevation acute coronary syndromes. *Am Heart J* 2005; **150**: 215–220.

11. Ferguson JJ, Califf RM, Antman EM *et al*. Enoxaparin vs unfractionated heparin in high-risk patients with non-ST-segment elevation acute coronary syndromes managed with an intended early invasive strategy: primary results of the SYNERGY randomized trial. *JAMA* 2004; **292**: 45–54.

12. Yusuf S, Mehta SR, Xie C *et al*. Effects of reviparin, a low-molecular-weight heparin, on mortality, reinfarction, and strokes in patients with acute myocardial infarction presenting with ST-segment elevation. *JAMA* 2005; **293**: 427–435.

13. Mehta SR, Eikelboom JW, Rupprecht HJ *et al*. Efficacy of hirudin in reducing cardiovascular events in patients with acute coronary syndrome undergoing early percutaneous coronary intervention. *Eur Heart J* 2002; **23**: 117–123.

14. Lincoff AM, Kleiman NS, Kereiakes DJ *et al*. Long-term efficacy of bivalirudin and provisional glycoprotein IIb/IIIa blockade vs heparin and planned glycoprotein IIb/IIIa blockade during percutaneous coronary revascularization: REPLACE-2 randomized trial. *JAMA* 2004; **292**: 696–703.

15. Antithrombotic Trialists' Collaboration. Collaborative meta-analysis of randomised trials of antiplatelet therapy for prevention of death, myocardial infarction, and stroke in high risk patients. *BMJ* 2002; **324**: 71–86.

16. Harker LA, Boissel JP, Pilgrim AJ, Gent M. Comparative safety and tolerability of clopidogrel and aspirin: results from CAPRIE. CAPRIE Steering Committee and Investigators. Clopidogrel versus aspirin in patients at risk of ischaemic events. *Drug Saf* 1999; **21**: 325–335.

17. Yusuf S, Zhao F, Mehta SR, Chrolavicius S, Tognoni G, Fox KK. Effects of clopidogrel in addition to aspirin in patients with acute coronary syndromes without ST-segment elevation. *N Engl J Med* 2001; **345**: 494–502.

18. Sabatine MS, Cannon CP, Gibson CM *et al*. Addition of clopidogrel to aspirin and fibrinolytic therapy for myocardial infarction with ST-segment elevation. *N Engl J Med* 2005; **352**: 1179–1189.

19. Chen Z, Collins R. Clopidogrel, Metoprolol Prove Their Worth in Treatment of Acute MI (COMMIT/CCS-2 trial). Proceedings of the ACC Scientific Session, Orlando FL, March 2005.

20. Kastrati A, Mehilli J, Schuhlen H *et al*. A clinical trial of abciximab in elective percutaneous coronary intervention after pretreatment with clopidogrel. *N Engl J Med* 2004; **350**: 232–238.

21. Mehilli J, Kastrati A, Schuhlen H *et al*. Randomized clinical trial of abciximab in diabetic patients undergoing elective percutaneous coronary interventions after treatment with a high loading dose of clopidogrel. *Circulation* 2004; **110**: 3627–3635.

22. Diener HC, Bogousslavsky J, Brass LM *et al*. Aspirin and clopidogrel compared with clopidogrel alone after recent ischaemic stroke or transient ischaemic attack in high-risk patients (MATCH): randomised, double-blind, placebo-controlled trial. *Lancet* 2004; **364**: 331–337.

23. Wallentin L, Lagerqvist B, Husted S, Kontny F, Stahle E, Swahn E. Outcome at 1 year after an invasive compared with a non-invasive strategy in unstable coronary-artery disease: the FRISC II invasive randomised trial. Fast Revascularisation during Instability in Coronary artery disease Investigators. *Lancet* 2000; **356**: 9–16.

24. Cannon CP, Weintraub WS, Demopoulos LA *et al.* Comparison of early invasive and conservative strategies in patients with unstable coronary syndromes treated with the glycoprotein IIb/IIIa inhibitor tirofiban. *N Engl J Med* 2001; **344**: 1879–1887.

25. Schwartz GG, Olsson AG, Ezekowitz MD *et al.* Effects of atorvastatin on early recurrent ischemic events in acute coronary syndromes: the MIRACL study: a randomized controlled trial. *Jama* 2001; **285**: 1711–1718.

26. Thompson PL, Meredith I, Amerena J, Campbell TJ, Sloman JG, Harris PJ. Effect of pravastatin compared with placebo initiated within 24 hours of onset of acute myocardial infarction or unstable angina: the Pravastatin in Acute Coronary Treatment (PACT) trial. *Am Heart J* 2004; **148**: e2.

27. Cannon CP, Braunwald E, McCabe CH *et al.* Intensive versus moderate lipid lowering with statins after acute coronary syndromes. *N Engl J Med* 2004; **350**: 1495–1504.

28. de Lemos JA, Blazing MA, Wiviott SD *et al.* Early intensive vs a delayed conservative simvastatin strategy in patients with acute coronary syndromes: phase Z of the A to Z trial. *Jama* 2004; **292**: 1306–1316.

CHAPTER 19

From guidelines to registries

Luigi Tavazzi

In the framework of patient-oriented research, observational research dominated the scene until the advent of randomized, controlled trials (RCTs) in large populations as the method of measuring efficacy/safety of therapeutic interventions. RCTs prevent numerous methodological biases that cannot otherwise be avoided. This point is not under discussion. This premise is important because many of the concerns about observational research derive from the inappropriate use of results of such research as proof of therapeutic efficacy. Observational research is complementary to randomized, controlled investigations and has specific well-defined methodologies, which can vary in relation to the aims of the research.

Tables 19.1 and 19.2 report some of the different features and aims of observational studies and RCTs. A short summary of the observational and interventional research performed in Italy in the area of acute coronary syndromes (ACSs) in the last 5 years may exemplify these concepts.

Systematic observational research in a country

The GISSI trials are population trials performed by a large network of cardiology centers in Italy. The first two trials addressed ST-segment elevation myocardial infarction (MI) (STE-ACS) in its acute phase [1,2], the third trial examined the subacute phase [3], and the fourth trial considered the postacute, chronic phase, focusing on prevention [4]. Alongside the RCTs at the end of the 1980s, a large nationwide observational study [the avoidable delay in acute myocardial infarction (AMI) treatment Survey] revealed that the main reason for the delay (at that time very long) in the patients' presentation was the patients' decision stage [5]. Public campaigns to modify this aspect were, therefore, needed.

Subsequently, an observational study was designed (the GISSI-Prognosis), in which 1489 postinfarct patients were enrolled by 65 centers that had been selected for being nationally representative [6]. The evaluation strategies were analyzed step by step. One important result was that the very strong prognostic significance of left ventricular dysfunction seemed to be undervalued during the decision-making, while the prognostic value of a "positive" stress test seemed to be overvalued, despite this having been shown to have very weak prognostic value in the large population of the GISSI 2 trial [7].

Table 19.1 The characteristics of efficacy studies (RCTS) and outcome studies.

RCTs	Outcome studies
Evaluate the effects of a single intervention on one or more measurable results	Examine complex interventions
Establish a cause–effect relationship between the intervention and the result	Establish an association between the procedures adopted and the results obtained
The care system is rigidly established	The care system is heterogeneous, without controls of the interventions
Patients	
Study homogeneous groups of subjects	Include all the subjects with a specific problem
Exclude complex patients and those with comorbid conditions	Include patients with comorbid conditions
Data	
Collected ad hoc	Routine
Tend to maximize compliance under consideration	Lack of compliance is one of the factors examined
Costs	
Very expensive	Usually less expensive
The costs do not match those of the real-life situation	The costs are those of the real-life situation

With the appearance and spread of primary angioplasty for AMI the problem arose of verifying whether the new therapeutic techniques were being implemented and what clinical impact they were having. From 1998 to 2003 three observational studies were carried out: one survey called BLITZ I [8], in which 1959 STE-ACS and non-ST-elevation acute coronary syndrome (NSTE-ACS) patients were enrolled in 2 weeks by 296 cardiology centers, and two outcome studies, one focusing on STE-ACS patients and the other on NSTE-ACS patients. The MISTRAL study [9] (3074 STE-ACS patients enrolled in 1 year by 47 centers and followed-up for 1 year) recorded the first approach to the patient with Acute MI (AMI) across the country, whereas BLITZ II [10] included NSTE-ACS patients (1888 patients enrolled in 2 weeks by 275 centers and followed-up for 1 month). In essence, the results of the MISTRAL study showed that there was no difference in mortality or major complications between patients treated invasively or conservatively, except among the patients treated within the first hour of entering hospital, in whom there was an advantage in favor of treatment and a lower rate of angina during the subsequent 1 year of follow-up in patients undergoing percutaneous coronary intervention (PCI) at presentation. BLITZ II (not yet published) pictured the contemporary management of Italian ACS patients: 67% underwent coronary angiography, 33% PCI, and 11% coronary artery bypass grafting

Table 19.2 Aims of observational research.

To monitor the results and costs of one's own activity

To outline an epidemiological profile (state of health, QoL) of a population of patients and of met/unmet health needs

To describe opinions (behaviors of patients and doctors)

To implement a (hopefully) permanent observatory of morbidity, mortality, and avoidable costs

To evaluate the practicability/transferability of research results

To evaluate adherence to guidelines and the impact of their application

To examine behavior and results in groups of patients excluded from trials and in those at higher risk of receiving inappropriate treatments/care

To identify subgroups of patients with different risk profiles (of events or of side effects)

To evaluate care profiles and compare the yields of different care strategies

To evaluate compliance with drug use over time

To record the "natural" dynamics of the use of therapeutic instruments (off-label applications, reduced use in favor of other drugs, etc.)

"Inductive" studies of little employed but useful therapeutic strategies (e.g. β-blockers in heart failure)

To highlight areas of greatest uncertainty, with the aim of generating ideas for research and for defining guidelines better

---

(CABG), with apparent overuse of resources in low-risk patients in hospitals with catheterization laboratory facilities and underuse in high-risk patients in hospitals without such facilities.

Finally, with the endorsement of the health authorities of the Region of Lombardy (the most heavily populated region in north Italy, with almost 10 million inhabitants), two studies on the appropriateness of myocardial revascularization were carried out. These studies showed an underuse of mechanical revascularization and, in about 2 years of follow-up, a higher incidence of events in eligible patients who inappropriately were not treated [11]. The availability of interventional centers and the number of interventions now carried out in Lombardy have more than doubled since those studies, the results of which contributed to the development of interventional cardiology in the region.

Observational research in ACS across the world

Acute coronary syndrome encompasses a continuum of conditions ranging from STE-ACS to NSTE-ACS and unstable angina. Large clinical trials performed in the last decade have produced data on the evolving therapeutic strategies for ACS, and clinical practice guidelines on the treatment of ACS have been founded on evidence from these studies. During the same period, several observational studies were performed, picturing the evolving state of the diagnostic and therapeutic approaches to ACS across the world.

Interregional differences

In spite of the similarity of the guidelines, observational studies have revealed remarkable differences in patients' characteristics, treatment strategies, and outcomes in different geographical and social areas. The diagnosis and therapy of ACS involve cultural, technical, organizational, and economic issues, and it is not surprising that these issues have different impacts in the various regions of the heterogeneous world in which we live. The probability that trial populations themselves do not represent the universe of real patients is higher in ACS than in other disease areas. Interregional differences in patients' risk profiles, together with imbalances in selecting patients for enrollment, may account for marked differences in outcome observed in trials [12,13] and in registries [14,15]. For instance, in the HERO-2 trial morbidity rates were 6.7% in western countries, 10.2% in eastern Europe, and 13.2% in Russia despite the patients having similar baseline characteristics and treatment [12]; in the TIME II trial mortality rates were 5.7% and 10.1% in North and South America, respectively [13]. The differences in risk profile for atherosclerotic disease in northeastern versus southern European populations is of specific relevance to the European Community public health policy [16].

Striking differences in therapeutic strategies, particularly reperfusion procedures and medication, were observed in surveys performed in the same period of time, around 1999–2001, such as EUROASPIRE [17], the PRAIS-UK [18], the EuroHeart Survey ACS [14], and BLITZ 1 [8]. Prominent variations were recorded among countries in the rate of coronary angiography and revascularization procedures in both STE-ACS and NSTE-ACS patients. Time to reperfusion, an important factor influencing outcome in STE-ACS patients, varies in relation to local organizational policies. The GRACE registry revealed that while the time between symptom onset and admission to an emergency department was somewhat longer in Europe than in the United States (152 versus 120 min), the "door to balloon" time was much longer in the United States than in Europe (158 versus 93 min) [19]. This was confirmed in the NRMI-2, which indicated a "door to balloon" time of about 2 h [20], while the recent EuroHeart Survey on Coronary Revascularization showed that the majority of STE-ACS patients undergoing primary PCI were treated within the advocated timeframe of 90 min [21]. This survey also confirmed huge differences among countries in the rates of invasive versus noninvasive strategies in patients with ACS. The ENACT Survey had already shown such heterogeneity [22]. For instance, the rate of cardiac catheterization in patients with unstable angina ranged from 19% in the United Kingdom to 68% in France. In Italy, surveys conducted in both STE-ACS and NSTE-ACS patients – the BLITZ I [8] and II [10] studies – showed important differences from center to center in the rates of revascularization that appeared to be more related to local practice than to the patients' characteristics or baseline risk. Similar findings were reported in other registries, including the OASIS [23], CRUSADE [24], ROSAI [25], and the more recent French FACT [26] registries. Moreover, in the FACT registry a relationship was noted between mortality rate and equipment of the hospital: 5.9% for the departments with an angioplasty facility, 11% for the departments with a coronary angiography, facility but without angioplasty and 13.8% for the departments without any interventional equipment [26].

In practice, it seems that guidelines are systematically ignored when catheterization facilities are available on site [10]. Marked interregional differences in evidence-based use of medications also emerged from the registries. In the GRACE registry glycoprotein (GP) IIb/IIIa inhibitors appeared to be more widely used in the United States than in Europe [27]. Conversely, although European guidelines did not advocate the use of low molecular weight heparin with fibrinolytic therapy, these drugs were being used in 60% of European STE-ACS patients [28]. The EuroHeart Survey on Coronary Revascularization confirmed the sizable proportion of high-risk patients and/or procedures in which GP IIb/IIIa receptor blockers were not being used [21]. Drugs with proven prophylactic effects are generally prescribed in European countries: anti-thrombotics and β-blockers more systematically than ACE-inhibitors and statins. Similar findings were also recorded in the CRUSADE registry [24].

Outcome in STE-ACS/NSTE-ACS and Q-wave and non-Q-wave MI

The in-hospital mortality of NSTE-ACS patients frequently, but not always, appears higher than in clinical trials [14]. Unlike STE-ACS the diagnosis of NSTE-ACS is often uncertain upon arrival at the hospital. Thus populations enrolled in observational studies may be more heterogeneous than those enrolled in trials. The "all-comers" philosophy of the former leads to the enrollment of more comprehensive populations into observational studies than into trials. The in-hospital mortality rate was 7% for STE-ACS patients, 2–4% for NSTE-ACS patients, and 11.8% in patients with an undetermined initial electrocardiographic pattern in the EuroHeart Survey ACS [14]. At 30 days the mortality rates were, respectively, 8.4%, 3.5%, and 13.3%. Thus, marked differences in mortality were recorded according to the initial electrocardiographic pattern. Differences were also noted according to the final diagnosis. The 30-day mortality rates were 11.1% in Q-wave myocardial infarction (QMI), 7.4% in non-Q-wave myocardial infarction (NQMI), and 1.7% in unstable angina [14]. Revascularization procedures were performed in 43.8% of STE-ACS and 30.8% of NSTE-ACS patients.

The GRACE registry reported different results. Death rates were 7.8% among patients with STE-ACS, 5.9% in those with NSTE-ACS, and 2.7% in patients with unstable angina (in 1999–2002). The 6-month post discharge death rates were 4.8%, 6.2%, and 3.6%, respectively [29]. Thus, the cumulative 6-month mortality was similar in STE-ACS and NSTE-ACS patients (12.6% versus 12.1%). Coronary interventions were performed during hospitalization in 49.4% of patients with STE-ACS, in 40.2% with NSTE-ACS, and in 25% of those with unstable angina. Lower event rates were observed in the Canadian ACS Registry, performed in the years 1999–2001, which enrolled 5312 ACS patients [30]. The in-hospital mortality rates were 4.9%, 2.5%, and 0.4% in the QMI, NQMI, and unstable angina groups, respectively. Reinfarction complicated 7.4% of QMI patients and 8.5% of NQMI patients. However, the mortality rate was high in the year following discharge: 10% in NQMI and 6.5% in QMI patients, with a cumulative mortality rate of 11.4% in QMI, and 12.5% in NQMI at 1 year. In adjusted analysis, NQMI was a significant risk factor for death (OR, 1.53; 95% CI, 1.19–1.97) [30]. Revascularization (either percutaneous or surgical) was performed in hospital in 23.5% of QMI and 18.7% of NQMI patients, and in 6.6% of both QMI and NQMI patients during the following year. In BLITZ I, in which 48% of the 1275 STE-ACS patients and 43% of the 580 NSTE-ACS patients enrolled underwent coronary angiography, the in-hospital and the 30-day mortality rates were, respectively, 7.4% and 9.4% for STE-ACS and 5.2% and 7.1% for NSTE-ACS [8].

Overall, these findings indicate a continuum of evolution of coronary artery disease through unstable phases with a potential difference of severity of the immediate outcome but a similar mid to long term outcome between STE-ACS/NSTE-ACS and QMI/NQMI patients.

Further evidence of this is the incidence rate of heart failure complicating ACS. There is a consistency in various observational studies indicating a similar rate of heart failure associated with the acute ischaemic event in both STE-ACS and NSTE-ACS and in both QMI and NQMI. In the GRACE registry, the heart failure rates among STE-ACS and NSTE-ACS patients were 15.6% and 15.7%, respectively, whereas heart failure was only half as frequent in patients with unstable angina (8.2%) [31]. The cumulative 6-month mortality of patients presenting with symptoms of congestion upon admission was 20.7% whereas it was 25.3% in those who developed symptoms afterward. In the ACS Canadian Registry, heart failure was observed in hospital in 17.4% of QMI patients and in 21.4% of NQMI patients [30]. In the EuroHeart Survey, ACS heart failure was reported upon admission in only 2% of both STE-ACS and NSTE-ACS patients, but the in-hospital rate of congestive heart failure was 27.7% in STE-ACS and 17.2% in NSTE-ACS patients [14]. Thus the gradient in severity between STE-ACS and NSTE-ACS patients reflected by the mortality rate among the EuroHeart Survey ACS patients was confirmed by the incidence of new onset heart failure. In a cohort of all residents of Olmsted County, MI, 1915 had an AMI between 1979 and 1998 (mean age 73 years); 41% of them experienced new onset heart failure (occurring during the first month), after the index event in 59% of patients, and after the first year in 34% [32]. Among these, three-quarters had a depressed left ventricular ejection fraction. The median survival after the onset of heart failure was 4 years, being 5.8 years in patients with preserved left ventricular function and 3.9 years in those with a depressed left ventricular ejection fraction. Interestingly, during the 20 years of observation, survival did not improve in these AMI-HF patients.

Risk stratification of ACS patients

Stratification of the risk of patients with ACS can be of practical value as an aid to guide clinical decision-making. The TIMI score is the stratification tool most used in trials and clinical practice [33]. It is a set of independent predictors of 14-day outcome based on the database of the TIMI 11B trial that enrolled NSTE-ACS and unstable angina patients. The TIMI score was validated and its predictive power confirmed in the ESSENCE trial [34]. In a more heterogeneous cohort of ACS patients enrolled in a registry during the year 1999–2000, the TIMI score failed to predict outcome, whereas a set of similar, but not identical, variables (the RUSH score) showed a better ability to predict cardiac events [35]. Recently, the GRACE group reported the results of an analysis performed in 17 142 ACS patients enrolled in 1999–2002 as a development cohort and 7638 patients enrolled in 2002–2003 as a validation cohort. They proposed a new score for bedside risk estimation of in-hospital mortality risk in patients with STE-ACS, NSTE-ACS, or unstable angina [36]. The same score showed a high diagnostic prediction for the 6-month mortality of patients hospitalized with ACS and discharged alive. If the predictive ability of this score is confirmed in other settings, clinicians will have new help, generated by observational research, to guide therapy in ACS.

However, the main concern remains that stratification scores are rarely used in practice. BLITZ II [10] and other registries [23,24] show that when catheterization laboratory facilities are available on site, invasive procedures are preferred to a conservative strategy, even in patients at lower risk. Hospitals without catheterization facilities struggle with restricted access to the procedures and should, therefore, be forced to stratify patients. However, in the hospitals participating in the BLITZ II study, functional stratification was carried out in only about 15% of patients [10]. Despite a high number of patients being transferred for coronary angiography and revascularization (about 40%), there was a marked underuse of the invasive strategy in patients at high risk, giving rise to what Di Chiara *et al.* called an "inverse" stratification, favoring low-risk patients [10].

The ACS patients undergoing revascularization included in the EuroHeart Survey on Coronary Revascularization, even after adjustment using the EuroSCORE, had low 1-year mortality rates: 7% in STE-ACS patients and 5% in those with NSTE-ACS or unstable angina [21]. However, it is of concern that markers of necrosis (known to be independent predictors of cardiac mortality and subsequent MI) were not measured after 39% of PCI procedures and two-third of CABGs.

Does adherence to guidelines really affect outcome?

This is one of the main questions that we expect to answer by observational research. The early survival of STE-ACS patients is improved by using guideline-recommended therapies. Analysis of the treatments and outcome of the more than 1.5 million patients with STE-ACS included in the National Registry of Myocardial Infarction in the United States over the last decade showed that improved adherence to guidelines was associated with a 16% reduction in early mortality [37]. Similar data were reported in population-based studies such as the Minnesota Heart Survey [38] and the Worcester Heart Attack study [39].

Limited data are available and less firm conclusions can be drawn on the relation between evidence-based care and outcome of the NSTE-ACS population. In fact, in longitudinal registries, such as GRACE and CRUSADE, despite a global increase in evidence-based therapies no changes in outcome were evident in the last few years and, conversely, despite substantial regional differences in treatments, outcome did not differ significantly across regions [40].

Observational research to gauge guideline incorporation into clinical practice and clinical quality improvement

Application of the official recommendations is easier and more successful in STE-ACS patients than in NSTE-ACS ones for several reasons. First, the diagnosis and the recognition of patients at high risk can be more difficult and made later in NSTE-ACS patients than in STE-ACS patients. Second, while treatments such as reperfusion and early administration of aspirin have been shown unequivocally to reduce mortality in STE-ACS patients, no acute treatment for NSTE-ACS has been found to reduce early mortality significantly. Thus, in spite of the common pathophysiological mechanism and similar long-term outcome, implementation of guidelines for the STE-ACS and NSTE-ACS populations may differ [41].

Quality improvement (QI) strategies should be planned on the basis of comprehensive information about contemporary patterns of care and adherence to the current recommendations obtained through the recent surveys and registries. Two pilot projects of QI were successfully carried out in the United States: the GAP and the GWTG projects. These showed a similar improvement in adherence to discharge care guidelines in STE-ACS patients [42,43]. Similar favorable results were found in a retrospective analysis of a registry of 3754 consecutive patients during the period 1999–2000 in the United States [38]. The nationwide version of the GWTG, launched by the American Heart Association, is ongoing [43]. It includes all patients with ACS and is focused on the discharge management of ACS patients, directly linking cardiologists with primary-care physicians through internet-based data collection in order to improve communication and postdischarge care. The CRUSADE registry represents an attempt at close collaboration between emergency department physicians and cardiologists to improve the care of high-risk-patients with ACS [24]. Chest-pain risk stratification protocols, standard admission orders reflecting ACC/AHA recommendations, and discharge treatment reminders should help to improve adherence to guidelines.

In summary, even in the presence of sound scientific evidence, regional differences in populations, physicians' knowledge, attitudes and beliefs, heterogeneity in structural and organizational aspects, and many other factors contribute to a lack of uniformity in medical practice. It is important to systematically record all this as a new field of epidemiology, the "epidemiology of (non)uniformity" in medicine. Different practice patterns are not necessarily all bad except one, but we must know to what patients' outcome they lead in order to help patients, providers, and purchasers to make sound decisions based on a deeper knowledge of the effects of different choices on a patient's life. This is the ultimate goal of observational clinical research.

References

1. Gruppo Italiano per lo Studio della Streptochinasi nell'Infarto Miocardio (GISSI). Effectiveness of intravenous treatment in acute myocardial infarction. *Lancet* 1986; **1**: 397–402.
2. Gruppo Italiano per lo Studio della Sopravvivenza nell'Infarto Miocardio. GISSI-2: a factorial randomised trial of alteplase versus streptokinase and heparin versus no heparin among 12,490 patients with acute myocardial infarction. *Lancet* 1990; **336**: 65–71.
3. Gruppo Italiano per lo Studio della Sopravvivenza nell'Infarto Miocardico. GISSI-3: effects of lisinopril and transdermal glyceryl trinitrate singly and together on 6-week mortality and ventricular function after acute myocardial infarction. *Lancet* 1994; **343**: 1115–1122.
4. Gruppo Italiano per lo Studio della Sopravvivenza nell'Infarto Miocardico. Dietary supplementation with n-3 polyunsaturated fatty acids and vitamin E after myocardial infarction: results of the GISSI-Prevenzione trial. *Lancet* 1999; **354**: 447–455.
5. GISSI-Avoidable Delay Study Group. Epidemiology of avoidable delay in the care of patients with acute myocardial infarction in Italy. A GISSI-generated study. *Arch Intern Med* 1995; **155**: 1481–1488.
6. Maggioni AP, Tavazzi L, Fabbri G *et al*. Epidemiology of post-infarction risk stratification strategies in a country with a low volume of revascularization procedures. GISSI-Prognosis Investigators. *Eur Heart J* 1998; **19**: 1784–1794.
7. Tavazzi L, Volpi A. Remarks about postinfarction prognosis in the light of the GISSI trials' experience. *Circulation* 1997; **95**: 1341.
8. Di Chiara A, Chiarella F, Savonitto S *et al*. Epidemiology of acute myocardial infarction in the Italian CCU network. *Eur Heart J* 2003; **24**: 1616–1629.
9. Steffenino G, Santoro GM, Maras P *et al*. In-hospital and one-year outcomes of patients with high risk acute myocardial infarction treated with thrombolysis or primary coronary angioplasty. *Ital Heart J* 2004; **5**: 136–145.
10. Di Chiara A, Fresco C, Savonitto S *et al*. Epidemiology of non ST elevation acute coronary syndromes in the Italian cardiology network. The BLITZ 2 study. *Eur Heart J* 2005 in press.
11. Filardo G, Maggioni AP, Mura G *et al*. The consequences of under-use of coronary revascularization; results of a cohort study in Northern Italy. *Eur Heart J* 2001; **22**: 654–662.
12. Simes J, White H, Marchner L *et al*. International differences in patients, care and outcomes associated with acute myocardial infarction: the HERO-2 trial. *Heart Lung Circ* 2003; **12**: A23.

13. Giuliano RP, Llevadot J, Wilcox RG *et al.* Geographic variation in patient and hospital characteristics, management and clinical outcomes in ST-elevation myocardial infarction, treated with fibrinolysis: results from in TIME–II. *Eur Heart J* 2001; **22**: 1702–1715.

14. Hasdai D, Behar S, Wallentin L *et al.* A prospective survey of the characteristics, treatments and outcomes of patients with acute coronary syndromes in Europe and the Mediterranean basin. *Eur Heart J* 2002; **23**: 1190–1201.

15. Fox KAA, Goodman SG, Anderson FA *et al.* From guidelines to clinical practice: the impact of hospital and geographical characteristics on temporal trends in the management of acute coronary syndromes. *Eur Heart J* 2003; **24**: 1414–1424.

16. Cardiovascular Disease in Europe. Euro Heart Survey and National Registries of Cardiovascular Disease and Patient Management 2004. www.euroheartsurvey.org.

17. Euroaspire II Study Group. Lifestyle and risk factor management and use of drug therapies in coronary patients from 15 countries. Principal results from EUROASPIRE II Euro Heart Survey Programme. *Eur Heart J* 2001; **22**: 554–572.

18. Collinson J, Flather M, Fox KAA *et al.* Clinical outcomes, risk stratification and practice patterns of unstable angina and myocardial infarction without ST elevation: prospective registry of acute ischaemic syndromes in the UK (PRAIS-UK). *Eur Heart J* 2001; **21**: 1450–1457.

19. Steg PG, Goldberg RJ, Gore JM *et al.* Baseline characteristics, management practices and in-hospital outcomes of patients hospitalized with acute coronary syndromes in the Global Registry of Acute Coronary Events (GRACE). *Am J Cardiol* 2002; **90**: 358–363.

20. Cannon CP, Gibson CM, Lambrew CT *et al.* Relationship of symptom-onset-balloon time and door to balloon time with mortality in patients undergoing angioplasty for acute myocardial infarction. *JAMA* 2000; **293**: 2941–2947.

21. Lenzen MJ, Boersma E, Bertrand ME *et al.* Management and outcome of patients with established coronary artery disease: the Euro Heart Survey on Coronary Revascularization. *Eur Heart J* 2005; **26**: 1169–1179.

22. Steg PJ, Iung B, Feldman LJ *et al.* Determinants of use and outcomes of invasive coronary procedures in acute coronary syndromes: results from ENACT. *Eur Heart J* 2003; **24**: 613–622.

23. Yusuf S, Flather M, Pogue J *et al.* Variations between countries in invasive cardiac procedures and outcomes in patients with suspected unstable angina or myocardial infarction without initial ST elevation. OASIS (Organization to Assess Strategies for Ischaemic Syndromes) registry Investigators. *Lancet* 1998; **352**: 507–514.

24. Bhatt DL, Roe MT, Peterson ED *et al.* Utilization of early invasive management strategies for high-risk patients with non-ST segment elevation acute coronary syndromes: results from the CRUSADE quality improvement initiative. *JAMA* 2004; **292**: 2096–2104.

25. De Servi S, Cavallini C, Dellavalle A *et al.* Non-ST elevation acute coronary syndrome in the elderly: treatment strategies and 30-day outcome. *Am Heart J* 2004; **147**: 830–836.

26. Dujardin JJ, Steg PG, Puel J *et al.* FACT: French national registry of acute coronary syndromes. Specific study of the French general hospital centers. *Ann Cardiol e Angiol* 2003; **52**: 337–343.

27. Klein W, Kraxner W, Hodl R *et al.* Patterns of use of heparin in ACS: correlates and hospital outcomes: the Global Registry of Acute Coronary Events (GRACE). *Thromb Haemost* 2003; **90**: 519–527.

28. Budaj A, Brieger D, Steg OG *et al.* Global patterns of use of antithrombotic and antiplatelet therapies in patients with acute coronary events (GRACE). *Am Heart J* 2003; **146**: 999–1006.
29. Goldberg RJ, Currie K, White K *et al.* Six-month outcomes in a multinational registry of patients hospitalized with an acute coronary syndrome (The Global Registry of Acute Coronary Events – GRACE). *Am J Cardiol* 2004; **93**: 288–293.
30. Yan AT, Tan M, Fitchett D *et al.* One-year outcome of patients after acute coronary syndromes (from the Canadian Acute Coronary Syndrome Registry). *Am J Cardiol* 2004; **94**: 25–29.
31. Steg PJ, Dabbous OH, Feldman LJ *et al.* Determinants and prognostic impact of heart failure complicating acute coronary syndromes. Observations from the Global Registry of Acute Coronary Events (GRACE). *Circulation* 2004; **109**: 494–499.
32. Hellerman JP, Jacobsen SJ, Redfield MM *et al.* Heart failure after myocardial infarction: clinical presentation and survival. *Eur J Heart Fail* 2005; **7**: 119–125.
33. Antman EM, Mc Cabe CH, Gurfinkel EP *et al.* Enoxaparin prevents death and cardiac ischemic events in unstable angina/non Q wave myocardial infarction. Results of the thrombolysis in myocardial infarction (TIMI) 11 B trial. *Circulation* 1999; **100**: 1593–1601.
34. Antman EM, Cohen M, Bernink PJ *et al.* The TIMI risk score for unstable angina/non ST elevation MI: a method for prognostication and therapeutic decision making. *JAMA* 2000; **284**: 835–842.
35. Gulati M, Patel S, Jaffe A *et al.* Impact of contemporary guideline compliance on risk stratification models for acute coronary syndromes in the registry of acute coronary syndromes. *Am J Cardiol* 2004; **94**: 873–878.
36. Eagle KA, Lim MJ, Dabbous OH *et al.* Validated prediction model for all forms of acute coronary syndrome. *JAMA* 2004; **291**: 2727–2733.
37. Rogers WJ, Canto JG, Lambrew CT *et al.* Temporal trends in the treatment of over 1.5 million patients with myocardial infarction in the US from 1990 through 1999. *J Am Coll Cardiol* 2000; **36**: 2056–2063.
38. Mc Govern PG, Jacobs DR, Shahar E *et al.* Trends in acute coronary heart disease mortality, morbidity and medical care from 1985 through 1997. The Minnesota Heart Survey. *Circulation* 2001; **104**: 19–24.
39. Goldber RJ, Yarzebski J, Lessard D *et al.* A two-decades (1975–95) long experience in the incidence, in-hospital and long-term case-fatality rates of acute myocardial infarction: a community-wide perspective. *J Am Coll Cardiol* 1999; **33**: 1533–1539.
40. Sinnaeve P, Van de Werf F. Global patterns of health care for acute coronary syndromes. *Curr Opin in Cardiol* 2004; **19**: 625–630.
41. Roe MT, Ohman M, Pollack CV *et al.* Changing the model of care for patients with acute coronary syndromes. *Am Heart J* 2003; **146**: 605–612.
42. Mehta RH, Montoye CK, Gallogly M *et al.* Improving quality of care for acute myocardial infarction: the Guidelines applied in practice (GAP) initiative. *JAMA* 2002; **287**: 1269–1276.
43. Mc Carthy M. US heart-guidelines strategy makes promising start. *Lancet* 2001; **358**: 1618.

Section nine:
Secondary prevention

CHAPTER 20

Secondary prevention after acute episode of patients presenting with nonpersistent ST-segment elevation

Michel E. Bertrand

Observational studies show that most recurrent cardiac events occur within a few months following the initial presentation of acute coronary syndromes (ACSs) [1,2]. Initial stabilization of a patient's clinical condition does not imply that the underlying pathologic process has stabilized. There are sparse data concerning the duration of the healing process of ruptured plaques. Some studies have shown sustained potential for rapid progression of culprit lesions in ACSs despite initial clinical stability on medical therapy) [3]. Increased thrombin generation has been observed for as long as six months following unstable angina or myocardial infarction. Angioscopic studies performed in the follow-up of myocardial infarction showed a persistent residual thrombus in 70% of patients successfully treated with thrombolysis) [4] and even at 18 months there are still 18% of residual thrombus in the infarct-related artery [5]. In addition, trials that examined efficacy of heparin in addition to aspirin reported an increase in clinical events after heparin withdrawal [6,7]. Nevertheless, in FRISC II, continuation of low molecular weight heparin was only beneficial in patients waiting for an invasive procedure.

Thus, it appears that patients stabilized after an acute episode should be treated with an adequate secondary prevention treatment. Since the patient is still shocked by the occurrence of the critical event and is particularly receptive to advices and recommendations, the time of hospital discharge is particularly appropriate to convey important messages. Time before discharge is the most adequate "teachable" period.

In the vast majority of cases, patients who have been treated for non-ST-segment elevation acute coronary syndromes (NSTE-ACSs) are restabilized. In this view, the recommendations for stable coronary artery disease patients should be applied. The European Society of Cardiology (ESC) guidelines for stable coronary artery disease are expected to be published within the last quarter of 2005. For the moment, one can recommend to modify lifestyle and risk factors and to prescribe a secondary prevention medical regimen.

Aggressive risk factor modification is warranted in all patients following diagnosis of ACS

Smoking. It is mandatory that patients quit smoking. Patients should be clearly informed that smoking is a major risk factor. The recent case–control INTER-HEART [8] study has clearly demonstrated that current smokers have three times more chances to develop a myocardial infarction when compared with nonsmokers: Odds ratio (OR) = 2.95 (95% CI, 2.72–3.20). A strong and graded relation was noted between number of smoked cigarettes/day and risk of myocardial infarction: the risk is multiplied by 4 if individuals are smoking more than 20 cigarettes/day and by 9 if they smoke more than 40 cigarettes/day. Referral to smoking cessation clinics is recommended and the use of nicotine replacement therapy should be considered.

Obesity. It is also an important risk factor and patients should be encouraged to follow an appropriate diet to lose weight. However, in the INTERHEART study [8], body mass index was related to risk of further myocardial infarction but this relation was weaker than that of abdominal obesity (waist/hip ratio). Abdominal obesity doubles the risk of acute myocardial infarction. Daily consumptions of fruits, vegetables, and moderate consumption of alcohol are protective.

Exercise. Moderate or strenuous physical exercise is useful. The risk to develop a myocardial infarction is decreased by 28% in comparison with sedentary individuals (OR: 0.72; 95% CI, 0.65–0.79). It is strongly recommended to have daily exercises, such as walking, jogging, or biking.

Blood pressure control. Blood pressure control should be optimized. In the INTERHEART [8] study, the risk of hypertension to develop a myocardial infarction is multiplied by 2.48 in comparison of normotensives (OR: 2.48; 95% CI, 2.30–2.68). It is necessary to maintain the blood pressure level at less than 130/80 mm Hg. The details of the antihypertensive treatment are beyond the scope of this chapter.

Lipid disorders. This should be tightly controlled. In the INTERHEART [8] study, ApoB/ApoA1 ratio can predict the risk of myocardial infarction (MI). There is no threshold, but it appears a graded relation with MI risk that is multiplied by 4.7 for the top versus the lowest quintile of ApoB/ApoA1. We will see that statins should be systematically prescribed but lipid measurements in the follow-up are needed to verify if the patients have reached the target.

Diabetes. It is a huge predictor of recurrent events (OR = 3.1; 95% CI, 2.77–3.42) and a tight control of hyperglycemia is absolutely mandatory in diabetics.

Long-term medical treatment

Five types of drugs are recommended for the secondary prevention of patients who experienced NSTE-ACS.

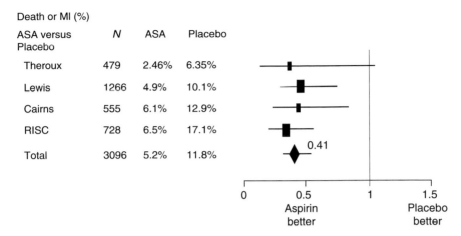

Death or MI (%)

ASA versus Placebo	N	ASA	Placebo
Theroux	479	2.46%	6.35%
Lewis	1266	4.9%	10.1%
Cairns	555	6.1%	12.9%
RISC	728	6.5%	17.1%
Total	3096	5.2%	11.8%

Figure 20.1 Benefits of aspirin over placebo in clinical trials.

Antiplatelet treatment

Aspirin should be prescribed (Figure 20.1). According to the antiplatelet trialists' meta-analysis, there is no advantage in higher doses of aspirin [9]. For patients with a history of MI, a mean of 27 months treatment results in 36 fewer vascular events per 1000 patients, including 18/1000 fewer nonfatal MI and 14/1000 fewer death with aspirin treatment [9].

Based on the results of the CURE trial, clopidogrel 75 mg should be prescribed for at least 9, possibly 12 months, and the dose of aspirin should be reduced to 75–100 mg [10].

The dual antiplatelet treatment, aspirin+clopidogrel, for 1 year has demonstrated a significant benefit in patients who underwent percutaneous coronary intervention (CREDO trial) [11]. There are no data, for the moment, supporting the concept to give the combination of aspirin + clopidogrel for more than 1 year. The CHARISMA trial will bring further information regarding that issue. Currently after 1 year, clopidogrel should be discontinued while aspirin is continued for life. Clopidogrel (75 mg/day) might replace aspirin in patients with gastro-duodenal disorders under aspirin. Clopidogrel is also superior to aspirin in patients who underwent coronary bypass surgery.

β-blockers. They improve prognosis in a patient after MI and should be continued after ACSs with increased levels of troponin signing the myocardial necrosis. However, patients with significantly impaired atrioventricular conduction, a history of asthma, or of acute left ventricular dysfunction should not receive β-blockers.

Lipid lowering therapy. This should be initiated without delay. HMG-CoA reductase inhibitors substantially decrease mortality and coronary events in patients with high, intermediate, or even low (<3.0 mmol/L) levels of LDL cholesterol (Heart Protection Study) [12]. Small subgroups of patients from PURSUIT, PRISM, PRISM-PLUS [13–15], and TACTICS [16] suggest that statins may provide an immediate benefit in ACSs but these data were non-randomized. The MIRACL trial [17] compared atorvastatin (80 mg daily given on average 63 h after admission and for 16 weeks) plus diet versus placebo in 3086 randomized patients. The primary endpoint (a composite endpoint of death, nonfatal MI, rehospitalization for worsening angina at 16 weeks) was marginally ($p = .0459$) positive: 14.8% versus 17.4% but robust endpoints, such as death/MI were similar in both groups (10.1% versus 10.9%). The difference in the primary endpoint was driven by rehospitalization for recurrent angina (6.2% versus 8.4%). In the RIKS-HIA registry (Register of Information and Knowledge about Swedish Intensive care Admissions), the 1 year -mortality rate was lower in patients with non-ST-elevation MI discharged with statin therapy than in the group without that treatment [18,19].

More recently, the Z phase of A to Z has compared two different strategies in patients with ACSs. The first was a conservative strategy including a late treatment (placebo for 4 months) followed by a moderate dose prescription of simvastatin (40 mg/day) for 2 years. The second group received an early (immediate) prescription of simvastatin: 40 mg/day during 1 month followed by 80 mg/day for 2 years. The study population included 40% of patients with STE-ACS and 60% with NSTE-ACS. There was no significant difference in the primary endpoint (a composite of cardiovascular death, infarction, stroke, and readmission for ACS), 16.7% conservative strategy versus 14.4% in the moderate strategy. At 4 months there was no significant difference of the primary endpoint but between 4 and 24 months there was a significant benefit in favor of the early and aggressive strategy (significant reduction of primary endpoint from 9.3% to 6.8%). There was also less cases of heart failure in the early and aggressive strategy, which also decreases the cardiovascular mortality significantly. Similar results were noted in the PRINCESS trial that was conducted in patients with STE-ACSs.

One can conclude the following four points:

1 As previously demonstrated in 4S study [20], LIPID [21], CARE [22], and HPS [12] patients with coronary artery disease and ACSs should systematically receive a treatment with statin, whatever be the baseline level of cholesterol, age, sex, or other conditions (Figure 20.2).

2 The benefit in the acute phase (<30 days) in terms of reduction of robust endpoints (death and MI) is still not established.

3 Nevertheless, statin treatment should be initiated as soon as possible and certainly before discharge. It has been clearly demonstrated that the adherence to statin treatment is greater if the patient was discharged under that treatment.

4 The PROVE-IT trial [23], like the A to Z trial, suggests the use of higher doses of statins at the price of slightly more muscular complications. These high doses are markedly lowering the level of LDL cholesterol and the dogma

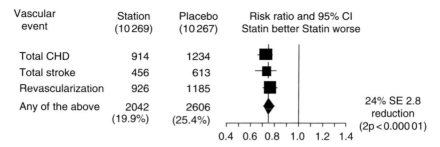

Vascular event	Station (10 269)	Placebo (10 267)	Risk ratio and 95% CI Statin better Statin worse	
Total CHD	914	1234		
Total stroke	456	613		
Revascularization	926	1185		
Any of the above	2042 (19.9%)	2606 (25.4%)		24% SE 2.8 reduction (2p < 0.00001)

Figure 20.2 Benefit of a systematic prescription of 40 mg of simvastatin to prevent major cardiac events (Heart Protection Study trial).

of "lower is better" tends to prevail. Nevertheless, the specific trials are ongoing to assess whether high doses are more effective than intermediate doses.

ACE inhibitors

The role for angiotensin converting enzyme (ACE) inhibitors in secondary prevention of coronary syndromes is now established.

Many randomized, multicenter, clinical trials have established the role of ACE inhibitors after MI: CONSENSUS-2 [24], AIRE [25], SAVE [26], TRACE [27], SMILE [28], CCS-1 [29], ISIS-4 [30], and GISSI-3 [31]. In the different trials, a careful analysis of the follow-up period showed that the recurrence of major ischemic events was significantly reduced. In AIRE [25], SOLVD (both trials involved treatment and prevention) [32], SAVE [26], and TRACE [27], a significant reduction of reinfarction was observed. A metaanalysis of 12 763 patients enrolled in SAVE [26], AIRE [25], TRACE [27], and SOLVD [32] showed that the risk of reinfarction was significantly decreased ($p = .0001$) by 21%.

Thereby, it was interesting to launch trials especially designed to assess the role of ACE inhibitors for secondary prevention of patients with coronary artery disease. Four trials have been performed: the QUIET trial [33] with quinapril, the HOPE (Heart Outcomes Prevention Evaluation) trial [34] with ramipril, the EUROPA trial [35] with perindopril, and the PEACE trial with trandolapril [36].

The HOPE study [34] showed a reduction of cardiovascular death from 8.1% to 6.1% (ARR, 2%; RR, 0.74; 95% CI, 0.64–0.87; $p < .001$) and MI (RR, 0.80; 95% CI, 0.70–0.90; $p < .001$) over 4–6 years [34].

The EUROPA trial [35] was a large (12 218 patients) clinical, prospective, double-blinded randomized controlled trial over 4 years in patients with established coronary artery disease without clinical symptoms of heart failure. The EUROPA trial [35] demonstrated that treatment with perindopril 8 mg was associated with a 20% relative risk reduction (RRR) ($p = 0.0003$) in the primary endpoint (cardiovascular death, nonfatal MI and cardiac arrest) (ARR (Absolute risk reduction), 2%, RRR, 0.80; 95% CI, 0.71–0.91; $p = .0003$).

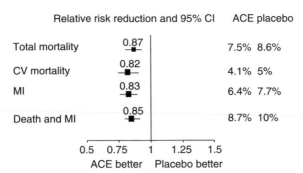

Figure 20.3 Metananalysis of four randomized clinical trials for secondary prevention in patients with stable coronary artery disease.

In the opposite the QUIET trial [33] ($n = 1750$ patients) was negative. The primary outcome (death, MI, resuscitated cardiac arrest, rehospitalization, and coronary revascularization) was the same in the placebo and the quinapril group: ARR, 0.7%, RRR, 1.04; 95% CI, 0.89–1.22; $p = .6$.

The PEACE trial [36] conducted in 8290 patients assigned to trandolapril (4 mg/day) or placebo showed no significant benefit. The incidence of the primary endpoint, (cardiovascular death, MI, or coronary revascularization) was 21.9% in the trandolapril group as compared with 22.5% in the placebo group: ARR, 0.6%; RRR, 0.96; 95% CI, 0.88–1.06; $p = .43$.

Thus, there are two positive [HOPE [34] and EUROPA [35]] trials and two negative trials [QUIET and PEACE [36]]. The two negative results might be explained by an underpowered study [QUIET [33]] and a too small dose of ACE inhibitor (trandolapril 4 mg/day) which was taken by only 51% of the trandolapril randomized population.

The metaanalysis of these four trials shows that ACE inhibitors determine a strong beneficial effect on total and cardiovascular mortality, MI, death and MI, need for revascularization, occurrence of new heart failure and stroke (Figure 20.3).

Thus, ace inhibitors should be prescribed in patients stabilized after an ACS.

Practical applications and conclusions

In 2000, the ESC launched a survey in 24 European countries and was able to collect the data from 10 484 patients with ACSs of whom 51% had NSTE-ACS. In 2004, a new survey was conducted in 30 countries and the preliminary data showed a significant improvement within the 4-year time span.

In 2000, 85% of patients with NSTE-ACS were discharged under aspirin, 73% with a β-blocker, 59% with an ACE inhibitor, and 53% with a statin. It is interesting to note that in 2004, these drugs are prescribed in 92%, 81%, 76%, and 78% of patients, respectively. These results are certainly encouraging but suggest an implementation program to still improve these figures.

References

1. van Domburg RT, van Miltenburg-van Zijl AJ, Veerhoek RJ, Simoons ML. Unstable angina: good long-term outcome after a complicated early course. *J Am Coll Cardiol* 1998; **31**: 1534–1539.
2. Theroux P, Fuster V. Acute coronary syndromes: unstable angina and non-Q-wave myocardial infarction. *Circulation* 1998; **97**: 1195–1206.
3. Kontny F. Reactivation of the coagulation system: rationale for long-term anti-thrombotic treatment. *Am J Cardiol* 1997; **80**: 55E–60E.
4. Van Belle E, Lablanche JM, Bauters C, Renaud N, McFadden EP, Bertrand ME. Coronary angioscopic findings in the infarct-related vessel within 1 month of acute myocardial infarction: natural history and the effect of thrombolysis [see comments]. *Circulation* 1998; **97**: 26–33.
5. Ueda Y, Asakura M, Yamaguchi O, Hirayama A, Hori M, Kodama K. The healing process of infarct-related plaques. Insights from 18 months of serial angioscopic follow-up. *J Am Coll Cardiol* 2001; **38**: 1916–1922.
6. Theroux P, Ouimet H, McCans J *et al*. Aspirin, heparin, or both to treat acute unstable angina. *New Eng J Med* 1988; **319**: 1105–1111.
7. RISC Group. Risk of myocardial infarction and death during treatment with low dose aspirin and intravenous heparin in men with unstable coronary artery disease. The RISC Group. *Lancet* 1990; **336**: 827–830.
8. Yusuf S, Hawken S, Ounpuu S *et al*. Effect of potentially modifiable risk factors associated with myocardial infarction in 52 countries (the INTERHEART study): case–control study. *Lancet* 2004; **364**: 937–952.
9. Antithrombotic Trialist Collaboration. Collaborative meta-analysis of randomised trials of antiplatelet therapy for prevention of death, myocardial infarction, and stroke in high risk patients. *BMJ* 2002; **324**: 71–86.
10. Yusuf S, Zhao F, Mehta SR, Chrolavicius S, Tognoni G, Fox KK. Effects of clopidogrel in addition to aspirin in patients with acute coronary syndromes without ST-segment elevation. *N Engl J Med* 2001; **345**: 494–502.
11. Steinhubl SR, Berger PB, Mann JT III *et al*. Early and sustained dual oral antiplatelet therapy following percutaneous coronary intervention: a randomized controlled trial. *JAMA* 2002; **288**: 2411–2420.
12. Collins R, Armitage J, Parish S, Sleight P, Peto R. Effects of cholesterol-lowering with simvastatin on stroke and other major vascular events in 20536 people with cerebrovascular disease or other high-risk conditions. *Lancet* 2004; **363**: 757–767.
13. PURSUIT Study investigators. Inhibition of platelet glycoprotein IIb/IIIa with eptifibatide in patients with acute coronary syndromes. The PURSUIT Trial Investigators. Platelet glycoprotein IIb/IIIa in unstable angina: receptor suppression using integrilin therapy. *N Engl J Med* 1998; **339**: 436–443.
14. PRISM investigators. A comparison of aspirin plus tirofiban with aspirin plus heparin for unstable angina. Platelet Receptor Inhibition in Ischemic Syndrome Management (PRISM) Study Investigators [see comments]. *N Engl J Med* 1998; **338**: 1498–1505.
15. PRISM-PLUS Study Investigators. Inhibition of the platelet glycoprotein IIb/IIIa receptor with tirofiban in unstable angina and non-Q-wave myocardial infarction. Platelet Receptor Inhibition in Ischemic Syndrome Management in Patients

Limited by Unstable Signs and Symptoms (PRISM-PLUS) Study Investigators [see comments]. *N Engl J Med* 1998; **338**: 1488–1497.

16. Cannon CP, Weintraub WS, Demopoulos LA *et al*. Comparison of early invasive and conservative strategies in patients with unstable coronary syndromes treated with the glycoprotein IIb/IIIa inhibitor tirofiban. *N Engl J Med* 2001; **344**: 1879–1887.

17. Schwartz GG, Olsson AG, Ezekowitz MD *et al*. Effects of atorvastatin on early recurrent ischemic events in acute coronary syndromes: the MIRACL study: a randomized controlled trial. *JAMA* 2001; **285**: 1711–1718.

18. Stenestrand U, Wallentin L. Early statin treatment following acute myocardial infarction and 1-year survival. *JAMA* 2001; **285**: 430–436.

19. Stenestrand U, Wallentin L. Early revascularization and 1-year survival in 14-days survivors of acute myocardial infarction: a prospective cohort study. *Lancet* 2002; **359**: 1805–1811.

20. 4S Investigators. Randomised trial of cholesterol lowering in 4444 patients with coronary heart disease: the Scandinavian Simvastatin Survival Study (4S). *Lancet* 1994; **344**: 1383–1389.

21. LIPID Study Group. Prevention of cardiovascular events and death with pravastatin in patients with coronary heart disease and a broad range of initial cholesterol levels. The Long-Term Intervention with Pravastatin in Ischaemic Disease (LIPID) Study Group. *N Engl J Med* 1998; **339**: 1349–1357.

22. Sacks FM, Pfeffer MA, Moye LA *et al*. The effect of pravastatin on coronary events after myocardial infarction in patients with average cholesterol levels. Cholesterol and Recurrent Events Trial Investigators. *N Engl J Med* 1996; **335**: 1001–1009.

23. Cannon CP, Braunwald E, McCabe CH *et al*. Intensive versus moderate lipid lowering with statins after acute coronary syndromes. *N Engl J Med* 2004; **350**: 1495–1504.

24. Swedberg K, Held P, Kjekshus J, Rasmussen K, Ryden L, Wedel H. Effects of the early administration of enalapril on mortality in patients with acute myocardial infarction. Results of the Cooperative New Scandinavian Enalapril Survival Study II (CONSENSUS II) [see comments]. *N Engl J Med* 1992; **327**: 678–684.

25. AIRE Investigators. Effect of ramipril on mortality and morbidity of survivors of acute myocardial infarction with clinical evidence of heart failure. The Acute Infarction Ramipril Efficacy (AIRE) Study Investigators. *Lancet* 1993; **342**: 821–828.

26. Pfeffer MA, Braunwald E, Moye LA *et al*. Effect of captopril on mortality and morbidity in patients with left ventricular dysfunction after myocardial infarction. Results of the survival and ventricular enlargement trial. The SAVE Investigators. *N Engl J Med* 1992; **327**: 669–677.

27. Kober L, Torp-Pedersen C, Carlsen JE *et al*. A clinical trial of the angiotensin-converting-enzyme inhibitor trandolapril in patients with left ventricular dysfunction after myocardial infarction. Trandolapril Cardiac Evaluation (TRACE) Study Group. *N Engl J Med* 1995; **333**: 1670–1676.

28. Ambrosioni E, Borghi C, Magnani B. The effect of the angiotensin-converting-enzyme inhibitor zofenopril on mortality and morbidity after anterior myocardial infarction. The Survival of Myocardial Infarction Long-Term Evaluation (SMILE) Study Investigators [see comments]. *N Engl J Med* 1995; **332**: 80–85.

29. Oral captopril versus placebo among 13,634 patients with suspected acute myocardial infarction: interim report from the Chinese Cardiac Study (CCS-1). *Lancet* 1995; **345**: 686–687.

30. ISIS-4: a randomised factorial trial assessing early oral captopril, oral mononitrate, and intravenous magnesium sulphate in 58,050 patients with suspected acute myocardial infarction. ISIS-4 (Fourth International Study of Infarct Survival) Collaborative Group. *Lancet* 1995; **345**: 669–685.

31. GISSI-3: effects of lisinopril and transdermal glyceryl trinitrate singly and together on 6-week mortality and ventricular function after acute myocardial infarction. Gruppo Italiano per lo Studio della Sopravvivenza nell'infarto Miocardico. *Lancet* 1994; **343**: 1115–1122.

32. The SOLVD Investigators. Effect of enalapril on survival in patients with reduced left ventricular ejection fraction and congestive heart failure. *N Engl J Med* 1991; **325**: 293–302.

33. Pitt B, O'Neill B, Feldman R *et al.* The QUinapril Ischemic Event Trial (QUIET): evaluation of chronic ACE inhibitor therapy in patients with ischemic heart disease and preserved left ventricular function. *Am J Cardiol* 2001; **87**: 1058–1063.

34. Yusuf S, Sleight P, Pogue J, Bosch J, Davies R, Dagenais G. Effects of an angiotensin-converting-enzyme inhibitor, ramipril, on cardiovascular events in high-risk patients. The Heart Outcomes Prevention Evaluation Study Investigators. *N Engl J Med* 2000; **342**: 145–153.

35. Fox KM. Efficacy of perindopril in reduction of cardiovascular events among patients with stable coronary artery disease: randomised, double-blind, placebo-controlled, multicentre trial (the EUROPA study). *Lancet* 2003; **362**: 782–788.

36. Pfeffer MA, Domanski M, Rosenberg Y *et al.* Prevention of events with angiotensin-converting enzyme inhibition (the PEACE study design). Prevention of Events with Angiotensin-Converting Enzyme Inhibition. *Am J Cardiol* 1998; **82**: 25H–30H.

37. SOLVD investigators. Effect of enalapril on mortality and the development of heart failure in asymptomatic patients with reduced left ventricular ejection fractions. The SOLVD Investigattors [published erratum appears in *N Engl J Med* 1992; **327**(24): 1768] [see comments]. *N Engl J Med* 1992; **327**: 685–691.

38. Collins R, Peto R, MacMahon S *et al.* Blood pressure, stroke, and coronary heart disease. Part 2, short-term reductions in blood pressure: overview of randomised drug trials in their epidemiological context [see comments]. *Lancet* 1990; **335**: 827–838.

39. Rabbani RTE. Strategies to achieve coronary arterial plaque stabilization. *Cardiovasc Res* 1999; **41**: 402–417.

40. Yusuf S, Kostis JB, Pitt B. ACE inhibitors for myocardial infarction and unstable angina. *Lancet* 1993; **341**: 829.

41. Dagenais GR, Yusuf S, Bourassa MG *et al.* Effects of ramipril on coronary events in high-risk persons: results of the Heart Outcomes Prevention Evaluation Study. *Circulation* 2001; **104**: 522–526.

CHAPTER 21

How to detect vulnerable plaque

Dirk Boese and Raimund Erbel

Introduction

Recent clinical and histopathological studies indicate that most of acute coronary syndromes are caused by rupture or erosion of a coronary atherosclerotic plaque with different degrees of superimposed thrombosis [1,2]. Different features of these rupture prone, vulnerable plaques could be identified. They tend to have a large lipidic necrotic core with a thin fibrous cap and signs of inflammation as well as positive remodelling. More than 80% of these plaques are clinically silent before rupture with luminal narrowing <70%, and nearly 70% has a stenosis less than 50% [2]. Due to vessel remodeling, coronary angiography cannot detect signs of early atherosclerosis unless the plaque excess 45–50% (Glagov phenomenon) [3]. Several invasive, catheter based and noninvasive imaging modalities were developed and approved in clinical practice to identify vulnerable plaques. In this chapter, we review the current status of invasive imaging techniques to detect vulnerable plaques in human coronary arteries. Beside the local parameters, systemic effects, such as systemic inflammation, also influence plaque stability especially in the coronary tree.

Angiography

In the recent years, coronary X-ray contrast angiography became the gold standard in the detection of luminal diameters and in the detection of severe coronary stenosis with high resolution and accuracy. However, it is not possible to identify vessel wall changes and plaque formation with this technique because angiography can only provide a negative image of the contrast-filled lumen. Remodeling processes make it difficult to assess the amount of atherosclerosis and may conceal early stages of atherosclerosis. Especially, in eccentric coronary lesions it may be difficult to estimate the amount of atherosclerosis and vessel dimensions with angiography alone. After plaque rupture, typical signs of thrombus formation or plaque ulceration after washout of debris may be described [4].

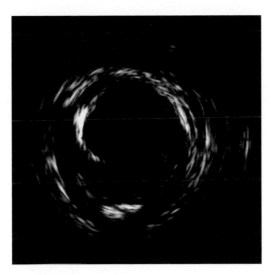

Figure 21.1 IVUS gray scale image of a ruptured plaque.

Intravascular ultrasound

Intravascular ultrasound (IVUS) is a catheter-based imaging technique that allows both imaging of the vessel dimensions and vessel wall characteristics. Whereas contrast angiography offers only a two-dimensional silhouette of the lumen, IVUS provides a real-time cross-sectional image of the vessel wall and allows tomographic measurements of the lumen area and plaque burden, as well as estimation of qualitative atherosclerotic plaque characteristics (Figure 21.1). The basic principle of IVUS is the conversion of electrical energy into sound waves, and the subsequent detection of reflected ultrasound waves or echoes by a transducer. The transducer converts the ultrasound energy back into electrical energy that is amplified, processed, and filtered to create a graphical image on IVUS console. Currently, there are two different IVUS catheter systems available. In the mechanical catheters, there is a single transducer rotating at 1800 rpm to generate a 360° image. For imaging of coronary arteries these catheters are available with frequencies between 30 and 40 MHz. The solid-state catheter system consists of an array of 64 transducer elements in a cylindrical pattern. These transducers are activated consecutively to create a cross-sectional image of the coronary vessel wall. IVUS reaches an axial resolution of 100–200 μm and a lateral resolution of 250 μm depending on imaging depth. IVUS is easy to use in daily clinical practice and provides a unique method for studying the morphology of atherosclerosis *in vivo*. However, IVUS cannot be used to detect and quantify specific histological plaque components. According to the ACC AHA task force, plaque components were divided by their echogenicity. Plaque structures that appear hypoechoic in the IVUS were called "soft" or "echolucent" plaques [5]. This is generally the result of high rate of lipid components with less collagen and elastin. However, echolucent areas within the plaque may also be caused by intramural hemorrhage. Plaques with a higher content of fibrous tissue appear more echogenic in the IVUS images. The echogenicity of the fibrous plaques is comparable with the surrounding adventitia. Calcified lesions appear as bright echos with "acoustic shadowing." Calcium deposits can be described qualitatively by their location in superficial and deep structures and by their circumferential extent [5,6].

Within recent years, some characteristics of vulnerable, rupture prone coronary plaques were identified by IVUS [7–12]. Lesions in proximal vessel segments with an expansive, positive remodeling are often associated with plaque rupture or erosion with consecutive acute coronary syndrome [10]. In these lesions the area-stenosis is less than 50% [10]. Especially, the atheromas and fibroatheromas (Stary IV/Va) with extensive echolucent areas, appeared to result from lipid-rich plaque structures with a thin fibrous cap, to be vulnerable and often associated with plaque rupture or erosion with consecutive acute coronary syndrome [13–15]. The amount of calcification visualized by IVUS is also an indicator of plaque vulnerability. Spotty superficial calcification with an arc of less 90° is often found in patients with acute myocardial infarction (AMI). Conversely, extensive calcification can be found more often in patients with stable angina [6].

Intravascular ultrasound is a unique tool to identify the morphological characteristics of vulnerable and rational plaques (Figure 21.1) in human coronary arteries, but the qualitative classification of different plaque components might be difficult and depends on the experience of the investigator. The sensitivity for detection of lipid-rich plaque components is quite low [16]. In addition, IVUS is limited by its resolution in the identification of thin fibrous caps with a thickness less than 110 μm especially in catheters with low frequencies. This might be a problem for the detection of so-called thin-cap fibroatheromas. Some technical artifacts, such as NURDS (nonuniform rotational distortions) or ring down artifacts may also reduce the quality of IVUS examination. However, IVUS is currently the only commercially available clinical technique providing real-time cross-sectional images of the coronary artery and enabling plaque visualization and demonstrating lipid cores, vessel remodelling, plaque ulceration, plaque thrombosis and hemorrhage [14,15].

IVUS – virtual histology

The virtual histology is a new imaging modality based on the IVUS technique for quantifying plaque composition. The radiofrequency signal that is underlying the conventional IVUS-grayscale image is analyzed using a spectral analysis and compared with a histological database. The virtual histology analyzing system can identify and quantify the different histological plaque components *in vivo*. It is possible to identify fibrous, fibrolipidic, lipidic-necrotic, and calcified plaque components with an accuracy ranging from 79.7% to 93%. This technique offers the possibility to identify vulnerable plaques not only by the IVUS criteria but also by the size of the lipid core and the amount of lipid and fibrolipidic tissue [17,18]. The analyzing software is integrated in the IVUS-console so that virtual histology analyses can be performed online in the catheterization laboratory. After semiautomatic contour detection, the profile and quantification of different plaque components are automatically performed by the software.

Recent studies have been able to demonstrate the relationship between arterial remodeling and plaque components. In plaques with a positive expansive remodeling, significantly more lipid-rich tissue might be found. Thin-cap fibroatheromas and fibroatheromas could be found in 100% of the plaques with positive remodeling, whereas plaques with negative remodeling appear to be more stable with a higher content of calcified and fibrous tissue [19]. Virtual histology offers potential to analyze the influence of systemic risk factors on plaque composition and vulnerability. The comparison with cardiovascular risk factors demonstrates a significant inverse correlation between HDL-cholesterol and the amount of lipidic-necrotic plaque components [20]. This suggests that HDL-cholesterol increase can influence (perhaps, reduce) the lipid core and, therefore, one of the characteristics of plaque vulnerability. The limitations of this technique are comparable with IVUS. At the present time, virtual histology is only available for solid-state catheters with a frequency of 20 MHz.

Elastography/palpography

The intravascular elastography is another invasive imaging technique based upon radiofrequency IVUS signal analysis which was developed in order to receive not only morphological but also functional parameters. IVUS elastography is based on the principle that different plaque components can be compressed differently during pressure changes in the cardiac circle depending on their histopathological composition. Several *in vitro* studies indicate that intravascular elastography can identify fibrous, fibrofatty, and fatty tissue by the local strain related to the pressure change induced by ultrasound signals at two defined pressure points in diastole [21,23,24]. The radial strain in fibrous tissue (0.27%) was lower than in fibrofatty (0.45%) and, fatty tissue (0.60%) [24]. The technique signals identify plaque vulnerability by high strain at the plaque surface and adjacent low strain regions. High strain characterizes unstable plaques and soft plaque components. A sensitivity of 88% and a specificity of 89% for the detection of vulnerable plaques has been described *in vitro* [25]. A threshold value of 1.26% strain was found. Plaques with high strain showed a significant higher amount of macrophages ($p < .006$) and lower content of smooth muscle cells ($p < .0001$) in the plaque surface than stable plaques [24]. Plaques that appear unstable with elastography had a thinner fibrous cap measured in histology than stable plaques ($p < .0001$) [24].

Intravascular palpography is a similar technique that focuses on strain measurements and assessment of mechanical properties at the luminal boundary of

Table 21.1 Potential of different imaging modalities in the detection of vulnerable plaque characteristics.

	Lipid core	Thin fibrous cap	Inflammation	Positive remodeling	Superficial calcification
Angiography	−	−	−	−	−
IVUS	+	+	−	+ + +	+ +
Virtual histology	+ + +	+	−	+ + +	+ + +
Palpography	+	+ +	+	+	+
OCT	+	+ + +	+ +	−	+ +
Thermography	−	−	+ + +	−	−
Angioscopy	+	+ +	−	−	−

the atherosclerotic plaque. Palpography is faster and more robust compared to elastography [23]. Three-dimensional intravascular palpography (Table 21.1) can not only provide elastograms of one-vessel cross-section but also of vessel segments. *In vivo* studies were able to demonstrate that patients with stable angina had significantly fewer deformable plaques per vessel (0.6 ± 0.6) than patients with unstable angina (1.6 ± 0.7) or AMI (2.0 ± 0.7): This supports the hypothesis that plaque vulnerability is not only a focal but also a multifocal process. A positive correlation between the level of high sensitive C-reactive protein as a marker of inflammation and the number of mechanically deformable plaques has been demonstrated [25]. However, the technique may be limited *in vivo* by the problem of cardiac contraction and movement of the catheter during the cardiac circle. This may lead to some errors in the correlation of the radiofrequency signals at different time points and may decrease the quality of strain information. The quality of this investigation may also be limited by the low radial resolution that reaches 500 μm. Nevertheless, three-dimensional intravascular palpography offers a promising tool for *in vivo* plaque characterization and identification of potentially vulnerable plaques.

Optical coherence tomography

The optical coherence tomography (OCT) measures the intensity of back-reflected infrared light, or optical echoes, to provide a tomographic visualization of the vessel wall and plaque structures. The OCT system uses fiber-optic interferometers coupled with a mid-infrared (wavelength, 1320 nm) light source. Measurements of the interferometer can be processed with a computer to produce cross-sectional or three-dimensional real-time images of the vessel wall. The main advantage of OCT compared with other catheter-based image modalities is the high resolution. OCT reaches an axial resolution of 2–30 μm and a lateral resolution of 5–30 μm [26–29]. Several *in vitro* studies indicate that OCT can clearly separate different plaque components and tissue types. Fibrous, fibrocalcific, and lipid-rich plaques can be divided qualitatively by their image characteristics with sensitivity between 71% and 98% and specificity between 92% and 97% [27]. Compared to high resolution IVUS, OCT has proved to be equivalent in detecting fibrous and calcified plaque structures. OCT measurements might more frequently identify echolucent regions corresponding to lipid-rich areas in the histology and thin fibrous cap [28–31]. Another advantage of the high resolution of OCT is the possibility to identify thin fibrous cap (<65 μm) overlaying atheromatous material [28]. In an *in vivo* study with 69 patients enrolled, the median value of the cap thickness in the culprit lesion was significantly ($p = .012$) lower in unstable patients (53 μm) or patients with an AMI (47 μm) than in patients with stable angina (102 μm) [28]. The frequency of thin-cap fibroatheromas, defined by a lipid-rich plaque with cap thickness less than or equal to 65 μm, was found more frequently in patients with an AMI (72%) than in unstable patients (50%) or patients with stable angina (20%) [29]. In another autopsy study, the ability of OCT to detect and quantify macrophage infiltration within the fibrous cap was demonstrated [30]. The presence of macrophages, identified by immunoperoxidase staining for CD68 was correlated with the OCT measurement. A sensitivity and specificity of 100% was achieved for identifying caps containing greater than 10% of CD68-positive macrophages within the imaged region [32]. A negative correlation between the amount of macrophages in the OCT and histological measurements of smooth muscle actin density could be revealed [32].

These data indicate that the OCT offers the feasibility to visualize plaque characteristics *in vivo*. The identification of vulnerable plaque characteristics, such as thin fibrous caps, lipid core, and local inflammation is promising for further application. Nevertheless, there are some limitations of this technique. Because the depth of penetration is limited to 1–2 mm, OCT can only visualize superficial plaque structures. For this reason, OCT cannot assess deeper lipid core or the external elastic membrane (EEM) to determine positive versus negative remodeling. Another limitation of OCT is that light is absorbed by blood. This requires displacement of the blood volume with saline or a proximal occlusion balloon during examination. In addition the rotation frequency of 6 rpm results in artefacts due to the lack of real-time visualization.

The short time window (2s) available for imaging while the blood is displaced makes it difficult to assess long vessel segments with OCT [30]. The system is not yet commercially available but further miniaturization, perhaps, down to 0.014 in. may facilitate clinical application.

Thermography

As previously mentioned, it is known that activated macrophages play an important role in the pathogenesis of acute coronary syndromes and cause a local inflammatory reaction that might enhance plaque vulnerability. Because the inflammatory reaction causes local heat production, the assessment of local temperature has been explored for the detection of local inflammatory processes in the vessel wall. *Ex vivo* studies in human carotid arteries after carotid endarterectomy have demonstrated a direct correlation between the temperature increase in the vessel wall and the amount of macrophages in the plaque indicating the ability to quantify inflammatory processes. An inverse correlation between temperature and the density of smooth muscle cells in the plaque surface was observed [33].

Several catheter-based thermistors have been developed for the measurement of temperature heterogeneity in human coronary arteries with the hypothesis to identify vulnerable plaques. Stefanadis *et al.* used a single thermistor with a diameter of 0.457 mm, a temperature accuracy of 0.05°C, a time constant of 300 ms, and a spatial resolution of 0.5 mm [34–36]. Temperature differences between the culprit lesion and healthy vessels were reported for patients with stable angina, unstable angina, and AMI. Temperature differences increased progressively from patients with stable angina (0.016±0.110°C) and unstable angina (0.683±0.347°C) to patients with AMI (1.472±0.691°C). Increased heterogeneity of temperature was observed more frequently in patients with AMI than in stable patients (67–20%). Patients with an increased temperature in the culprit lesion had higher adverse cardiac event rates after successful percutaneous coronary intervention (PCI) [36–38]. Lipid-lowering therapy could demonstrate a reduction in temperature heterogeneity supporting an antiinflammatory effect of statin therapy [34]. Schmermund *et al.* used another thermography catheter design with a self-expanding basket of five nitinol arms and a thermocouple on each arm as well as in the center of the basket. Temperature differences between the vessel wall (arms of the basket) and the flowing blood (central thermocouple) were measured in 19 patients. Temperature difference ranges from 0.14°C to 0.36°C and was quite lower than previously reported by Stefanadis *et al.* [35,39] with a considerable overlap in temperature recordings between stable and unstable patients. Nevertheless, thermal heterogeneity was found more frequently in patients with unstable angina than in patients with stable angina [39].

Intracoronary thermography gives a more functional insight into coronary artery disease by identifying inflammation in the vessel wall. It may be limited by the overlap in temperature heterogeneity between stable and unstable presentation of atherosclerosis and by individual variations of temperature heterogeneity. Furthermore, there is no clear evidence that temperature differences are related to specific plaque vulnerability or a general inflammation process. In addition, actual catheter designs are limited in clinical practice because they require contact with the vessel wall, and their use may therefore cause vessel injury.

Angioscopy

Angioscopy allows visualization of the inner vessel surface and the atherosclerotic plaque with the use of fiber optics. Atherosclerotic plaques can be divided by their color in white or yellow plaques [40]. The plaques that appear white in angioscopy were mostly stable plaques with a high content of fibrous tissue [40]. Yellow plaques consist of lipid-rich plaque structures with a thin fibrous cap and were generally considered as vulnerable plaques [40,41]. Yellow plaques were predominantly found in the culprit lesion of patients with AMI (90%) with subsequent thrombus formation (81%) [42]. The thrombus found on ruptured plaques in AMI patients was mainly white representing platelet rich thrombus. In some patients, a mixture of white and red thrombus (fibrin/erythrocyte-rich) could be found [43–48]. In serial follow-up studies, white thrombus could still be observed in greater than 50% of the AMI patients 1 month after infarction [43,44]. In patients with AMI, yellow vulnerable plaque could not only be found in the infarct-related vessels but also equally in the noninfarct-related vessels (3.7 ± 1.6 versus 3.4 ± 1.8), indicating a pan coronary process of plaque vulnerability [42]. It has been demonstrated that lipid-lowering therapy with atorvastatin has a positive effect on plaque color and morphology in serial angioscopy examination [47]. The intensity of yellow color had decreased significantly within the statin-treated patients correlating to the change in the LDL-levels after 6 months ($r = 0.81$, $p < .0001$) [47]. In addition, the identification of ruptured yellow plaques with subsequent thrombosis is correlated with an adverse outcome after coronary intervention [49].

Nevertheless, angioscopy can only assess the surface of plaque. Deeper characterization of plaque morphology or composition and deeper plaque structure is missing. Moreover, the technique may be limited by the subjectivity of color interpretation that requires further development, that is, automated analysis systems. The current angioscopy systems needs blood free vessel segments, achieved by a proximal occlusion balloon or continuous flushing with saline, to enable visualization of the coronary vessel wall. Both, balloon occlusion and flushing may induce complications and limit the method to research applications. Current catheter designs with a diameter between 3 F and 5 F do not allow angioscopy of small vessels. In addition, very proximal segments cannot be explored.

Near infrared spectroscopy/Raman spectroscopy

The near infrared spectroscopy and the Raman spectroscopy utilize different sources of energy (infrared light/laser) for identification and classification of several tissue types within human coronary arteries by their chemical composition. Both techniques are limited to *in vitro* studies at the moment: further development and validation are needed [50–53].

References

1. Libby P. Current concepts of the pathogenesis of the acute coronary syndromes. *Circulation* 2001; **104**(3): 365–372.
2. Falk E, Shah PK, Fuster V. Coronary plaque disruption. *Circulation* 1995; **92**(3): 657–671.

3. Glagov S, Weisenberg E, Zarins CK, Stankunavicius R, Kolettis GJ. Compensatory enlargement of human atherosclerotic coronary arteries. *N Engl J Med* 1987; **316**(22): 1371–1375.
4. Ambrose JA, Winters SL, Stern A *et al.* Angiographic morphology and the pathogenesis of unstable angina pectoris. *J Am Coll Cardiol* 1985; **5**(3): 609–616.
5. Mintz GS, Nissen SE, Anderson WD *et al.* American College of Cardiology clinical expert consensus document on standards for acquisition, measurement and reporting of intravascular ultrasound studies (IVUS). A report of the American College of Cardiology Task Force on Clinical Expert Consensus Documents. *J Am Coll Cardiol* 2001; **37**(5): 1478–1492.
6. Ehara S, Kobayashi Y, Yoshiyama M *et al.* Spotty calcification typifies the culprit plaque in patients with acute myocardial infarction: an intravascular ultrasound study. *Circulation* 2004; **110**(22): 3424–3429
7. Zamorano J, Erbel R, Ge J *et al.* Spontaneous plaque rupture visualized by intravascular ultrasound. *Eur Heart J* 1994; **15**(1): 131–133.
8. Kearney P, Erbel R, Rupprecht HJ *et al.* Differences in the morphology of unstable and stable coronary lesions and their impact on the mechanisms of angioplasty. An *in vivo* study with intravascular ultrasound. *Eur Heart J* 1996; **17**(5): 721–730.
9. Jeremias A, Ge J, Erbel R. New insight into plaque healing after plaque rupture with subsequent thrombus formation detected by intravascular ultrasound. *Heart* 1997; **77**(3): 293.
10. Birgelen von C, Klinkhart W, Mintz GS *et al.* Plaque distribution and vascular remodeling of ruptured and nonruptured coronary plaques in the same vessel: an intravascular ultrasound study *in vivo. J Am Coll Cardiol* 2001; **37**(7): 1864–1870.
11. Ge J, Chirillo F, Schwedtmann J *et al.* Screening of ruptured plaques in patients with coronary artery disease by intravascular ultrasound. *Heart* 1999; **81**(6): 621–627.
12. Gossl M, von Birgelen C, Mintz GS *et al.* Volumetric assessment of ulcerated ruptured coronary plaques with three-dimensional intravascular ultrasound *in vivo. Am J Cardiol* 2003; **91**(8): 992–996.
13. von Birgelon C, Klinkhart W, Mintz GS *et al.* Plaque distribution and vascular remodeling of ruptured and nonruptured coronary plaques in the same vessel: an intravascular ultrasound study *in vivo. J Am Coll Cardiol* 2001; **37**(7): 1864–1870.
14. Ge J, Baumgart D, Haude M *et al.* Role of intravascular ultrasound imaging in identifying vulnerable plaques. *Herz* 1999; **24**(1): 32–41.
15. Erbel R, Ge J, Gorge G *et al.* Intravascular ultrasound classification of atherosclerotic lesions according to American Heart Association recommendation. *Coron Artery Dis* 1999; **10**(7): 489–499.
16. Di Mario C, Gorge G, Peters R *et al.* Clinical application and image interpretation in intracoronary ultrasound. Study Group on Intracoronary Imaging of the Working Group of Coronary Circulation and of the Subgroup on Intravascular Ultrasound of the Working Group of Echocardiography of the European Society of Cardiology. *Eur Heart J* 1998; **19**(2): 207–229.
17. Nair A, Kuban BD, Tuzcu EM, Schoenhagen P, Nissen SE, Vince DG. Coronary plaque classification with intravascular ultrasound radiofrequency data analysis. *Circulation* 2002; **106**(17): 2200–2206
18. Böse D, Schmermund A, Margolis P *et al.* Intravascular ultrasound radiofrequency analysis identifies plaque composition: virtual histology. *Eur Heart J* 2004; **6**(Suppl): 211A.
19. Rodriguez-Granillo GA, Serruys PW, Garcia-Garcia HM *et al.* Coronary artery remodelling is related to plaque composition. *Heart* 2005, in press.

20. Böse D, Schmermund A, Margolis P *et al*. Intravascular ultrasound radiofrequency analysis identifies plaque composition depending on risk factors: *in vivo* virtual histology. *Am J Cardiol* 2004; **94**(6, Suppl. 1): 163.

21. Schaar JA, Regar E, Mastik F *et al*. Incidence of high-strain patterns in human coronary arteries: assessment with three-dimensional intravascular palpography and correlation with clinical presentation. *Circulation* 2004; **109**(22): 2716–2719.

22. Schaar JA, de Korte CL, Mastik F *et al*. Intravascular palpography for high-risk vulnerable plaque assessment. *Herz* 2003; **28**(6): 488–495.

23. de Korte CL, Cespedes EI, van der Steen AF, Pasterkamp G, Bom N. Intravascular ultrasound elastography: assessment and imaging of elastic properties of diseased arteries and vulnerable plaque. *Eur J Ultrasound* 1998; **7**: 219–224.

24. de Korte CL, Pasterkamp G, van der Steen AF, Woutman HA, Bom N. Characterization of plaque components with intravascular ultrasound elastography in human femoral and coronary arteries *in vitro*. *Circulation* 2000; **102**(6): 617–623.

25. Schaar JA, De Korte CL, Mastik F *et al*. Characterizing vulnerable plaque features with intravascular elastography. *Circulation* 2003; **108**(21): 2636–2341.

26. Fujimoto J, Boppart S, Tearney G, Bouma B, Pitris C, Brezinski M. High resolution *in vivo* intra-arterial imaging with optical coherence tomography. *Heart* 1999; **82**: 128–133.

27. Yabushita H, Bouma BE, Houser SL *et al*. Characterization of human atherosclerosis by optical coherence tomography. *Circulation* 2002; **106**: 1640–1645.

28. Jang IK, Bouma BE, Kang DH *et al*. Visualization of coronary atherosclerotic plaques in patients using optical coherence tomography: comparison with intravascular ultrasound. *J Am Coll Cardiol* 2002; **39**: 604–609.

29. Jang IK, Tearney GJ, MacNeill B *et al*. *In vivo* characterization of coronary atherosclerotic plaque by use of optical coherence tomography. *Circulation* 2005; **111**(12): 1551–1555.

30. Tearney GJ, Yabushita H, Houser SL *et al*. Quantification of macrophage content in atherosclerotic plaques by optical coherence tomography. *Circulation*. 2003; **107**: 113–119.

31. Gerckens U, Buellesfeld L, McNamara F, Grube E. Optical coherence tomography (OCT). Potential of a new high-resolution intracoronary imaging technique. *Herz* 2003; **28**(6): 496–500.

32. Tearney GJ, Yabushita H, Houser SL *et al*. Quantification of macrophage content in atherosclerotic plaques by optical coherence tomography. *Circulation* 2003; **107**: 113–119.

33. Casscells W, Hathorn B, David M *et al*. Thermal detection of cellular infiltrates in living atherosclerotic plaques: possible implications for plaque rupture and thrombosis. *Lancet* 1996; **347**: 1447–1451.

34. Stefanadis C, Toutouzas K, Vavuranakis M *et al*. Statin treatment is associated with reduced thermal heterogeneity in human atherosclerotic plaques. *Eur Heart J* 2002; **23**: 1664–1669.

35. Stefanadis C, Diamantopoulos L, Vlachopoulos C *et al*. Thermal heterogeneity within human atherosclerotic coronary arteries detected *in vivo*: a new method of detection by application of a special thermography catheter. *Circulation* 1999; **99**: 1965–1971.

36. Stefanadis C, Toutouzas K, Tsiamis E *et al*. Increased local temperature in human coronary atherosclerotic plaques: an independent predictor of clinical outcome in patients undergoing a percutaneous coronary intervention. *J Am Coll Cardiol* 2001; **37**: 1277–1283.

37. Stefanadis C, Vavuranakis M, Toutouzas P. Vulnerable plaque: the challenge to identify and treat it. *J Interv Cardiol* 2003; **3**: 273–280.
38. Diamantopoulos L. Arterial wall thermography. *J Interv Cardiol* 2003; **16**(3): 261–266.
39. Schmermund A, Rodermann J, Erbel R. Intracoronary thermography. *Herz* 2003; **6**: 505–512.
40. Mizuno K, Miyamoto A, Satomura K *et al.* Angioscopic coronary macromorphology in patients with acute coronary disorders. *Lancet.* 1991; **337**(8745): 809–812.
41. Uchida Y, Nakamura F, Tomaru T *et al.* Prediction of acute coronary syndromes by percutaneous coronary angioscopy in patients with stable angina. *Am Heart J* 1995; **130**(2): 195–203.
42. Ueda Y, Asakura M, Hirayama A, Komamura K, Hori M, Komada K. Intracoronary morphology of culprit lesions after reperfusion in acute myocardial infarction: serial angioscopic observations. *J Am Coll Cardiol* 1996; **27**(3): 606–610.
43. Asakura M, Ueda Y, Yamaguchi O *et al.* Extensive development of vulnerable plaques as a pan-coronary process in patients with myocardial infarction: an angioscopic study. *J Am Coll Cardiol* 2001; **5**: 1284–1248.
44. Van Belle E, Lablanche JM, Bauters C, Renaud N, McFadden EP, Bertrand ME. Coronary angioscopic findings in the infarct-related vessel within 1 month of acute myocardial infarction: natural history and the effect of thrombolysis. *Circulation* 1998; **97**: 26–33.
45. Ueda Y, Asakura M, Yamaguchi O, Hirayama A, Hori M, Kodama K. The healing process of infarct-related plaques. Insights from 18 months of serial angioscopic follow-up. *J Am Coll Cardiol* 2001; **38**(7): 1916–1922.
46. Ueda Y, Hirayama A, Kodama K. Plaque characterization and atherosclerosis evaluation by coronary angioscopy. *Herz* 2003; **6**: 501–504.
47. Takano M, Mizuno K, Yokoyama S *et al.* Changes in coronary plaque color and morphology by lipid-lowering therapy with atorvastatin: serial evaluation by coronary angioscopy. *J Am Coll Cardiol* 2003; **42**(4): 680–686.
48. Ueda Y, Ohtani T, Shimizu M, Hirayama A, Kodama K. Assessment of plaque vulnerability by angioscopic classification of plaque color. *Am Heart J* 2004; **148**(2): 333–335.
49. White CJ, Ramee SR, Collins TJ *et al.* Coronary thrombi increase PTCA risk. Angioscopy as a clinical tool. *Circulation* 1996; **93**(2): 253–258.
50. Wang J, Geng YJ, Guo B *et al.* Near-infrared spectroscopic characterization of human advanced atherosclerotic plaques. *J Am Coll Cardiol* 2002; **39**(8): 1305–1313.
51. Moreno PR, Lodder RA, Purushothaman KR, Charash WE, O'Connor WN, Muller JE. Detection of lipid pool, thin fibrous cap, and inflammatory cells in human aortic atherosclerotic plaques by near-infrared spectroscopy. *Circulation* 2002; **105**(8): 923–927.
52. Romer TJ, Brennan JF, Schut TC *et al.* Raman spectroscopy for quantifying cholesterol in intact coronary artery wall. *Atherosclerosis* 1998; **141**: 117–124.
53. Romer TJ, Brennan JF III, Puppels GJ *et al.* Intravascular ultrasound combined with Raman spectroscopy to localize and quantify cholesterol and calcium salts in atherosclerotic coronary arteries. *Arterioscler Thromb Vasc Biol* 2000; **20**: 478–483.

CHAPTER 22

Local versus systemic prevention treatment

Mario Togni and Bernhard Meier

Introduction

The lack of linear relation between stenosis severity and the probability of developing an acute coronary syndrome (ACS) is well recognized [1]. Indeed the majority of plaques leading to acute myocardial infarction are not of angiographic significance and it has been for quite a while now that we have started looking at the coronary artery plaque (or any vascular plaque for that matter) in a more differentiated way. Not every plaque means clinical trouble, and there is clinical trouble in determining whether a plaque has a potential for myocardial infarction and death and if it will result in a loss of quality of life. The active or vulnerable plaque represents the former. It is characterized by activated macrophages, a dearth of smooth muscle cells at the surface (and hence a thin and brittle cap), and an abundance of inflammatory cells producing enzymes such as metalloproteinases eroding the cap further. The nonobstructive plaque with a thick fibrous cap may be a nuisance but it is not a real threat. It is characterized by a robust surface with abundant smooth muscle cells and few inflammatory cells or macrophages. It may even harbor a protective potential as it often represents a scar over a tear in the arterial wall. This scar may be even less rupture prone than the normal endothelium, not unlike the callus after a bone fracture.

A plethora of terms have emerged dealing with the subject of plaque vulnerability. They encompass thin-cap fibroatheroma, plaque erosion, plaque rupture, plaque sealing, plaque passivation, and plaque stabilization [2]. New terms are being coined as this chapter is being written. The saying of Thomas Sydenham (1624–89): "A man is as old as his arteries" [3] has proved pertinent once again. Tiny accidents in coronary or cerebral arteries decide between life and death. They will continue to happen but it is our goal and within our reach to reduce their numbers and push them back to old age. Research, knowledge, and techniques described in this chapter continue to empower us further in the struggle with the vulnerable plaque.

Systemic and local plaque passivation by drugs

Systemic administration

Lipid modification

Modest reduction in plaque dimension by statin therapy has been described but remains unconfirmed [4]. The fact that statins are of paramount clinical benefit both in primary and secondary prevention points to a multifaceted mode of action. The supposed pleiotropic effects of statins include reorganization of the plaque with relative diminution of the lipid rich core, deflammation by thickening of the fibrous cap and decreasing of foam cells and activated or apoptotic macrophages, enhancement of endothelial function resumption, and antiplatelet activity. Some of these actions are immediate and some take time. This explains that randomized trials vary in terms of first appearance of the clinical benefit of statins. Some of these pleiotropic effects have been substantiated in animal trials, such as the number of macrophages and matrix metalloproteinase-1 expression with reciprocal collagen content increase [5]. Some emerge from clinical studies using intravascular ultrasound and variables, such as the hyperechogenicity index and plaque volume [6]. Finally, some were suggested by otherwise unexplained promptness or extent of clinical benefits suggesting mechanisms beyond cholesterol reduction [7].

Alternative lipid lowering agents (nicotinic acid, ezetimibe) have yet to produce similar data. However, it can be conjectured that they also lead to plaque passivation via cholesterol lowering and other avenues. Finally, increasing high density lipoprotein cholesterol may, by itself, reduce the risk of plaque rupture. It can be achieved by niacin, antioxidant vitamins on top of statins [8], or simply by vigorous and regular physical exercise.

Antithrombosis

Both superficial plaque erosion and penetrating plaque rupture expose extracellular matrix to the blood stream. This leads to platelet activation by platelet adhesion molecules and tissue factors. Platelet adhesion leads to platelet aggregation and goes hand in hand with activation of the clotting cascade. This orchestrates atherothrombosis. It goes without saying that part of it can be prevented by antiplatelet agents or anticoagulation. Even once the process has started, it can be stopped or abated by antithrombotic therapy. Whether this represents an additional passivating effect of the vascular wall [9] or whether the effect is limited to the thrombus remains to be elucidated.

Platelet aggregability can be reduced mainly by four different pathways. For over 100 years acetylsalicylic acid has been available orally. It reduces the synthesis of thromboxane A_2 from arachidonic acid by blocking cyclooxygenase. More recently, thienopyridines, such as ticlopidine and its successor clopidogrel, have been introduced to block the adenosin-diphosphate-P_2Y_{12} receptor. The most potent platelet inhibitors are unfortunately only available for intravenous use. They are abciximab, eptifibatide, and tirofiban. They directly block glycoprotein receptors IIb/IIIa. This prevents, quite powerfully, that any of the approximate 100 000 such receptors per platelet interlink with one end of a fibrinogen molecule of which the other end might then bind to such a receptor of another platelet leading to permanent connection of the two thrombocytes. Finally, thrombin is a potent platelet activator apart from being the key element in the coagulation cascade leading to fibrin clots.

Acetylsalicylic acid has an excellent record of preventing first or subsequent atherothrombotic events in virtually all risk groups [10]. Even in the setting of acute myocardial infarction where plaque rupture has already happened and a thrombus has already formed, acetylsalicylic acid proved beneficial with an efficacy comparable to that of streptokinase [11]. A metaanalysis showed a reduction of mortality from 11.5% to 9.2% with significant effects also on reinfarction, vascular death, or stroke [10]. The effect was comparable with doses of 75–1500 mg with less bleeding at lower dosages. Additional platelet inhibition can be obtained by adding clopidogrel. The effect starts within hours if a bolus is used or within days without a bolus [12]. Recent data in stroke patients even suggest that acetylsalicylic acid may no longer be required when clopidogrel is employed [13]. The beneficial effect of clopidogrel has also been corroborated by its supremacy over acetylsalicylic acid alone in randomized trials in ACSs. The more conspicuous effect in patients undergoing percutaneous coronary interventions (PCI) (the ultimate model of plaque rupture) points to its pivotal role in such high risk situations [14,15]. The effect seems to augment when clopidogrel treatment is pursued for 1 year suggesting a secondary prevention apart from the acute event reduction around the intervention [15]. Based on this, some suggest lifelong use, others consider the benefit not significant enough to be worthwhile [16].

The effect of the costly intravenous direct glycoprotein IIb/IIIa inhibitors could only be brought out in the context of an acute intervention or a positive troponin [17] and their role has been relegated to these circumstances and high-risk patients (e.g. diabetics). In particular, the anticipated supremacy of abciximab also inhibiting the Mac 1 and the vitronectin receptors that are instrumental in the apoptosis of vascular smooth muscle cells, induced by the macrophage colony stimulating factor activated macrophages [18], did not materialize in clinical trials so far.

The coagulation pathway leading to the red component of the thrombus can be inhibited or modified at several levels. Both internal and external activation of the coagulation pathways merge at the activation of factor X to factor Xa. The external pathway requires factors V, VII, and IX for this. They are vitamin-K dependent and can be blocked by warfarin and similar oral drugs (all necessitating monitoring of the international normalized ratio). Factor Xa can be inhibited by the intravenous drug fondaparinux and partially by low molecular weight heparins, also applicable subcutaneously. The latter require the presence of antithrombin III (AT III) as does unfractionated heparin.

Both heparins exert their main action in thrombin inhibition. The debate whether low molecular weight heparins are superior to unfractionated heparin appears to be put to rest by draw in the SYNERGY trial [19]. Whether new trials will bring out the theoretical advantage of low molecular weight heparins in terms of more direct inhibition of the factor Xa and reduced risk of thrombocytopenia remains to be seen.

Thrombin inhibition without AT III can be achieved intravenously by hirudin and alike (e.g. bivalirudin) or orally by melagatran (i.e. the oral precursor ximelagatran). Thrombin inhibition is the last and most logical point of interference (comparable with glycoprotein IIb/IIIa inhibition in platelet aggregation). Thrombin (also known as factor II) activates the formation of fibrin from fibrinogen. Fibrin can be broken down to its split products by intravenous fibrinolytics as the last resort in plaque passivation.

Calcium antagonists

The capabilities to reduce lipid oxidation and foam cell formation together with increased transmembrane calcium transport attach a prominent antiatherogenic and plaque smoothening role to calcium antagonists. For amlodipine, a second-generation dihydropyridine, some clinical benefits in patients with high cardiovascular risk have been demonstrated [20].

Angiotensin-converting enzyme inhibitors

Angiotensin fosters oxygen-free radical production. Its inhibition is therefore likely to improve plaque stability. Moreover, angiotensin converting enzyme inhibitors have been shown to mitigate endothelial dysfunction and decrease macrophage and smooth muscle cell lipoxygenase activity. Atherosclerosis in general could be slowed with these compounds in animal models. Clinical trials in high-risk patients and patients with ACSs showed benefit from such drugs that appeared to be more marked than would have been predicted by the induced decrement in blood pressure [21].

Other compounds

The highly promising oral antioxidants, in particular some of the vitamins, have turned out total failures in clinical trials looking at the atherothrombotic event prevention in various risk groups. Nonetheless, clear-cut benefit of a Mediterranean type diet [22] and the still open debate of the usefulness of a cocktail of vitamin B_6, vitamin B_9, and vitamin B_{12} to lower homocysteine keep the interest in such compounds alive. Oral immunosuppression with corticosteroids [23] and rapamycin [24] represent a more robust approach to plaque passivation showing some promise without, however, being unequivocal.

Local delivery

The era of catheter-based local drug delivery to premedicate or postmedicate plaques bound to rupture or already ruptured plaques has passed in spite of the alluring concept of achieving high onsite concentrations without risking systemic side effects. Impediments to its success were the cumbersome techniques using sweating balloons, enclosing tandem balloons, microneedle injections, etc., many of these requiring prolonged episodes of absent coronary flow [25]. Trying to maintain flow during drug application made the instruments even more complex, expensive, and difficult to handle. Despite a trial showing reduction of restenosis with local enoxaparin [26], the concept has not been further pursued, not even in conjunction with PCIs providing a compelling reason for introducing catheters into the coronary arteries.

In addition, drug eluting stents have all but monopolized the attention of interventional cardiologists. This type of local drug delivery is easy on the side of the operator, necessitating no additional effort and introducing no added discomfort or risk for the patient. Heparin was used first with no apparent advantage [27]. Then came dexamethazone, showing some benefit in initially unstable patients [28]. The dam broke with the first publications of clinical trials with stents eluting rapamycin (sirolimus) or paclitaxel. Although their extent of plaque stabilization was limited to reduction of restenosis, an annoying yet benign event, they are about to raid the arena of coronary stenting. The gross mechanical impact of stent implantation at the very site camouflages the plaque passivation effect (if there is any) of these compounds. More interestingly, it will have to be followed if the eluting drug stabilizes plaques further downstream at least for a certain time [29].

Plaque sealing by balloon angioplasty

Rationale

Coronary plaque sealing by balloon angioplasty is based on two major concepts [30]. First, experience with millions of balloon angioplasty procedures has shown that apart from an acute risk of vessel occlusion lasting for a few hours after the end of the procedure, or the discontinuation of heparin, there is virtually no risk of a later occlusion causing a myocardial infarction. Even in the case of a restenosis (occurring in about one-third of balloon angioplastics), the intimal proliferation causing the renarrowing is smooth and elastic, virtually precluding endothelial rupture and subsequent thrombosis. The second concept is that it appears more important to prevent plaque rupture by whatever means available than to just normalize impeded blood flow. In other words, the hemodynamical significance of the stenosis is only of secondary importance. The potential for plaque erosion, fissure, or rupture is the salient point. It implies myocardial infarction or death while the degree of narrowing just impacts on the presence and degree of angina pectoris, a nuisance but no threat.

Hitherto the focus in indications and clinical evaluation of coronary angioplasty has been on hemodynamical significance of the stenoses rather than on its prognostic impact (myocardial infarction and mortality). The fact that pertinent trials failed to show a prognostic benefit of balloon angioplasty [31] is not a valid proof that it lacks prognostic impact. Perhaps indications need to be expanded to glean the full benefit of the procedure. We should realign our target and include the mechanical approach to seal potentially dangerous plaques that are not yet hemodynamically significant without relenting on the effort to remove significant narrowings and thereby the nuisance of angina, limitations in physical activity, and need to consume medications with side effects.

The distinction between a stable and an unstable plaque resides in the thickness of the fibrous cap [32,33]. The thick fibrous cap with several layers of smooth muscle cells but few inflammatory cells separating the lumen from the macrophages in the plaque may be a spontaneously occurring event. On the other hand, it is also typical for a coronary plaque that had been subjected to balloon angioplasty, irrespective of the fact whether a restenosis occurred or not. Hence, balloon angioplasty offers itself to induce a stable plaque, that is, to seal a potentially or actually unstable plaque. Angioplasty of the significant but prognostically irrelevant plaque is universally accepted, angioplasty of the prognostically menacing but hemodynamically nonsignificant plaque is not. This clearly has to be reconsidered.

Clinical background

Already, the preclinical animal studies of Andreas Gruentzig, the inventor of coronary angioplasty, unveiled the potential of balloon to first cause plaque rupture but then induce sealing of the site (Figure 22.1) [34]. Editorial comments have conjectured that balloon angioplasty should indeed bring forward proliferation of smooth muscle cells producing plaque-smoothening proteins, rendering the plaques less rough and less rupture prone, strengthening the fibrous cap, and regulating the synthesis of interstitial collagen. They emphasized that plaque sealing might be more important than restoration of normal flow, and the stimulation of intimal proliferation dreaded because of its role in restenosis might have a prognostically beneficial side to it [29,34–36]. Useful clinical data first emerged with a Japanese study specifically examining the infarct potential of a site successfully subjected to balloon angioplasty [37]. Over 300 patients who suffered an infarction within 7 years after balloon angioplasty of a coronary lesion, which had showed a good result at a 6-month follow-up angiogram, underwent an additional coronary angiography. The dilated lesion could be exculpated in 99.3% of instances. This testifies to the clinical impression that balloon angioplasty sites may cause angina due to restenosis but do not typically cause infarction. The clinical follow-up of over 3000 patients in an American registry of balloon angioplasty corroborates this. Whether or not restenosis occurred, there was no difference in mortality over 6 years [38]. Restenosis is thus an annoyance often requiring an additional intervention but it is not a prognostically important problem. The concern that the 30% risk of restenosis after balloon angioplasty may forfeit a potential gain of plaque sealing by balloon dilatation appears invalidated by this study. Moreover, nonsignificant lesions harbor a small risk for restenosis, to be estimated at 10% or less even without using a stent. Likewise, the risk of

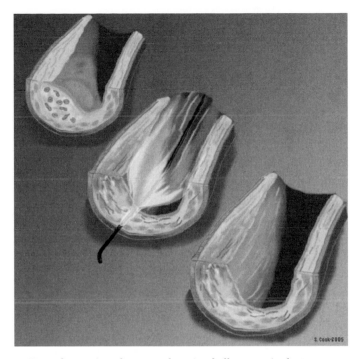

Figure 22.1 Non-obstructive plaque undergoing balloon angioplasty.

abrupt closure is minute (about 2%) when dealing with nonsignificant sten-oses. Most of abrupt closures nowadays can be bailed out by implanting a stent. In addition to this, the concept becomes even more appealing by the possibility to save costs if plaque sealing of a nonsignificant lesion is done con-currently with angioplasty of one or several significant lesions (utilization of same material).

Some publications appear to advise against coronary plaque sealing [39,40]. However, these two trials were not designed to show a potential benefit of dilating nonsignificant stenoses. These lesions were dilated incidentally while dilating significant lesions or because they were apparently considered responsible for symptoms (i.e. clinically significant). The only randomized trial addressing this subject was designed to show that hemodynamically nonsig-nificant lesions will not benefit from balloon angioplasty over the first 2 years [41]. While there was indeed no benefit to the patients subjected to balloon angioplasty with or without stenting in the light of a lesion that had a normal fractional flow reserve (as proof of lack of hemodynamic significance), there was no disadvantage either. An alternate conclusion to the one by the authors that angioplasty should be omitted for such lesions could have been that it harbors no risk for the patient and may still prove beneficial during longer follow-up. It could also be mentioned that the time and money invested in the assessment of hemodynamic significance could have been invested into the treatment of the stenosis without adding much acute risk to the patient but with a good probability to save the patient from a later intervention to that lesion, let alone from a prognostically important clinical event.

It has been iteratively shown that about two-thirds of infarctions are caused by a lesion with less than 50% diameter narrowing and 86% by a lesion with less than 70% of diameter narrowing (still unlikely to be hemodynamically significant) [42]. Using this as an argument to approach nonsignificant stenoses interventionally, these papers have often been misquoted. They do not assign a particularly high risk for infarction to nonsignificant lesions. The sheer number of nonsignificant lesions compared with that of significant lesions is responsible for the fact that abundant nonsignificant lesions, rather than the rare significant lesions, are the typical causes of myocardial infarction. Indeed, the individual risk of a lesion increases with its stenosis diameter with the exception of subtotal and total lesions. They are often well collateralized or subtend to already infarcted myocardium. Therefore, they may be devoid of the risk of a subsequent infarction. In the impossibility of predicting whether a nonsignificant lesion seen during a coronary angiogram will cause a cardiac event in the future, it appears justified to proceed with angioplasty for those positioned in a strategically important region (i.e. in a large proximal coronary artery). The goal is to prevent catastrophic events. Similar experiences on a larger scale were made in a registry of 189 consecutive patients with 203 moderate lesions. Thirty-six lesions had an abnormal fractional flow reserve and underwent PCI mostly with stenting; 45 of 165 lesions with a normal fractional flow reserve underwent PCI; and 120 did not. Mortality and infarction rate was 0 in patients undergoing PCI but 4% and 2%, respectively, in those being treated conservatively. Whether the four patients who died and the two who suffered a nonfatal myocardial infarction would have escaped their fate had they been subjected to PCI cannot be determined. First it was not a randomized trial and second the cohorts were small (Fisher *et al.* communication at the SCAI meeting 2003).

Role of stents

Stents have not been initially considered in the concept of plaque sealing by coronary angioplasty. Although initially conceived to remedy abrupt closure, stents have overall failed to prognostically impact on the outcome of coronary angioplasty [43]. Undoubtedly, they salvaged some dire situations during and immediately after PCIs. On the other hand, this initial prognostical advantage is lost during early follow-up because of subacute stent thrombosis to catch up with the initially higher rate of infarctions and deaths occurring with plain balloon angioplasty. What remains is a significant reduction in need for reintervention, a lifestyle type of a problem. Even this reduction seems to be fully exploited with a stenting rate of 20% or even less according to a metaanalysis [43]. The risk of subacute thrombosis, virtually unknown to balloon angioplasty but inherent with stenting, casts a shadow on plaque sealing by angioplasty if stents are employed. Notwithstanding, the community of interventional cardiologists have moved entirely to stenting as the sine qua nonmodality of PCI. Embarking on treating nonsignificant lesions, the aspect of doing a "perfect job" appears even more crucial. Hardly an interventional cardiologist is ready to refrain from implanting a stent under such circumstances, albeit for all the wrong reasons. Hence, in real life it is moot to further investigate the potential of plaque sealing with balloon angioplasty because balloon angioplasty has long been doomed and replaced by stenting. If stents were used judiciously (in 20% or less of the cases, that is), there would be no problem. Using them in 100% of cases, probably means giving up the prognostic advantage of plaque sealing of nonsignificant lesions for at least the first 2 years. A nonsignificant lesion has about a 2% risk of abrupt closure over the subsequent 2 years [44], which corresponds to the risk of subacute stent thrombosis in the first weeks.

Role of drug eluting stents

Compared with bare stents, drug eluting (active) stents further reduce the need for reintervention, thereby improving the comfort for the patients. However, they again failed to better the prognosis after the procedure. The incidence of subacute thrombosis is comparable with that of bare stents. The points raised in the section above are valid for drug eluting stents as well. Even so, the advent of drug eluting stents appears to intrigue interventional cardiologists to include nonsignificant lesions into their interventional treatment plan. A first report has already appeared showing impeccable results in a small series treating lesions of a stenosis diameter less than 50% with active stents [45].

Identification of vulnerable plaques

There are several techniques to assess the vulnerability of a coronary artery plaque [33,46–49]. It is unlikely that any of these techniques will reach routine application. First, they are costly in spite of their limited specificity and sensitivity. Second, they provide a snap-shot assessment. Should the plaque prove stable when assessed, there is no guarantee that it will remain stable in the future. Third, some of them are invasive and fraught with intrinsic risks. Fourth, an invasive assessment carries the risk of mechanically destabilizing an initially stable plaque. Fifth, mechanical plaque scaling can be performed with less logistic investments than the assessment. Sixth, if several assessment technologies are used, it is highly likely that some suspicion of instability remains and mechanical plaque sealing will be done, anyhow. Hence, the instances of such an assessment obviating the need for an intervention will be scarce in contrast to the measurement of the fractional flow reserve.

Perspectives

While the research interest in assessing the vulnerability of a plaque has gained a dramatic momentum in the past years, it is likely that the interventional treatment of nonsignificant plaques will catch up and overpass the research aspect. Knowledge gained from the intricate assessment methods will be used for justification of the treatment in general. However, it will hardly bring about routine tools for the cardiac catheterization laboratory. The hemodynamic assessment of a lesion has already played a minor part in the busy catheterization laboratory. In the future, it will be relegated to the academic playground while inserting a drug eluting stent at first sight even for mild (most probably not hemodynamically significant) lesions. What has been introduced as plaque sealing by balloon angioplasty will turn into standard treatment of angiographically conspicuous lesions in addition to a hemodynamically relevant lesion or as sole target in a patient having been sent to the catheterization laboratory for suspicion of coronary artery disease. These lesions may in fact account for a new upturn in coronary angioplasty case numbers after the recent plateau phase. Although many authors attribute to drug eluting stents a potential to expand the indications toward the realm of coronary artery bypass surgery, they may expand the indication field more toward the early coronary artery disease, that is, than the nonsignificant lesions. After all, drug eluting stents have failed to significantly ameliorate the safety of the procedure, a prerequisite to set out on a crusade into the territory of cardiac surgery.

The argument that there are so many nonsignificant plaques so that it is impossible to go after them mechanically will continue to be raised. It is hardly valid when confining mechanical plaque sealing to the proximal thirds of the major coronary arteries and to lesions of at least 50% narrowing diameter. This restricts the potential targets to a few per average patient [50]. And then again, it would be like apprehending a pickpocket but letting him run on the basis that this one might perhaps not steal again and that there are more of them out there, anyhow.

References

1. Ambrose JA, Tannenbaum MA, Alexopoulos D *et al.* Angiographic progression of coronary artery disease and the development of myocardial infarction. *J Am Coll Cardiol* 1988; **12**: 56–62.
2. Fuster V, Badimon L, Badimon JJ *et al.* The pathogenesis of coronary artery disease and the acute coronary syndromes. *N Engl J Med* 1992; **326**: 242–250.
3. Garrison F, Sydenham T. *Bull New York Acad Med* 1928; **4**: 993.
4. Vaughan CJ, Gotto AM, Jr, Basson CT. The evolving role of statins in the management of atherosclerosis. *J Am Coll Cardiol* 2000; **35**: 1–10.
5. Aikawa M, Rabkin E, Okada Y *et al.* Lipid lowering by diet reduces matrix metalloproteinase activity and increases collagen content of rabbit atheroma: a potential mechanism of lesion stabilization. *Circulation* 1998; **97**: 2433–2444.
6. Schartl M, Bocksch W, Koschyk DH *et al.* Use of intravascular ultrasound to compare effects of different strategies of lipid-lowering therapy on plaque volume and composition in patients with coronary artery disease. *Circulation* 2001; **104**: 387–392.

7. Schwartz GG, Olsson AG, Ezekowitz MD *et al.* Effects of atorvastatin on early recurrent ischemic events in acute coronary syndromes: the MIRACLE study: a randomized controlled trial. *JAMA* 2001; **285**: 1711–1718.

8. Brown BG, Zhao XQ, Chait A *et al.* Simvastatin and niacin, antioxidant vitamins, or the combination for the prevention of coronary disease. *N Engl J Med* 2001; **345**: 1583–1592.

9. Spratt J, Camenzind E. Plaque stabilisation by systemic and local drug administration. *Heart* 2004; **90**(12): 1392–1394.

10. Antithrombotic Trialist's Collaboration. Collaborative meta-analysis of randomised trials of antiplatelet therapy for prevention of death, myocardial infarction, and stroke in high risk patients. *BMJ* 2002; **324**: 71–86.

11. Randomised trial of intravenous streptokinase, oral aspirin, both, or neither among 17,187 cases of suspected acute myocardial infarction: ISIS-2. ISIS-2 (Second International Study of Infarct Survival) Collaborative Group. *Lancet* 1988; **2**: 349–360.

12. Cadroy Y, Bossavy JP, Thalamas C *et al.* Early potent antithrombotic effect with combined aspirin and a loading dose of clopidogrel on experimental arterial thrombogenesis in humans. *Circulation* 2000; **101**: 2823–2828.

13. Diener HC, Bogousslavsky J, Brass LM *et al.* Aspirin and clopidogrel compared with clopidogrel alone after recent ischaemic stroke or transient ischaemic attack in high-risk patients (MATCH): randomised, double-blind, placebo-controlled trial. *Lancet* 2004; **364**: 331–337.

14. Mehta SR, Yusuf S, Peters RJ *et al.* Effects of pretreatment with clopidogrel and aspirin followed by long-term therapy in patients undergoing percutaneous coronary intervention: the PCI-CURE study. *Lancet* 2001; **358**: 527–533.

15. Steinhubl SR, Berger PB, Mann JT III *et al.* Early and sustained dual oral antiplatelet therapy following percutaneous coronary intervention: a randomized controlled trial. *JAMA* 2002; **288**: 2411–2420.

16. Eriksson P. Long-term clopidogrel therapy after percutaneous coronary intervention in PCI-CURE and CREDO: the "Emperor's New Clothes" revisited. *Eur Heart J* 2004; **25**: 720–722.

17. Boersma E, Harrington RA, Moliterno DJ *et al.* Platelet glycoprotein IIb/IIIa inhibitors in acute coronary syndromes: a meta-analysis of all major randomised clinical trials. *Lancet* 2002; **359**: 189–198.

18. Monroe VS, Kerensky RA, Rivera E *et al.* Pharmacologic plaque passivation for the reduction of recurrent cardiac events in acute coronary syndromes. *J Am Coll Cardiol* 2003; **41**: 23S–30S.

19. Ferguson JJ, Califf RM, Antman EM *et al.* Enoxaparin vs unfractionated heparin in high-risk patients with non-ST-segment elevation acute coronary syndromes managed with an intended early invasive strategy: primary results of the SYNERGY randomized trial. *JAMA* 2004; **292**: 45–54.

20. Pitt B, Byington RP, Furberg CD *et al.* Effect of amlodipine on the progression of atherosclerosis and the occurrence of clinical events. PREVENT Investigators. *Circulation* 2000; **102**: 1503–1510.

21. Fox KM. Efficacy of perindopril in reduction of cardiovascular events among patients with stable coronary artery disease: randomised, double-blind, placebo-controlled, multicentre trial (the EUROPA study). *Lancet* 2003; **362**: 782–788.

22. de Lorgeril M, Salen P, Martin JL *et al.* Mediterranean diet, traditional risk factors, and the rate of cardiovascular complications after myocardial infarction: final report of the Lyon Diet Heart Study. *Circulation* 1999; **99**: 779–785.

23. Versaci F, Gaspardone A, Tomai F *et al.* Immunosuppressive therapy for the prevention of restenosis after coronary artery stent implantation (IMPRESS Study). *J Am Coll Cardiol* 2002; **40**: 1935–1942.

24. Brara PS, Moussavian M, Grise MA *et al.* Pilot trial of oral rapamycin for recalcitrant restenosis. *Circulation* 2003; **107**: 1722–1724.

25. Esente P, Kaplan AV, Ford JK *et al.* Local intramural heparin delivery during primary angioplasty for acute myocardial infarction: results of the local PAMI pilot study. *Catheter Cardiovasc Interv* 1999; **47**: 237–242.

26. Kiesz RS, Buszman P, Martin JL *et al.* Local delivery of enoxaparin to decrease restenosis after stenting: results of initial multicenter trial: Polish-American Local Lovenox NIR Assessment study (The POLONIA study). *Circulation* 2001; **103**: 26–31.

27. Serruys PW, van Hout B, Bonnier H *et al.* Randomised comparison of implantation of heparin-coated stents with balloon angioplasty in selected patients with coronary artery disease (Benestent II). *Lancet* 1998; **352**: 673–681.

28. Liu X, Huang Y, Hanet C *et al.* Study of antirestenosis with the BiodivYsio dexamethasone-eluting stent (STRIDE): a first-in-human multicenter pilot trial. *Catheter Cardiovasc Interv* 2003; **60**: 172–178.

29. Hodgson JM, Bottner RK, Klein LW *et al.* Drug-eluting stent task force: final report and recommendations of the working committees on cost-effectiveness/economics, access to care, and medicolegal issues. *Catheter Cardiovasc Interv* 2004; **62**: 1–17.

30. Meier B, Ramamurthy S. Plaque sealing by coronary angioplasty. *Cathet Cardiovasc Diagn* 1995; **36**: 295–297.

31. RITA-II. Coronary angioplasty versus medical therapy for angina: the second Randomised Intervention Treatment of Angina (RITA-2) trial. RITA-2 trial participants. *Lancet* 1997; **350**: 461–468.

32. Libby P. Molecular bases of the acute coronary syndromes. *Circulation* 1995; **91**: 2844–2850.

33. Kolodgie FD, Virmani R, Burke AP, *et al.* Pathologic assessment of the vulnerable human coronary plaque. *Heart* 2004; **90**(12): 1385–1391.

34. Schneider J. Andreas Grüntzig – wie alles anfing. *Infobl Dt Ges Kardiol* 1995; **2**: 30–32.

35. Weissberg PL, Clesham GJ, Bennett MR. Is vascular smooth muscle cell proliferation beneficial? *Lancet* 1996; **347**: 305–307.

36. Lafont A, Libby P. The smooth muscle cell: sinner or saint in restenosis and the acute coronary syndromes? *J Am Coll Cardiol* 1998; **32**: 283–285.

37. Saito T, Date H, Taniguchi I *et al.* Outcome of target sites escaping high-grade (>70%) restenosis after percutaneous transluminal coronary angioplasty. *Am J Cardiol* 1999; **83**: 857–861.

38. Weintraub WS, Ghazzal ZM, Douglas JS, Jr *et al.* Long-term clinical follow-up in patients with angiographic restudy after successful angioplasty. *Circulation* 1993; **87**: 831–840.

39. Ischinger T, Gruentzig AR, Hollman J *et al.* Should coronary arteries with less than 60% diameter stenosis be treated by angioplasty? *Circulation* 1983; **68**: 148–154.

40. Mercado N, Maier W, Boersma E *et al.* Clinical and angiographic outcome of patients with mild coronary lesions treated with balloon angioplasty or coronary stenting. Implications for mechanical plaque sealing. *Eur Heart J* 2003; **24**: 541–551.

41. Bech GJW, De Bruyne B, Pijls NHJ *et al.* Fractional flow reserve to determine the appropriateness of angioplasty in moderate coronary stenosis: a randomized trial. *Circulation* 2001; **103**: 2928–2934.

42. Falk E, Shah PK, Fuster V. Coronary plaque disruption. *Circulation* 1995; **92**: 657–671.

43. Brophy JM, Belisle P, Joseph L. Evidence for use of coronary stents. A hierarchical bayesian meta-analysis. *Ann Intern Med* 2003; **138**: 777–786.

44. Ellis S, Alderman E, Cain K *et al.* Prediction of risk of anterior myocardial infarction by lesion severity and measurement method of stenoses in the left anterior descending coronary distribution: a CASS Registry Study. *J Am Coll Cardiol* 1988; **11**: 908–916.

45. Hoye A, Lemos PA, Arampatzis CA *et al.* Effectiveness of sirolimus-eluting stent implantation for coronary narrowings <50% in diameter. *Am J Cardiol* 2004; **94**: 112–114.

46. Pasterkamp G, Falk E, Woutman H, Borst C. Techniques characterizing the coronary atherosclerotic plaque: influence on clinical decision making? *J Am Coll Cardiol* 2000; **36**: 13–21.

47. Badimon JJ, Fuster V. Can we image the "active" thrombus? *Arterioscler Thromb Vasc Biol* 2002; **22**: 1753–1754.

48. Casscells W, Naghavi M, Willerson JT. Vulnerable atherosclerotic plaque: a multifocal disease. *Circulation* 2003; **107**: 2072–2075.

49. De Korte CL, Schaar JA, Mastik F *et al.* Intravascular elastography: from bench to bedside. *J Interv Cardiol* 2003; **16**: 253–259.

50. Rioufol G, Finet G, Ginon I *et al.* Multiple atherosclerotic plaque rupture in acute coronary syndrome: a three-vessel intravascular ultrasound study. *Circulation* 2002; **106**: 804–808.

Conclusions

This book has outlined the pathophysiologic mechanisms, clinical presentations, and diagnostic methods used in acute coronary syndromes. Acute therapeutic options and secondary prevention methods that have been recently updated by the European Society of Cardiology, the American College of Cardiology, and the American Heart Association are presented by international authorities.

The advances in interventional cardiology are currently pushing the envelope and miniaturization of medical instrumentation seems to be the way of the future. In balance, however, we realize that atherosclerosis and the resulting acute syndromes are systemic diseases that are strongly influenced by metabolic and hemodynamic factors. The recent breakthroughs in medical therapy are dramatic and the impact on survival and myocardial infarction are highly significant, results not achieved by interventional means alone. Therefore it is imperative that all physicians caring for patients with acute coronary syndromes couple the acute care with aggressive follow-up care outlined in this volume and in more detail in recent guidelines.

Whether local therapy of unobstructed arteries will provide additional prophylactic protection as suggested in the concluding chapter, of course, remains speculative although interesting to interventional cardiologists.

Important questions for the near future are as follows

- Will aggressive medical therapies to prevent thrombosis, to produce dramatic LDL reduction, to reverse cholesterol transport, and to reduce inflammation and oxidative stress make plaque instability and its clinical consequences rare or just postpone events to a later stage of life?
- Will mechanical revascularization methods become less necessary or will local intravascular interventions become part of the future practice?
- Will diagnostic methods be developed to detect impending acute coronary syndromes before they occur?
- How will changes in medical technology impact optimal methods for caring for such patients?

The answers to these questions and others will dramatically change the future face of cardiovascular medicine.

Index

Note: page numbers in *italics* refer to figures, those in **bold** refer to tables.